COMPLETE
HOLISTIC CARE
AND
HEALING
FOR HORSES

THE OWNER'S VETERINARY GUIDE
TO ALTERNATIVE METHODS AND REMEDIES

Mary Brennan, DVM

with Norma Eckroate

Trafalgar Square Publishing
North Pomfret, Vermont

First published in 2001 by
Trafalgar Square Publishing
North Pomfret, Vermont 05053

Printed in Hong Kong

DISCLAIMER

This book is not to be used in place of veterinary care and expertise. The authors and publisher shall have neither liability nor responsibility to any person or entity with respect to any loss or damage caused or alleged to be caused directly or indirectly by the information contained in this book. While the book is as accurate as the authors can make it, there may be errors, omissions, and inaccuracies.

Library of Congress Cataloging-in-Publication Data

Brennan, Mary L.
     Complete holistic care and healing for horses : the owner's veterinary guide to alternative methods and remedies / Mary Brennan with Norma Eckroate.
          p. cm.
Includes bibliographical references (p.).
ISBN 1-57076-045-4 (hardcover)
     1. Horses—Diseases—Alternative treatment. 2. Holistic veterinary medicine. I. Eckroate, Norma, 1951- II. Title.

SF951.B84 2001
636.1'089—dc21   00-053239

Cover and book design by Carrie Fradkin
Typeface: Trump Medieval and FF Scala Sans

Color separations by Tenon & Polert Colour Scanning Ltd.

10 9 8 7 6 5 4 3 2 1

Acknowledgments

First, and most importantly, I thank all the horses that have provided me with the inspiration and determination to continue supporting their health needs by exploring new avenues in veterinary medicine. These paths of discovery were only made possible because of the support of my husband, Andy, who was always there to encourage, help with research, and make suggestions. Another person I wish to thank is my assistant, Elizabeth Ruggiero, who, while driving with me to our daily veterinary calls, listened to me for countless hours as I developed the book. Her advice was invaluable, and her patience, remarkable.

A special thank-you goes to my dogs, Lily and Babette, who faithfully stayed by my side, night after night, year after year, as I worked on this book. They never complained about hearing new versions, being covered up with papers, or having research books spread all over the house.

I sincerely appreciate Norma Eckroate's courage in helping me write a book about an animal species with which she had very little experience. During the writing process she was able to turn what seemed like a limitation into a great asset by making sure that even the most inexperienced reader would be able to understand what was written.

I also wish to thank Caroline Robbins and Martha Cook for their wonderful ideas, persistence, and great assistance, during the publishing process.

Table of Contents

Part I

HOLISTIC VETERINARY TREATMENTS AND REMEDIES

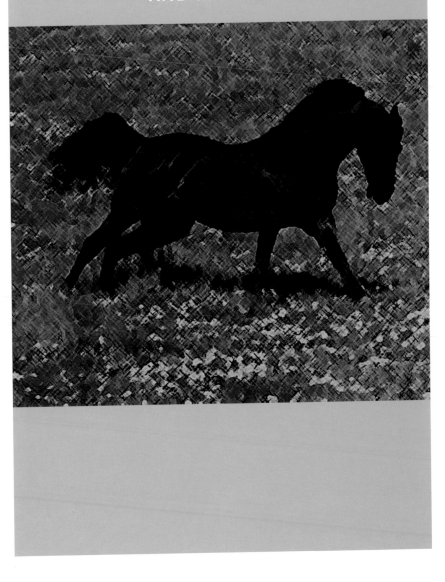

I A New Standard For Your Horse's Health

Is it possible to find an animal that better embodies the majesty of nature than the horse? We admire horses for their beauty and spirit, but by domesticating them, we have altered their relationship with the natural environment. Diet, hoof care, stabling and being ridden are just a few examples of ways in which the horse's life has been changed by his interaction with humans.

As many of us return to more natural ways of living, so, also do we seek more natural methods to handle and care for the animals we have domesticated. Holistic veterinary care is part of that trend. The term "holistic" denotes a view of the patient as a whole being—body, mind, and spirit. A holistic approach tends to be more detailed, emphasizing study of the whole horse, including his environment, his diet, and even his mental well-being. This emphasis on details often results in earlier diagnosis of disease based on subtle signs that might otherwise go unnoticed. Conventional veterinary medicine tends to focus more on symptoms that become notice-able only after a health problem has already developed. Thus in-depth examination by a holistic veterinarian is often worth the extra time it takes.

The treatments a holistic veterinarian uses are often referred to as "alternative" treatments. (The term "complementary" treatment is commonly used in England.) Both terms imply that these treatments are different from those used by conventional doctors, but the term complementary suggests that these approaches are meant not to replace traditional medicine but to allow for additional options. Some of these alternative treatments, such as herbal medicine and acupuncture, have been used throughout recorded history, though acupuncture was known only in the East until the last two centuries. But now, along with other alternative methods such as chiropractic, homeopathy, and magnetic therapy, they are gaining in popularity.

Conventional veterinary medicine is sometimes referred to as "traditional" or "allopathic" medicine. (Although the term "allopathic" is used to refer to the general practice of conventional medicine, its strict meaning is "opposed to homeopathy.") It relies to a great extent on pharmaceutical medications and is generally more invasive than alternative methods. Pharmaceutical drugs can be amazingly effective; however, even when a health problem is successfully treated by a pharmaceutical medication, there is a possibility that a negative side effect will develop, leading to further health concerns. The holistic veterinarian may decide either that a health problem is best treated by conventional medicine, or that an alternative method is likely to be the most efficacious. She may also determine that a combination of conventional medicine and alternative treatments is in order. In short, the holistic veterinarian has at her disposal all of the treatment possibilities of conventional medicine as well as a host of natural methods.

Alternative treatments are growing in popularity for a number of reasons, such as:

- They are effective.
- They are less expensive than many conventional treatments.
- They can be used on race and show horses in many cases when conventional drug therapies are not permitted.
- They can be effective in treating some common medical problems that may be unresponsive to conventional therapies. Among these conditions are the inability to sweat (anhidrosis), liver disease, navicular syndrome, and ringbone.

As trainers and owners have got to know my work, they have become aware that I work with horses using the more in-depth approach that characterizes holistic medicine. When a horse suddenly develops a poor attitude toward work, they call me in to make sure that a medical problem is not the cause. Many times I find that a misaligned spine—and the resulting discomfort or pain—is the reason for a sudden attitude change or refusal to perform. After a chiropractic adjustment, the horse returns to his normal self. Even very old injuries or problems are often still treatable with alternative methods. I always try to improve a condition even if it has existed for ten years. An owner often knows exactly when her horse was injured or a problem started and is able to give a concise history. I frequently hear things like, "He caught his head in a fence eight years ago and has not wanted to take the right lead ever since." I'm always so delighted when I am able to correct these long-standing problems because it's so sad to see an animal suffering.

The holistic approach greatly increases our ability to treat the horse and allows us to carry out treatment in a manner that is less invasive and more natural. Acupuncture rebalances the horse's body, allowing it to heal itself. Chiropractic realigns the spine, returning the body to its normal position. Homeopathy works on a highly sensitive level and stimulates the body to produce its own reaction against a particular ailment. These are just a few examples of alternative therapies covered in this book. Others are: acupressure, aromatherapy, Bach Flower Remedies, magnets, and massage. In the chapters that follow, I'll explain each of them (with complete lists in the appendix), and discuss how your horse might benefit from them. But first, let's review some of the signs that can alert you to a potential health problem in your horse.

THE SUBTLE SYMPTOMS OF ILLNESS

Owners are with their horses all the time; often they just don't see signs of deteriorating health. These signs can be so subtle and develop so gradually that they go unnoticed until the problem becomes serious. Even in young horses warning signs such as uneven gaits, lack of energy, or

SIGNS OF WELLNESS AND ILLNESS

Signs of Well-being	Symptoms of Illness
Good energy, even in an old horse	Lethargy (poor energy, or lack of energy)
Healthy skin and shiny coat	Dry and scaly skin, bald patches, mane or tail loss, dull coat, lighter hair color
Bright and clear eyes	Dull, cloudy, or sunken eyes
Correct weight	Overweight or underweight
No digestive problems	Recurring colic, chronic diarrhea, foul odor of manure, difficulty maintaining weight
Good temperament	Irritability

1.1

weight loss are common, but these small, often imperceptible signals that indicate a decline in health are sometimes difficult to measure. Astute veterinarians and owners, however, know that even a subtle change can be a symptom of a bigger problem brewing. What are the small changes that might signal a decline in health? Let's look at some criteria (fig. 1.1).

The symptoms of illness listed here are indications that the body is not properly digesting and assimilating nutrients, eliminating toxins and other wastes, or dealing with the stresses imposed on it. When your horse's body is overwhelmed by too many of these factors, it becomes sluggish; it is unable to operate efficiently. Any of these symptoms can be precursors of a health problem down the road. All too often I see horses with arthritis, cancer, laminitis, and other debilitating diseases. These conditions do not develop overnight. A well planned diet and a holistic approach to treatment is an excellent way to help maintain health and correct a health problem before it is even detectable—and before irreversible damage is done.

There are many ways that alternative treatments can help in achieving this new standard of health. Acupuncture, for example, is commonly used to successfully treat equine health problems, but it has also been found effective in maintaining health. Dr. Are Thorson, a Norwegian who is a leading pioneer in veterinary acupuncture, makes monthly visits to horse barns. He checks all of the horses and gives acupuncture treatments to those whose who require it. Owners have found a significant decrease in common problems such as colic and unsoundness among these horses. The routine acupuncture not only keeps the horses in excellent health but enables many horses to maintain a stressful performance schedule without breaking down. The cost of the monthly acupuncture treatments is a small investment considering the reduction in health problems and the larger veterinary bills owners would accrue if a serious problem arose. There is much to be gained by adopting preventive maintenance in which health problems are treated before they are outwardly visible. The regular acupuncture treatments correct imbalances in the body's energy system that, in turn, supports all the rest of the body's functions.

Alternative treatments can also be extremely helpful in correcting behavioral problems that are linked to discomfort or pain. Chiropractic adjustments often result in amazing improvements in behavior. For example, a horse whose first cervical vertebra is out of alignment may frighten easily because he cannot move his neck to see properly. When the vertebra is adjusted and the horse once again has a full range of motion, the spookiness often disappears.

One of my clients has a wonderful stable in South Carolina where she teaches children riding and takes them to competitions in dressage and eventing. Most of the children would not be able to have a horse except for Jill, who finds "diamonds in the rough." She takes horses that no one else wants and turns them into successful children's show horses.

Recently, Jill discovered a lovely paint gelding being sold at an auction where horses are usually destined for the slaughterhouse. She couldn't understand why such a nice horse was being sold at such a cheap price. When Jill examined him, she found that he wouldn't allow anyone to touch his head or the top area of his neck, but she decided to take a chance and purchased the horse for a young teenage girl.

When I was called to check the horse, Jill told me that he was difficult to handle and I probably would not be able to examine or adjust him. I started by doing a chiropractic adjustment low on his neck, just to let him know what I was going to do. Working my way up slowly, I was able to gain his trust, and finally, with no resistance from the horse, I adjusted the first cervical vertebra. A loud crack sounded as the badly misaligned vertebra slipped into place. The gelding immediately lowered his head, sighed, and put his head in my arms, wanting to be rubbed. Jill and the horse's new owner were astounded to find that the horse would allow touching anywhere on his head, ears, or neck — in fact, he truly enjoyed it. This is just one of the many examples of how miraculous the right treatment can be.

In Chapter Three, I will explain in more detail a number of alternative treatments that are being used increasingly in equine health care today. In

Chapter Four, I will discuss the conventional treatments that I use when necessary. It is the careful balance of these two methods that results in true holistic health care for the horse.

Let's review the way that many health problems evolve. When confronted with toxins, wastes, and stress, the body does its best to detoxify through normal channels — the liver, spleen, and kidneys. If these organs are overloaded or in a weakened state, other organs, including the skin, will begin to show toxic changes. The symptoms of illness that are listed in *Signs of Wellness and Illness* on page 5 indicate that the body is engaged in a battle to rid itself of excess toxins.

The immune system may also be affected by excessive toxicity. Chronic or long-term detoxification will deplete the immune system, which is the body's defensive shield against illness. A strong immune system wards off invading bacteria, viruses, allergens, and carcinogens, but it can be weakened or compromised by a build-up of toxins in the body caused by the side effects of medications and vaccinations; preservatives and additives in feed; chemicals and pollution in the air, water, and soil; or psychological stresses. Then, when the horse's body is attacked by any of these invading agents, the overburdened immune system is unable to defend the body and illness results.

In the remainder of this chapter, we will look at some of the sources of stress in greater detail.

ANTIBIOTICS, STEROIDS AND OTHER MEDICATIONS AND MEDICAL PROCEDURES

Overuse of medications is commonplace in today's world. In fact, there is now a term for the health risks associated with the overuse of medications. Iatrogenic disease means "physician induced" illness, usually as a result of long term negative side effects from the use of pharmaceutical drugs. The drugs used in conventional medicine often interfere with the body's natural defenses. Many are designed specifically for the purpose of suppressing the body's own natural responses. Repeated use of such pharmaceuticals often leaves the immune system in a weakened and ineffective state, unable to cope with further stresses and therefore open to new diseases or infections.

Some horse owners misuse drugs by administering leftover medications that were prescribed in the past. If you have leftover medication, do not give it again unless specifically directed to do so by your veterinarian. Prescription medications are given for specific problems, and in specific potencies and dosages. Also, many medications are given in a course, meaning that they are to be given for a certain period of time in the prescribed dosage. To be effective, the whole course must be completed at that time.

Any medication alters the body's natural balance (though natural remedies such as homeopathics and Bach Flower Remedies act on a deeper, more subtle level and do not alter this balance as much as pharmaceutical medicines). For example, oral antibiotics, such as those given by tablet or paste, kill many of the bacteria used for food digestion along with the disease-producing bacteria. The job of the antibiotic is to kill bacteria—it doesn't know the difference between the "good" bacteria the body needs and the "bad" bacteria that are causing an infection. Because of this, a dull, dry hair coat, poor appetite, decrease in performance ability and cranky attitude are sometimes noticed as signs of inadequate digestion long after the antibiotic treatment has been completed.

Many people involved with performance horses, which require a high level of exercise on a constant basis, have begun, whenever possible, to avoid antibiotics altogether to help prevent these and other side effects. Instead, they give immune stimulants to boost the immune system and allow the body to fight off infection by

itself. An example of this is the common respiratory infection faced by many horse owners each winter. Weanlings and yearlings seem to be particularly prone to respiratory illnesses. In the past, the first signs of a runny nose were vigorously treated with antibiotics. But the horses treated with antibiotics often had recurrences of the respiratory problems during the winter. Immune stimulants, when used instead of antibiotics, cause the body's natural defenses to respond, and the immune system is able to better protect the body against future challenges.

In fact, antibiotics are commonly prescribed for many health problems when the body would be better off dealing with the infection without them. In his book, *Natural Health, Natural Medicine*, Andrew Weil, M.D., says:

> Antibiotics are powerful medicine that should be reserved for situations that demand them, for instance, when the immune system cannot contain a bacterial infection or when a bacterial infection establishes itself in a vital organ like the heart, lungs, or brain. Another strong reason to be cautious about overuse of antibiotics is the possibility of selectively breeding new strains of antibiotic-resistant, more virulent bacteria. Even people who are aware of that danger seldom realize that frequent use of antibiotics can lead in the long run to weakened immunity. [1]

There are cases for which antibiotics are necessary and can be used effectively, but each case must be carefully examined before prescribing them.

Another common type of medication is the family of drugs known as corticosteroids, which are widely used for treatment of allergies, inflammatory conditions, and autoimmune dis-

---

[1] *Andrew Weil, M.D.,* Natural Health, Natural Medicine *(Boston: Houghton Mifflin Company, 1990), p. 192.*

eases. They are available as pills, injections, and topical creams. I rarely use corticosteroids because of their many negative side effects.

Dr. Weil also warns us about this family of pharmaceutical drugs:

> Steroids cause allergies and inflammation to disappear as if by magic. In fact, the magic is nothing other than direct suppression of immune function. I have no objection to giving these strong drugs for very severe or life-threatening problems, but even then I think they should be limited to short-term use: no more than two or three weeks. I deplore prescription of steroids for illnesses of mild or moderate severity or for months and years at a time.[2]

The side effects of corticosteroids are the same for horses as for people: weight gain, increased appetite, and increased urination, among others. Unfortunately the use of these drugs has grown more widespread during recent years because of the increase in allergy problems and the relatively few methods of treatment available. I realize that there are severe cases where corticosteroids must be utilized, such as acute shock; in most cases, however, I prefer to thoroughly investigate the problem first by looking at the cause of the symptoms. If the problem is an allergy, then I seek the underlying cause that has weakened the immune system, allowing it to react in this manner. Certain horses have genetic deficiencies that are associated with the immune system. Some of these immune problems are just deficiencies, whereas others are actual autoimmune or self-destroying syndromes.

I also use X-rays, tranquilizers, and anesthetics sparingly because they can be stressful for the body to detoxify. Excessive stress should be avoided whenever possible in order to keep the immune system healthy. When it is necessary to take X-rays or use a tranquilizer, I assist the horse with the detoxification process by giving a homeopathic remedy.

Vaccinations affect the immune system by stimulating a particular part of it to form an antigen for each of the diseases for which your horse is vaccinated. The antigen acts as a memory for the body and triggers a very fast response to protect the body when it is exposed to that particular disease. When vaccines are given, depending on the type of vaccine, the protection process can take as long as two weeks to become fully active. If many vaccines are administered at once, the immune system is kept "busy" responding to all of the vaccines and may therefore be unable to function efficiently. A good guideline is to give vaccines one at a time and at least two weeks apart to avoid overburdening the immune system and lessen the possibility of side effects. At present, vaccines are the only known effective protection against some specific diseases such as encephalomyelitis and rabies.

CHEMICALS IN THE FOOD CHAIN

In the last few decades there has been increased awareness of the toxins in our environment that adversely affect our sources of food and water. Most soil used for growing crops is treated with chemical fertilizers that break down into various chemical elements that are then selectively absorbed by plants. Occasionally this selective absorption results in a toxic concentration of a chemical in grains or hay, which can cause a horse to become ill. The level of toxicity from fertilizers in crops varies depending on the weather conditions during the growing season.

Another problem with crops is the use of pesticides. Residue from these chemicals remains on the crops when harvesting occurs. And, of course, the fertilizers and pesticides can eventu-

2 Ibid., p. 193.

ally affect our groundwater supplies. Even minute amounts of these chemicals that build up in soil and groundwater over time can have deleterious results.

In her book *Nontoxic, Natural and Earthwise*, environmental researcher Debra Lynn Dadd gives the following statistics:

In the United States, almost 2 billion pounds of pesticides are applied to our land every year, including food crops. In 1987, an EPA [Environmental Protection Agency] report ranked pesticides in food as one of the nation's most serious health and environmental problems. Pesticides are among the most deadly of chemicals: according to a report from the National Academy of Sciences, 30 percent of commercially used insecticides, 50 percent of herbicides, and 90 percent of fungicides are known to cause cancer in animal studies. Ironically, pesticides aren't even doing their job. Since they were first developed after World War II, pesticide use has increased ten times; during that same period, crop losses due to insects has doubled. Often less than .1 percent of the chemicals applied to crops actually reach target pests. Pesticides used in agriculture have contaminated nearly all the air, water, soil, and living beings of the entire planet. [3]

A newspaper article on this subject adds the following information:

Insect resistance to pesticides is also increasing. Currently, 600 of the most significant pests, including insects, weeds and plant diseases, are resistant to one or more classes of chemicals that had been developed to control them. Excessive use of toxic chemicals has also produced the unwanted result of creating pests out of species that had not previously caused any noticeable harm. "Spider mites are now a problem worldwide as a direct result of the use of DDT, which killed their natural enemy," [Sheila] Daar added. [4]

There are some encouraging signs, however. In place of chemicals, organic farmers use techniques such as crop rotation, disease-resistant crops, nontoxic products, and beneficial insects like ladybugs, spiders, lacewings and parasitic wasps that feed on the problem insects. More environmentally friendly farming techniques are also being used by a growing number of farms that are not certified as organic. We must also challenge governments around the world to continue doing more to respect our earth and its precious resources. (See the Appendices VII and VIII for books and organizations that offer more information on these issues.)

CHEMICAL HAZARDS IN STABLES AND BARNYARDS

As parts of the world become more environmentally conscious, there is increased public recognition of the dangers associated with the hazardous chemicals that we have used around our animals for decades. These chemicals are everywhere, it seems. I'm amazed at the way people continue to use the same pesticides, cleaning compounds, and other chemically questionable products with abandon. Horses and other animals may ingest or inhale these chemicals, causing yet another stress on the detoxification system and the immune system. Because of the widespread use of pesticides and other chemicals, it is wise to avoid letting your horse

3 *Debra Lynn Dadd, Nontoxic,* Natural and Earthwise, *(Jeremy P. Tarcher, Inc., 1990) p. 77.*
4 *Karen Dardick, "No Pests No Poisons," Los Angeles Times, June 14, 1992, p. K11.*

graze in any area that you are not certain is uncontaminated by such toxins.

Many fly repellents contain pesticides or other chemical solutions that cause some horses to develop itchy skin, dry flaky areas, or hives. Usually it is the long-term effect of these pesticides that is my major concern, but every now and then I treat a horse for a serious immediate reaction caused by this type of chemical poisoning.

Fortunately, there are now safer insecticides that use pyrethrin—a natural product obtained from flowers—as the active ingredient, but even pyrethrin can be toxic if your horse is overexposed or allergic to it. A number of books are now available on natural gardening and yard care, giving environmentally safe methods and products as alternatives to the chemicals that can be poisonous. Remember, though, that even products with natural ingredients such as pennyroyal, eucalyptus, and citronella must be used with caution because some animals have allergic reactions to them.

Carcinogenic and other toxic chemicals are found in cleaning products as well as paints and solvents. When you scrub down your barn aisle, stall, or driveway, a residue of the cleanser often remains. Chemicals in that cleanser might then be absorbed by your horse's skin, ingested, or harmful to hooves. Carefully check the labels of products you use around the stable and use natural products whenever possible.

SMOG, LEAD, AND OTHER ENVIRONMENTAL CONTAMINANTS

Sometimes it's hard to diagnose a problem that is stressing the immune system. This is the situation I encounter when working on an allergy case that is unresponsive or only partially responsive to therapy. Often I find that the problem is environmental pollution, such as smog. Allergic responses to environmental pollution are common, but they frequently go unrecog-

nized. As I question them, owners often realize that their horses were fine before they moved to an urban area, or that their condition improves when they are taken away from the city. The allergic reactions, however, usually recur within twenty-four hours of returning home. (Of course, this is true only when they travel to an area free of smog.)

Another hazard that is being investigated is the long-term effect of lead poisoning on both people and animals. One study concluded that lead contamination in our soil is the cause of many health problems. The amount of lead in the soil is high primarily in neighborhoods near major highways. This lead contamination, a frightening remnant from the days when "leaded" gasoline was standard, serves as another reminder that unsafe industrial and manufacturing practices can haunt us for years to come.

When I lived in Los Angeles, my horse Silver had an allergy problem caused by environmental pollution, so I understand the frustration experienced by my clients. Some animals are less able to handle this kind of toxic burden on the system, probably due to genetics. I have had good results in treating these animals with a combination of homeopathy and acupuncture, plus other remedies I mention in the listing under Allergies in Part Three of this book. Of course, the best solution is the drastic one of moving to a smog-free environment. That's the one I opted for when I moved away from Los Angeles.

EMOTIONAL ISSUES

In humans, the link between emotions and health has become an accepted truth in medicine. A new field of medicine, called psychoneuroimmunology, studies the interconnections between the mind (psycho), the nervous system (neuro), and the immune system (immunology). All of us who love horses know that, much like people, they are affected by changes in their environment, illness of a loved one, and the emotional well-being of the owner. Even a horse show or a long trailer ride can cause stress to a horse. These emotionally stressful situations can also be eased by alternative methods like homeopathies and Bach Flower Remedies.

If these emotional issues can result in a suppressed immune response for a person, there is every reason to believe that the same is true for horses.

IDENTIFYING STRESSES ON THE IMMUNE SYSTEM

There are many theories that attempt to explain the increase in immune deficiencies in recent years, and there may not be just one answer. When a horse suffers from an immune deficiency, the cause could be a single agent or a combination of agents. In an effort to pinpoint the underlying cause and eliminate it if possible, I start by taking a thorough history.

In addition, I review factors in the horse's food and environment that might be a source of toxins or allergies. The horse's vaccination history is reviewed, and, if necessary, I prescribe a nosode. Nosodes, which are described more fully in Chapter Four, are similar to homeopathic remedies; they are sometimes used to negate side effects from previous vaccinations. Next I record all grooming products that are used on the horse, from shampoo to fly spray, as well as the type of brushes.

Then I investigate the stable environment including bedding, cleaning products, and feed and water containers. I ask the owner about other possible negative influences, such as emotional upsets in the home. I know that my horse Charlie is extremely sensitive to my mood, and his behavior changes when I become upset. The same is true of my dogs. In particular, my white toy poodle, Lily, often has digestive problems and a poor appetite if I'm upset.

All phases of the horse's life are considered to have a bearing on his health and are integrated into the final diagnosis. Needless to say, the current complaint is strongly considered; however, as in the case of treatment of allergies and other reactions, the root cause of the problem must be found and dealt with, if possible, so a recurrence can be prevented.

The owner of a large racehorse-training barn was very astute when he noticed a gradual loss of color in the horses' coats. After a few weeks, their coats also began to look dull. In trying to pinpoint the cause, his first assumption was a deficiency in the diet. Blood samples were taken from a number of horses. They showed normal blood cell levels and blood chemistry balances. Even though the ration the horses were eating was completely balanced with vitamins and minerals, the owner decided to add additional supplements to the diet to see if they would make a difference. When this didn't improve the color and quality of the coats, I was consulted. This particular farm was already using mostly non-toxic products so the job of elimination was made easier. They had also already sent the grain and hay to a laboratory to test for the presence of toxins, and no toxins were found. Unfortunately, there are types of toxins for which no tests are currently available. So, with no further laboratory tests available, I used applied kinesiology muscle testing to check the feed and found that the grain was the culprit. Whether the reason was a toxin that was not found in the testing or a mold or bacteria, we will never know. However, once the grain was replaced, the horse's coats returned to their normal color and a healthy shine within a week.

The consideration of the entire horse and a thorough investigation into the root cause of a health problem is important to understand the symptoms. Most conventional veterinarians don't approach a problem like this in a holistic manner; therefore, their approach is more limited and may be less effective. Instead, in a situation like this one, a drug is usually prescribed or a coat conditioner suggested. But with the irritant still present—the grain in this case—the problem with the coats would not have been eliminated.

Keep in mind that it is crucial to implement the holistic approach from the very beginning of the diagnostic process. Otherwise, an owner may not remember all of the important details, starting at the onset of the problem that may serve as clues in diagnosis. As time passes, the horse's already sensitized immune system may begin overreacting to other things in addition to the original irritant, thus making it difficult to sort out a clear history and pinpoint the true cause of the problem. Although the holistic approach may seem to be more time consuming initially, in most cases the results are both more immediate and longer lasting than those attained using only conventional methods.

2 Holistic Veterinary Care

HOLISTIC VERSUS CONVENTIONAL VETERINARY MEDICINE

Holistic veterinarians care for their patients by combining all the resources, technology, and treatments of conventional medicine with a wide range of more natural, alternative methods. Not only does this give us a wider variety of treatment possibilities but it often provides a safer and healthier method of treatment. Dr. Andrew Weil, one of the leading holistic medical doctors today, refers to this mix of alternative and conventional methods as "integrative medicine" since it truly integrates all of the valid treatment options available.

Horse owners seek out holistic veterinarians for a variety of reasons, but the most common one is that conventional veterinary medicine alone has not kept their horses in the desired state of health. In most cases, when I diagnose a horse's problems I am able to identify one or more alternative treatments that are warranted. I prescribe conventional treatments such as pharmaceutical drugs or surgery only when there is no viable alternative treatment.

My objective in practice has always been to get the horse well using the safest, most effective method possible. Please note that speed is not one of my objectives. Although holistic treatment can sometimes bring fast results, it often works more gradually. Except in the case of emergencies, faster is not always better. Holistic veterinarians are thorough and leave no steps out of the diagnostic process. The goal of holistic veterinary treatment is long-term good health and soundness.

I was asked to examine a two-year-old Thoroughbred in training to be raced. The colt had great potential and had been started very slowly, but he would stay sound only about two weeks at a time before another injury would occur. When I examined the colt, I found very little structurally wrong. But his acupuncture points told a different story. The acupuncture points associated with the liver were extremely sensitive, and several other acupuncture points indicated extreme stress. I treated his liver with acupuncture and homeopathy. The colt was also given a Bach Flower Remedy to alleviate stress.

Following these treatments, he was able to train for four months at the farm and then be moved to train at a racetrack without a recurrence of the soundness problem.

This case demonstrates another advantage of holistic medicine. Most alternative methods of treatment were established before laboratory testing was available. They rely on diagnostic methods that are totally different from those used in conventional medicine. This is especially helpful when regular diagnostic methods do not provide enough answers. For instance, a veterinary acupuncturist uses pulse diagnosis to check energy meridians for deficiencies and can palpate to check for sensitive acupuncture points. A veterinarian who treats with homeopathy uses the horse's most important or guiding symptoms to determine the homeopathic remedy to be given. The need for chiropractic adjustments is determined by an in-depth palpation of the horse, although X-rays are sometimes also used.

It is this broader range of available diagnosis and treatment methods that first interested me in holistic medicine. Using conventional veterinary medicine I found that many medical problems were either not treatable or required drug therapy that was potentially harmful to the horse. Andy, a three-year-old Oldenburg gelding, was brought to me because of training problems. Six months previously Andy had been found cast (stuck lying down) in his stall. After his rescue, Andy had returned to dressage training but was very resistant and uncooperative. His owner was very upset since Andy had always loved his training sessions and showed great promise as an event and dressage horse.

Extensive testing and X-rays had revealed no problems so Andy was put on phenylbutazone (commonly known as "bute"), a non-steroidal anti-inflammatory drug, for a few weeks. The drug helped a little and was continued for two months, but phenylbutazone can cause inflammation of the stomach lining. Eventually it seemed to be affecting Andy's appetite so it was discontinued. At this point Andy's training was suspended and he was rested for four months. When he was returned to training, he seemed even worse and did not even tolerate grooming. He was brought to me as a last resort.

During my examination of him, Andy revealed that he was extremely sensitive and very intolerant to pain. His neck, thoracic area, sacrum, pelvis, and coccyx vertebrae were out of alignment. In addition, he had sensitivity over the spleen, stomach, and liver acupuncture points. I gave Andy a chiropractic adjustment that realigned his spine, sacrum, and pelvis. Then I treated him with acupuncture. The acupuncture helped relax Andy's muscles and balance his acupuncture meridians. Within three days Andy was feeling better, and he was more willing to work when ridden. His back was no longer sore to the touch and he was enjoying his grooming sessions again. After two treatments Andy was training normally and has not required further treatment.

I like to see results before judging the effectiveness of different forms of treatment. Andy's rapid recovery with holistic methods compared to his lack of progress with many weeks of conventional treatment confirmed for me the effectiveness of holistic medicine in this case.

While I have seen dramatic physical changes with holistic medicine, the positive results go even further. Most alternative methods also address the mental well-being of a horse. This is another aspect of holistic medicine that is a tremendous advantage when treating an animal. Horses are susceptible to a full range of emotional disturbances; many of them are tied to stresses in the environment surrounding them. An increasing number of horses seem to be affected by stress, particularly those that maintain rigorous show schedules or training regimens. The horse often becomes so stressed that he becomes physically ill.

Little Joe, a yearling Quarter Horse, was very successful in his early show career as a halter horse (shown in hand). The show schedule increased in the autumn when the weather was turning cold. Being hauled in a trailer for four to six hours—a common occurrence in the United States—and spending the night in strange places can be very stressful and traumatic to a horse, especially a young one.

The added impact of colder weather increased the stress on his immune system and Little Joe became ill with a respiratory infection. He was treated with antibiotics for one week and then returned to showing another week later when the symptoms were gone. Within a few weeks, the respiratory infection returned, and Little Joe was treated with antibiotics again. He lost weight and took three weeks to recover this time. As soon as he was better, he was taken to a show and was ill when he returned home again. After a third treatment with antibiotics, Little Joe was not shown any more. Once he had recovered, he was sold.

His new owner gave him some time to rest, but after a few months Little Joe still had not gained weight and had a dry, dull hair coat. He seemed lethargic and was often cranky and difficult to handle. Then the new owner called me in to do a holistic exam. I explained that the excessive stress from horse shows had not allowed this young horse to fully recover from one illness to the next, and his system had finally experienced a deficiency that it could not overcome. I treated Little Joe with acupuncture and homeopathy and within a week noticed a tremendous difference. His appetite returned, his energy improved, and his coat started to shine. After three treatments he had returned to normal health.

FINDING A HOLISTIC VETERINARIAN

Just because a veterinarian advertises that he is "holistic" does not mean he is well versed in a range of conventional and alternative treatment options. When you are evaluating the qualifications of a holistic veterinarian, ask about his affiliations with professional associations, years of experience, and which specific alternative methods are his specialties. Several associations of holistic veterinarians are listed in Appendix VIII.

If you are unable to find a holistic veterinarian in your area, it is possible to work long distance with a veterinarian who prescribes homeopathy, herbs, and Bach Flower Remedies as long as you have a consulting veterinarian locally to do examinations and any necessary tests for an accurate diagnosis. The long-distance veterinarian will require information obtained by the "hands on" veterinarian. If you choose to pursue this type of arrangement, be sure that your local veterinarian is agreeable to working in this manner. Another option is to find a holistic veterinarian who is willing to travel to areas where a holistic veterinarian is not available. Many holistic veterinarians do this, but they usually require a group of horses to make the trip viable.

While it was once standard for veterinarians to make farm visits, today many horse owners take their horses to the veterinarian because the veterinarian has a greater amount of diagnostic equipment and other services available at the clinic. The cost is lower for owners since they don't have to pay for the veterinarian's travel time, and veterinarians find it both more convenient and more cost effective.

Regardless of whether you choose conventional or holistic health care, it's important to find a veterinarian that both you and your horse like. Once you have narrowed the field of acceptable veterinarians, here are some additional questions to ask the veterinarian or clinic staff over the phone:

- When are your hours?
- What happens if my horse requires emergency treatment? Do you provide 24-hour care? (Some veterinarians handle their own emergencies, and others make referrals to an emergency hospital.)
- How many veterinarians are on your staff and what are their qualifications? Are they male or female? (Many horses are more comfortable with one gender or the other.)
- How do you feel about an owner getting a second opinion from another veterinarian in case of a major health problem?
- What are your payment policies? (Very few veterinarians offer credit, but many take credit cards and checks, with some also honoring equine insurance programs. Always include insurance information in your horse's records so your veterinarian has it in case of emergency when you are unavailable.)

The practice of getting a second opinion from another veterinarian has become more common in recent years. Each veterinarian views this in a different light, which is why it is advisable to ask the veterinarian's views on this topic before committing your horse to his care. A doctor who is secure and open-minded will encourage an owner to seek further advice from other sources when the case at hand is difficult, or may make a referral to a specialist. If you plan to get a second opinion, let your veterinarian know of your decision early on, because you may save the cost of repeat lab work or diagnostic expenses.

Once you have gone through the basic checklist, it's time to get down to the finer details. At this point you will need to meet the veterinarian (or talk to him on the phone if it's a long distance). If you are planning to take your horse to the clinic for treatment, you should make note of the way it is run. Here are a few considerations about the clinic itself:

- Is the outside clean and well kept?
- Is your first overall impression favorable?
- Is the receptionist friendly and helpful?
- Is the inside of the clinic clean?
- Are the employees neat and reasonably clean?
- Do you like the way the staff handles the horses?
- Are any signs posted specifying clinic policies that don't match your own needs?

The general condition of the clinic facility can be a reflection of the standards of the veterinary practice itself. If the clinic is designed for your horse's comfort and safety, you will probably find that the staff members are caring and thoughtful people who practice progressive medicine.

If your horse has special needs (a stallion stall, rubber mats on the floor, isolation), check to be sure they can be accommodated. Not all veterinarians have a full range of highly technical diagnostic machines such as the ECG (electrocardiograph) machine, ultra sound, or fiberoptic devices, but most have X-ray capability along with other basic equipment. If your horse requires a special type of diagnostic equipment, which an otherwise desirable veterinarian does not have, the clinic may be able to arrange a referral for that particular test. Referrals are common in veterinary practice just as in human medicine, and most veterinarians will not hesitate to refer to a colleague who specializes in a particular field.

THE VETERINARY EXAMINATION

Whenever possible, you should be present when your horse is examined. For one thing, you will be available to answer any questions that might assist the veterinarian in making a diagnosis. If you cannot be present, write down any pertinent information that the veterinarian might need including age, breed, main complaint, the diet you are feeding and how much, and what your horse's exercise program is. Include as much detail concerning the main problem as possible (especially if it is not an obvious one). You should also arrange to be available if needed for a phone consultation during or after the exam. Remember that most veterinarians speak to dozens of clients a day, so your veterinarian may not recall all of the information you told him in a previous phone conversation.

If you know that your horse is difficult to handle, be sure to inform the veterinarian so he can be prepared. The horse may need to be restrained or given a sedative. One of my worst experiences in practice resulted from an owner's failure to tell me about her gelding's recent treatment by another veterinarian. The owner simply stated that the horse was not moving correctly and she thought he needed a chiropractic adjustment. The horse was very tense and had muscle spasms down his back, so I suggested acupuncture instead to relieve the spasms. The owner agreed, and I got out the needles.

Most horses do not notice when acupuncture needles are placed, but this horse did not even let me get close to placing a needle. He started rearing and striking with his front feet, intent on avoiding any treatment. Fortunately, after years of practice, my reflexes are quick, and I was able to avoid being kicked—but it was too close for comfort. When I asked the owner why this horse suddenly reacted so violently, she told me he had just completed a treatment that called for three painful injections a day and had become very difficult to handle when injections were attempted. She had not warned me about this dangerous behavior, and she refused to

allow me to use any further restraint, or to tranquilize the horse so I was not able to treat him. There are two things to be learned from this situation. First, the veterinarian should always be warned about any potential for dangerous behavior, and second, the veterinarian must always be informed about the horse's medical history— especially any recent medical problem that might influence the choice of treatment.

It is important to know all the behavioral patterns your horse can exhibit. When examined by the veterinarian many horses become nervous and aggressive. Often the owner's presence helps to reassure and calm the horse, as well as making the owner aware that her horse might behave in an unruly manner when being treated. In case the owner ever has to administer first aid, this knowledge will forewarn her to take precautions if difficult behavior is anticipated.

Watch the way your horse is handled during the examination. Of course, if your horse is excited or resists the exam, then more restraint may be required. However, an experienced veterinarian will have methods to hold and restrain your horse that will not cause harm. Occasionally a horse will be so frightened or uncooperative that a sedative will have to be used. Only rarely is this necessary, but when it is, your veterinarian can administer an effective and safe tranquilizer.

THE ROUTINE CHECKUP

The annual checkup is the only time I see many of my patients, so I always give them a complete physical exam prior to administering any regularly scheduled treatment. It is particularly important to do a careful exam on horses approaching old age, in order to catch developing health problems. Occasionally for a horse of 15 years and older, I suggest laboratory blood work as well so that a baseline of that horse's normal values can be on record in case any problems arise in the future. In some cases I suggest this blood work regardless of the horse's age, particularly if the horse competes regularly. Then, if the horse has a health problem, medical attention can be more prompt.

Each veterinarian conducts an exam differently. I like to palpate, or feel, the entire horse, starting at the tip of the nose and working my way back to the tail. I give special attention to the teeth, checking for infected gums, broken teeth, hooks (sharp points on the molars), and uneven wear. These disorders interfere with a horse's ability to chew properly resulting in incomplete breakdown of food before it's swallowed. When food is chewed insufficiently, the horse's digestive system cannot extract the necessary nutrients that cause him to lose weight, and might even cause him to colic. When I detect any of these dental problems, the horse's teeth should be "floated"—a procedure that evens and shapes the teeth with a rasp (dental float). All dentistry work should be performed by a veterinarian, or a certified dental technician.

The same attention should be given to the ears, checking the outside as well as the inside. In climates where parasites are prevalent, the outside of the ears and tips should be checked for evidence of scratching or fly bites, and the insides for signs of ticks or fungal infections. Because a moist, humid climate increases the incidence of fungal infections, these problems often show up in the summer. Early detection helps prevent damage to the ear as well as avoiding a deep-seated infection.

I examine the rest of the body in a similar fashion, checking the skin, the hair coat quality, body weight, and muscle condition. The coat should be bright and glossy and I also take note of the hair color. Is it the same as always, or has a black horse turned brown? This type of change can be a warning sign of a health problem. Is the horse moving normally? Is his overall attitude depressed or defensive? Has his behavior changed? If the horse's weight is excessive, diet alternatives are discussed and possible contributing medical problems are evaluated. Many times, the first indications of glandular disorders such as hypothyroidism are a coat that becomes dull and sometimes changes color, and an increase in weight.

I also palpate the acupuncture points for any sensitivity. Then I run my hands down the legs and check for soreness or swelling. Detecting early tendon or ligament inflammation can prevent a more serious future condition. Hooves are also checked for condition, shape, and shoe set. In addition the leg conformation is assessed. If any conformation defects are noted, the owner is informed so any necessary preventive steps can be taken or certain exercises that might aggravate a problem area can be avoided.

Checking for external as well as internal parasites is always part of the exam. If parasites are not properly controlled, internal damage can occur, feed is not properly absorbed, and your horse's overall health and performance ability can be affected. Parasites can even cause death due to intestinal perforations, colic, and aneurysms. An effective worming program is very important.

I check for internal parasites, like large strongyles, through a fecal sample, which is either brought in by the owner or obtained from the horse during the exam. If excessive egg counts are found, the worming schedule is reviewed. I discuss various solutions and control measures that will work best for the needs of the horse. Fortunately, internal parasites are less commonly seen than they used to be because wormers are readily available in paste form, and most horse owners are aware that strict routine worming is necessary.

Worming programs will vary depending on where you live, the number of horses on the farm, and the living and pasture conditions. If horses have been kept on the same pasture for many years and have not been regularly wormed, the ground will become saturated with parasite eggs which horses can pick up as they graze or shift through the dirt. In some older facilities, the ground may be saturated with parasite larvae so you may have to worm your horse even more often to prevent parasite buildup.

If you live in a warm, humid climate, your worming program must be even more aggressive since parasites thrive in this type of climate. Cold winter weather breaks the parasite cycle, even though cold temperatures do not get rid of them entirely. You should have fecal checks done regularly until you and your veterinarian can assess the parasite load in your horse and determine the correct interval for worming.

The worming program will also depend on the individual horse's needs. Some horses have a history of insufficient worming or have had no worming at all. These horses may have suffered internal damage due to parasite migration and may colic with even low levels of parasite infestation.

During the exam I also always discuss the diet. If a change of diet is necessary, I discuss the options with the owner, including available feed, supplements, and electrolytes (see Chapter Five).

Any potential problem is addressed in the yearly exam, treating it the same as a human's annual physical exam. My objective is to keep your horse's health at optimum performance.

OTHER HEALTH CARE PROFESSIONALS

Until recent years, horse trainers and farriers were the only horse-care professionals an owner could consult other than veterinarians. As our desire to improve health care for our equine companions has grown, the range of professionals has expanded to include nutritionists, dentists, equine massage therapists, and animal communicators and behaviorists.

The procedure for selecting any of these professionals is similar to that outlined previously for choosing a veterinarian. Don't be shy about checking out any health care professional you are considering to treat your horse. At the very least, you can investigate the reputation of the person you are considering by asking people whose opinion you respect. Your veterinarian is a good source of information. Fellow horse owners, tack shops, and horse trainers may also be able to give you leads. Be aware that in some of the United States, and in the United Kingdom, there are specific laws regulating what equine professionals can and cannot do legally.

Finally, your own skill at interviewing prospective professionals will be important in determining if the person is someone you can trust.

3 Alternative Treatments

Many of the alternative healing methods used by humans have been adopted by veterinarians and other equine health-care professionals. In this chapter I will describe the most common treatments in use today, including acupuncture, acupressure, aromatherapy, Bach Flower remedies, chiropractic, herbs, homeopathy, hydrogen peroxide therapy, lasers, magnetic therapy, massage therapy, and the training and healing systems known as TTEAM and TTouch.

In many cases, I advise the combination of several treatments. For instance, herbal remedies, acupuncture, and homeopathy can all be utilized simultaneously. If a serious condition warrants a pharmaceutical drug or invasive medical procedure, the addition of complementary alternative remedies can make the difference that leads to successful treatment and speedy recovery.

ACUPUNCTURE AND MOXIBUSTION

Interest in the 4,000-year-old Chinese healing art of acupuncture has increased over the last thirty years. The dramatic health benefits that can be derived from acupuncture are becoming widely known and veterinarians have taken notice. In the United States, the International Veterinary Acupuncture Society (IVAS) teaches veterinarians the theory and application of acupuncture and also certifies veterinarians in the field of acupuncture. Attendance at this course has increased steadily each year. If you want to find a qualified veterinary acupuncturist, ask if he or she has been trained and certified by the IVAS.

The general public has been exposed to veterinary acupuncture in magazine and newspaper articles and television talk shows, leading to greater acceptance of this form of treatment. Nevertheless, misconceptions about the safety, effectiveness, and comfort of acupuncture have made some owners reluctant to consider it as a treatment for their horses. I am still pleasantly surprised when a new client asks about acupuncture as a treatment option for his or her horse. Usually the request is prompted by the experience of a friend or relative who has received acupuncture treatments and was pleased with the results. Interestingly, many of

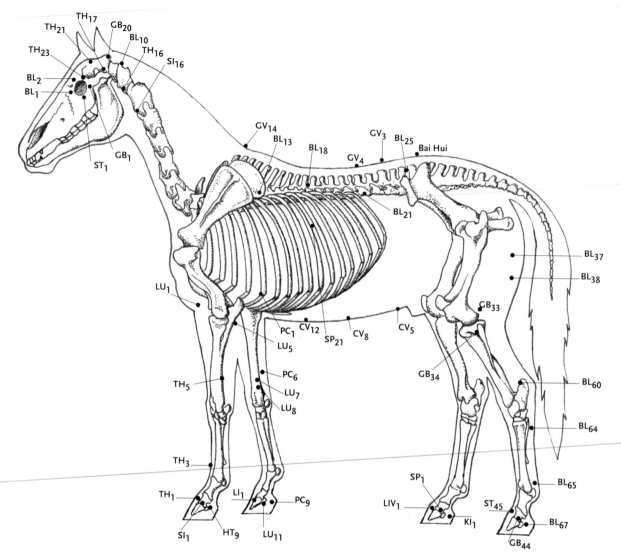

3.1 *Commonly used acupuncture points on the horse's body.*

my clients whose horses receive acupuncture eventually seek acupuncture for themselves when they observe the improvement in the horse's condition.

Acupuncture is one of the most fascinating modalities within Eastern medicine. It is a constant source of discovery and learning for me, since I have repeatedly seen how the simple insertion of a needle can influence the entire physiology of the body. An acupuncturist's goal is not only to relieve a patient's symptoms, but to balance the energy system of the entire body so the underlying problem will not recur. As a result of this rebalancing, owners often notice that not only has the original problem disappeared, but the horse seems more energetic and happy.

Acupuncture is also becoming increasingly popular with horse owners who compete because it usually allows continued performance without having to resort to the use of drugs, which are often banned in competition. In addition, some trainers find that the horse's attitude is greatly improved by acupuncture, and they request an energy-balancing treatment before major shows. Whatever the application, acupuncture is providing competitors with an alternative form of treatment to keep their horses in top form.

During an acupuncture treatment, hair-thin needles are inserted into the skin at locations known as acupuncture points (see fig. 3.1). The needles typically are inserted from 1/10 inch to 4/10 inch (0.3 to 1 centimeter) deep, although some procedures require the needles to be inserted much deeper. The number and placement of needles will vary depending on the particular symptoms or condition being treated. Most acupuncture treatments take from five to twenty minutes once the needles are in place, and the horse experiences very little discomfort when the needles are inserted.

The acupuncture points are specific places along lines of energy, known as the *meridian lines*, each of which corresponds to specific functions of the body. When there is a problem in an area of the body, the energy that flows through that area is decreased or sometimes even totally blocked. The insertion of the metal needle at the acupuncture point stimulates the energy, causing an increase or return of the flow. Re-establishment of the normal energy flow increases circulation and stimulates nerves, allowing the area previously depleted of energy to return to normal functioning.

The acupuncture treatment also causes the release of endorphins—substances in the brain which have opiate-like and analgesic properties. Occasionally this leads to sleepiness.

Many horses find this sensation very pleasant, even horses who react badly to needles when being inoculated often tolerate acupuncture surprisingly well. One Thoroughbred gelding that I treated regularly for back problems normally had a fractious disposition and was hard to handle. After the first needle was inserted, however, he would always fall sound asleep in the cross-ties, presenting no problems during treatment.

Enhancing the Acupuncture Treatment

In addition to the insertion of needles, some conditions benefit from extra stimulation to further enhance the acupuncture treatment. This can be achieved through the use of electrical stimulation, moxibustion, or acupressure.

Electrical stimulation is incorporated into an acupuncture treatment by using small clips that are attached to the acupuncture needles. The clips emit minute electrical impulses that increase the effect of the needles. These impulses are very small and often are not even noticed by the patient.

Another treatment used either in conjunction with acupuncture or on its own is moxibustion, which is also referred to as "moxa." Moxibustion is especially good for enhancing healing because it increases circulation to the area being treated. Although it is applied to many conditions, moxa is particularly effective in treating arthritic horses because it simultaneously applies heat over painful areas and stimulates the acupuncture point. In moxibustion the herb mugwort can be used in several different ways to further stimulate the acupuncture points being treated. The herb is available in a loose form, which is usually burned in a special holder which is held over the acupuncture needles that have been inserted by the veterinarian (see fig. 3.2).

In another technique, called *punk moxa,* small pieces of burning mugwort are attached to the top of the acupuncture needles.

A third method of moxibustion does not involve the use of acupuncture needles. This technique referred to as *indirect moxibustion* is easy and can be done by anyone, not just acupuncturists. It is a safe method of treatment so long as you exercise the precautions noted below. Indirect moxibustion is done with mugwort that has been shaped into a stick about one half-inch in diameter and ten inches long (about 10 mm and 25 cm).

INDIRECT MOXIBUSTION

Caution: Moxibustion involves the use of a flame and the burning of an herb. Do not do indirect moxibustion inside a barn or near any flammable material.

1. Light the end of the stick with a candle or match. It is usually slow to light. A butane fireplace lighter works well for this.

2. Hold the moxa stick about one half-inch above the acupuncture point you want to treat.

3. Move the stick in small circles over the general area of the point you are treating for two to five minutes. It is important to keep the stick constantly moving because it burns very hot, and you do not want to cause any discomfort to the horse. Caution: Do not allow the moxa stick to make direct contact with the horse's body.

4. Continue the treatment by repeating Steps 2 and 3 on additional acupuncture points.

If your horse has a recurring problem and is being treated with acupuncture, ask your veterinarian if indirect moxa treatments would be helpful. If so, he can show you the specific areas to treat and may be able to provide the moxa stick.

When to Use Acupuncture

There is a broad range of clinical indications for acupuncture in the equine. It is best known for the treatment of spinal disorders, particularly disc problems, but many other skeletal problems such as arthritis, navicular disease, and joint inflammation can be greatly improved by acupuncture.

In addition to performance-related problems, a wide variety of physiological disorders can also be treated with acupuncture. Pulmonary edema (heaves), allergies, anhidrosis (inability to sweat), kidney failure, liver problems, muscle atrophy, nerve injuries, Wobbler Syndrome, and reproductive disorders are among the conditions responsive to acupuncture. You will see a detailed description of the health ailments that can be treated with acupuncture in Part Three of this book.

Many veterinarians examine the acupuncture points either to detect conditions that may otherwise go unnoticed or to confirm a suspected diagnosis. There are hundreds of acupuncture points that can be used for diagnostic purposes. Like many veterinarians, I usually check the bladder meridian first because the acupuncture points along this meridian represent many of the organs and systems of the body. This meridian starts at the inside corner of the eye, runs up through the eyebrow over the top of the head, down the neck to the withers, along the back, and descends down the hind leg ending at the hoof. The points along the back—about three to

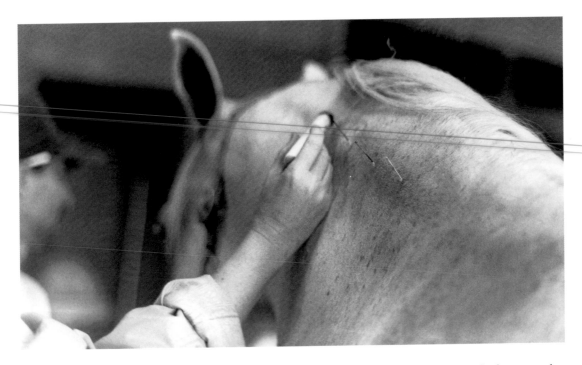

3.2 *A horse undergoing a moxibustion treatment. The veterinarian is using a moxibustion stick of mugwort that is burning on one end over the inserted acupuncture needles.*

four inches (seven to ten centimeters) from the midline of the back—correspond to the main organs of the body, including the heart, lungs, and liver.

When examining the acupuncture points, I find the meridian, then gently run my fingers along it to locate the exact points. The points feel like small indentations and any soreness or heat in them indicates the possibility of a problem. For instance, a horse that appears to have a sore back may actually be experiencing tenderness at the acupuncture points associated with the liver, which are located where the rear of the saddle and most of the rider's weight rest. The veterinarian must differentiate a sensitive acupuncture point from the possibility of a local injury to be sure the sensitivity is associated only with the point. Other acupuncture points may also be checked. I usually check many of the points located on the legs, particularly if the horse is lame.

Acupuncture is also used for cosmetic reasons. It is becoming very popular to use acupuncture to decrease the neck size of certain breeds of halter horses (horses shown in hand), making the neck appear thinner. This process has been successful with both young and mature horses. At least three treatments are required for maximum results, and occasionally the treatment must be repeated to maintain the results. The reduction of scar tissue surrounding injuries is another cosmetic use for acupuncture.

There are many other applications for acupuncture, and it is often used by holistic veterinarians together with conventional treatments. The specific acupuncture points can be used to help pinpoint a diagnosis or to see if an old problem is flaring up again. A good example is a horse that hemorrhages from the nose when raced. Sometimes the bleeding occurs in small amounts in the lung during workouts and can be difficult to detect. By checking the lung acupuncture points for sensitivity the veterinarian can monitor the severity of the problem and treat it when necessary with a combination of conventional medicine, acupuncture, homeopathy, and herbs.

One of the first cases in which I used acupuncture stands out among the many in which I have seen dramatic results. Perhaps it was because I was still a little skeptical, but the striking results in this case wiped away any doubts in my mind concerning the role of acupuncture in a holistic veterinary practice. When I arrived at the barn, a twenty-year-old horse was led out slowly, walking as though all of his legs were sore and he was stepping on eggshells. The old Thoroughbred had more things wrong with his legs than usually seen in one horse. He had one of each major leg ailment—bowed tendon, ringbone, and navicular disease—in addition to a number of huge scars in various places on his legs. There was even a steel pin still in one of his hocks. His function in life had been to carry young riders safely around a hunter course of low jumps, teaching them to compete. His trainer told me that his performance had gradually worsened.

My heart went out to this big 17-hand horse, but I didn't have much hope that his condition could be improved with any kind of treatment. Conditions like his usually lead to permanent lameness. Still, I decided to try acupuncture to see if I could at least alleviate some of his pain. I explained to the trainer that occasionally a horse gets worse for a few days after an acupuncture treatment and then improvement is noted. A few days later, I called to check on his progress, and the trainer told me that he had stepped out of his stall perfectly sound the day after his acupuncture treatment and had been jumping well ever since. The horse stayed sound for six months and then was re-treated. I was truly amazed that one acupuncture treatment

could result in such marked improvement and last so long.

Many physiological conditions such as kidney disorders, elevated liver enzymes, viruses, glandular imbalances, and allergies can also respond to acupuncture. Let's take allergies as an example. Appaloosas are prone to allergies, particularly during the spring and summer. One client of mine grew tired of seeing his favorite horse so uncomfortable, with runny eyes, crusty skin, and a chronic nasal discharge. I treated the horse with acupuncture three times, and his symptoms disappeared for the remainder of the summer. The following year the symptoms returned but were only half as severe. One acupuncture treatment was required to relieve the horse from allergy symptoms for the rest of that year. With each passing year, the horse's symptoms continued to decrease until, eventually, he no longer needed treatment.

Even when no symptoms of illness are present, I often check the meridians during an exam, just to make sure none of them are deficient. This is especially helpful for older horses. If a meridian is deficient, I recommend acupuncture treatment to prevent the development of an illness due to this decrease in energy. Although the old saying, "If it's not broken, don't fix it", has merit, sometimes regular maintenance can help prevent a full-scale breakdown.

As the replacement cost of well-trained and well-bred horses continues to climb, many are being used long past fifteen years of age. Acupuncture often can help these older horses continue to perform to the best of their ability. Most of us don't realize when our horses are in pain, and we may not attribute a training problem to pain unless the horse is noticeably lame. Many older horses have mild arthritis, and treatment combining acupuncture, herbs, and homeopathy can make them feel like a younger horse. My own 19-year-old Thoroughbred has an incredible attitude change after acupuncture treatment, having a "can-do-whatever-you-ask" frame of mind. I often hear from owners that their horses display a similar attitude improvement after treatment, even when their horses don't have major health problems.

How Acupuncture Affects Behavior

Owners frequently notice an immediate effect on behavior after an acupuncture treatment. Since acupuncture causes the release of endorphins, many horses associate the acupuncture with pleasurable feelings. Often, very difficult horses calm down immediately when the acupuncture treatment is started. After a treatment, horses may show a markedly calm disposition and a good attitude. The combined benefits of treating the problem area and the endorphin release can make a great difference in a horse's personality.

Each horse has an ideal point in time after the treatment when acupuncture seems to have the greatest impact. For some, it is the day after, and for others, up to five days after a treatment. When owners want a horse to feel particularly good for a competition, I recommend that at least one acupuncture treatment be done a month or so prior to the show. This way the owner can monitor the results and determine the optimum timing for a treatment before the show. Behavior, attitude, and overall energy are affected by an acupuncture treatment. After one treatment, you will have an idea of the results to expect.

Caution: Only a qualified acupuncturist should ever attempt acupuncture. The principles of acupuncture are complex and require considerable training.

*For a map of the points, and a list of the points that can be stimulated by the layman using acupuncture instead of acupuncture, please see the *Acupuncture/Acupressure Appendix I* on p. 291.

NAET

Acupressure, in conjunction with muscle testing (see p. 148), is used to identify allergies in a technique known as NAET, which stands for Nambudripad's Allergy Elimination Technique. Dr. Devi S. Nambudripad, who lives in California, developed the system and teaches it to health care practitioners.

First the allergen (or allergens) is identified through muscle testing. While holding the allergen against the patient, acupressure is applied to specific points on several meridians one at a time in a specific sequence. The key to a successful treatment is having a practitioner who knows the procedure well and who has a large variety of substances (possible allergens) to test on the horse. The technique is not painful, has no side effects, and is very effective. It may require more than one treatment. For more information, and how to order Dr. Devi S. Nambudripad's book explaining NAET, *Say Goodbye to Illness,* on the World Wide Web, see Appendix VII.

For additional methods of healing based on principals similar to acupuncture, see the next section on acupressure, *Acupuncture/Acupressure Appendix I,* and lasers on p. 44.

ACUPRESSURE

Acupressure, which is similar to the Japanese technique known as Shiatsu, is another variation on the theme of acupuncture. Instead of using a needle to stimulate the specific points, in acupressure a hard firm pressure is applied with the fingers. Acupressure is a safe method for owners to use. If you don't hit the precise acupuncture point you can't do any harm.

If you are like so many of the owners I know, you may wish there was more you could do yourself to help your horse maintain good health or recover from an illness. Acupressure may be just the answer. You can learn to do acupressure

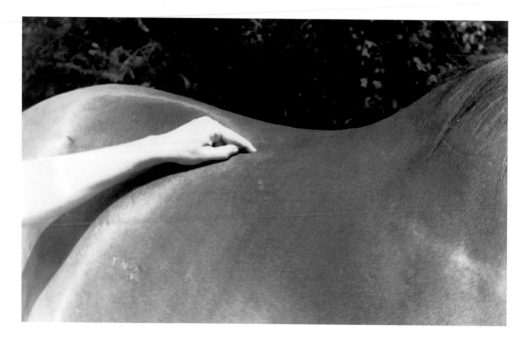

3.3   *Stimulating acupuncture points with a technique called acupressure—a firm pressure applied with the fingers—is an excellent way for owners to help their horses. Bladder meridian points are easy to locate and safe to treat. Here is BL_{18} , which is associated with the liver and may increase the appetite in stressed horses.*

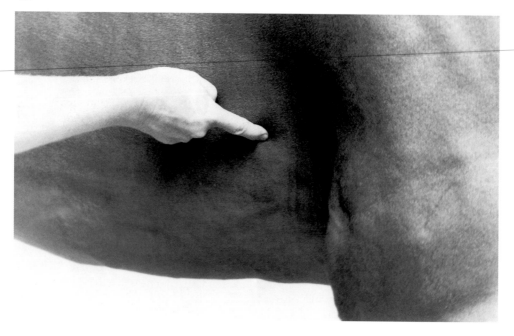

3.4 *Some acupuncture points are easier to locate than others. The first point on the pericardium meridian—PC_1—located behind the elbow may take some practice. Stimulating this point is helpful for treating hoof problems.*

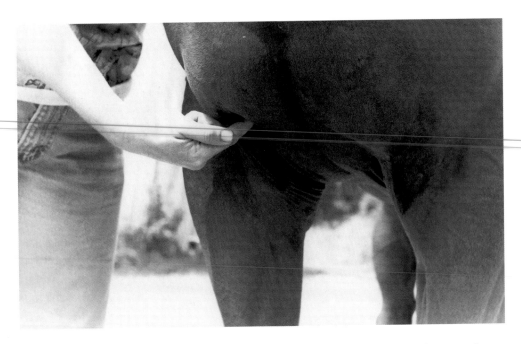

3.5 *Here is point LU$_1$ located on the front of the chest in a small depression in the pectoral muscle. Applying acupressure on LU$_1$ aids in the treatment of respiratory viruses, heaves, and chest and shoulder pain.*

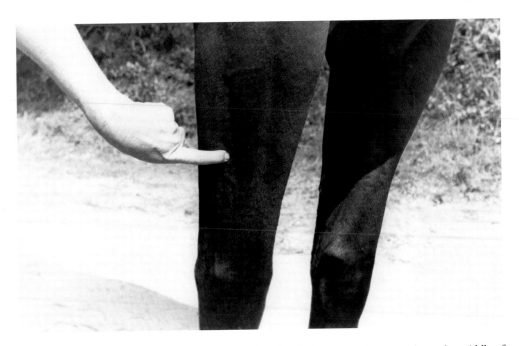

3.6 *Point TH$_5$ is located on the outside of the front leg in the crease that runs down the middle of the leg between the lateral and common digital extensor tendons, about 3 inches (8 cm) above the knee. Stimulation of TH$_5$ will help in the treatment of laminitis, tendonitis, navicular disease, and increase circulation to a healing leg injury.*

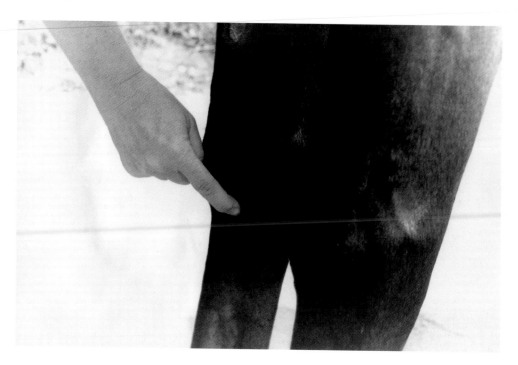

3.7 *LU₇, located on the inside of the front leg, has many important applications in treatment. Acupressure on this point is used for knee, neck, and tooth pain; it's helpful for coughs; and it supports treatment of large intestine problems, particularly constipation.*

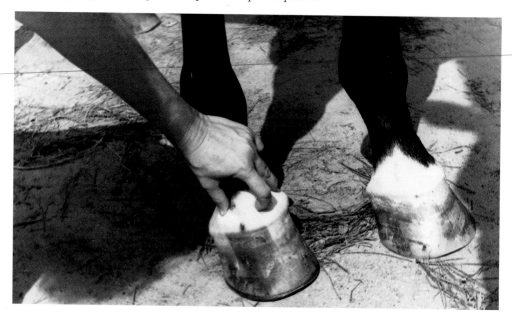

3.8 *These are three common points to stimulate around the coronary band: SI₁, on the outside, is used to treat laminitis and ringbone; TH₁, in the middle, helps with problems involving the hoof and can also be useful for treating gas colic and fever; LI₁, on the inside, aids the treatment of laminitis and ringbone, as well as upper respiratory illness.*

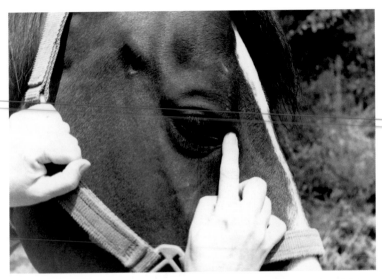

3.9 BL_1 is located slightly above the inside corner of the eye. Stimulation assists in healing eye problems. **Caution:** This is not a point for the use of moxibustion.

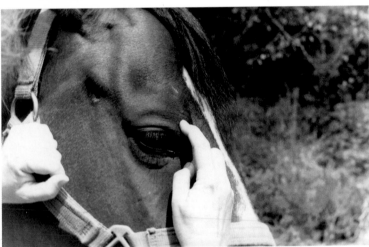

3.10 BL_2 is at the inside edge of the horse's "eyebrow" and can aid in circulation to the eye during the treatment of eye problems or head trauma.

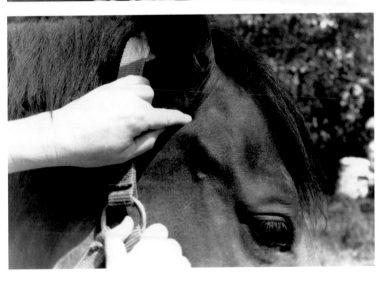

3.11 TH_{17} is found in the depression about 1/2 inch (1 cm) below the ear. It's commonly used for aiding all problems affecting the ear.

by following a few simple guidelines. Best of all, you don't need to buy any equipment. All you need is a positive attitude, willing spirit, and the techniques you'll learn on these pages.

An acupressure treatment can be done in minutes. Among the many positive benefits of acupressure treatments are:

- stimulating the immune system
- aiding the functioning of the lymph system
- promoting circulation of blood and nutrients throughout the body and the removal of toxins
- promoting relaxation and a feeling of contentment
- reducing pain and discomfort
- calming a nervous horse
- decreasing the heart rate

Acupressure can be extremely helpful in relieving health problems such as digestive upsets, arthritis, and muscle spasms. It can also be used to calm a horse after a traumatic injury, medical treatment, or emotional upset. Older horses and those who are chronically ill can benefit from acupressure.

I once treated a horse being shown in hand in the stallion classes at Quarter Horse shows. He had a recurring inflammation in his coffin joint, which caused a slight lameness. Even though he would be sound after an acupuncture treatment at home, the long trips in the trailer seemed to aggravate the condition again and he would turn up lame at the show. So I taught the owner how to use acupressure to improve circulation in the leg and suggested that he treat the horse when he arrived at the show. With the improved circulation, the coffin joint inflammation decreased, and the lameness disappeared.

Acupressure is based on the same principles as acupuncture, except that acupressure can be done by an owner with a minimum of instruc-

tion. Just as with acupuncture, acupressure affects the entire body system and significant improvements can often be seen after only one or two treatments. Although the results from acupressure are not as dramatic as seen with acupuncture, similar benefits can be achieved—especially when a specific treatment is repeated a few times. (When a horse is receiving acupuncture treatments, I often suggest that owners use acupressure as an adjunct to stimulate the energy between acupuncture treatments.) The use of acupressure often shortens healing time in half and it is another way you are empowered to help your horse through a difficult time.

There are other benefits to the acupressure treatment as well. It's a time you and your horse can spend together, bonding and focusing on his health and well-being. The therapeutic benefits of touch through massage, laying on of hands healing, and other touch oriented modalities have been documented in the healing of both people and animals. The human/animal bond is fortified and reinforced with every caring word, thought, and touch. Acupressure combines the healing power of touch with the ancient healing method of acupuncture.

*Part Three of this book contains a detailed list of treatments for many common horse ailments. In it I have laid out the specific acupressure points which you can use to treat different medical conditions. A complete list of these acupressure points and related information is available in the *Acupuncture/Acupressure Appendix I*. There are also charts showing you exactly where each pressure point is situated on the body of the horse.

AROMATHERAPY

Until recently scents have been used mainly in perfumes and bath oils, but the use of essential oils in healing is now gaining increased popular acceptance. Aromatherapy is one of the oldest forms of healing and preventive treatment, dating back to ancient Egypt. Much was forgotten and lost through the centuries, but in the 1920s aromatherapy developed a following in Europe. Herbalists and other natural healers revived the art of treating with essential oils derived from plants, and today the popularity of aromatherapy is once again expanding.

In his best-selling book, *Perfect Health*, Dr. Deepak Chopra explains why aromatherapy works:

The language of taste is limited to sweet, sour, salty, bitter, astringent, and pungent. The nose, on the other hand, understands a vast vocabulary of smells, amounting to about ten thousand different odors if you have a well-trained beak. The odors that can be detected by the nose must first dissolve in the moisture of the nasal tissue and are then passed on by specialized olfactory cells straight to the hypothalamus in the brain....The fact that smells go straight to the hypothalamus is very significant, for this tiny organ is responsible for regulating dozens of bodily functions, including temperature, thirst, hunger, blood sugar levels, growth, sleeping, waking, sexual arousal, and emotions such as anger and happiness. To smell anything is to send an immediate message to "the brain's brain," and from it to the whole body. At the same time, the message of an odor goes to the brain's limbic system, which processes emotions, and to an area called the hippocampus, the part of the brain responsible for memory, which is why smells bring back past memories so vividly. [1]

In addition to the therapeutic value of their scents, essential oils used in aromatherapy have other healing properties. Some are antiseptic or bactericidal, and others work against viruses. These oils work with the body to promote healing by stimulating and supporting the body's own healing abilities. Essential oils are often used in conjunction with other forms of natural healing such as herbs and homeopathics.

Dr. Chopra has found aromatherapy to be a helpful adjunct to other natural treatments both for specific conditions and for general relief from stress. He also notes that some patients who did not respond to other treatments for conditions such as migraine headache, back pain, skin rash, and insomnia were helped by aromatherapy. [2]

If you are in doubt about the effectiveness of essential oils, try a bath with a particular essential oil and notice how you feel afterward. Recently, a friend was visiting and complained of so much stress that she had not been sleeping well. After a long tiring day, she was still unable to sleep so I made her a warm bath with the essential oil hops, an excellent relaxer before bed. Although she had previously tried warm baths, they had not helped her relax enough to go to sleep. She stayed in the bath for such a long time that I became concerned and knocked on the door to check on her. She said the bath was so relaxing she wanted to stay and savor the relief. She slept soundly that night and has used aromatherapy baths ever since to combat the stress in her life.

Essential oils are inhaled through the lungs where the fumes then cross over into the bloodstream and are carried throughout the body.

[1] *Deepak Chopra, M.D.,* Perfect Health: The Complete Mind/Body Guide, *(Harmony Books, 1991) p. 152.*

[2] *Ibid., p.154*

Some essential oils can also be absorbed through the skin. However, the inhaling method has been found to be the most reliable and is suggested unless a lung problem is present. If you are skeptical that the smell of a particular essential oil can cause a physical reaction, remember that smelling salts and ammonia have been commonly used to revive people who have fainted or are about to faint.

Just as a certain perfume may appeal to you more than another or may change to a different odor on your skin, essential oils interact with each horse's body chemistry differently, so you should experiment with several different ones. The horse's diet is one of the factors that influence this interaction.

Essential oils are sold in health food stores, usually in a bottle that allows one drop out at a time, or with an eye dropper-type lid. They can be inhaled, or used with direct application as a compress, poultice, or massage oil. Caution: Many essential oils are extremely potent and must be handled carefully.

*In the *Horse Ailments* section of this book (Part Three), I have included aromatherapy and recommendations for specific essential oils where appropriate, in the treatment of a problem. (NOTE: Some essential oils, such as peppermint, may influence drug-screening tests. It is not possible to predict which ones will, so make sure you have not used these oils for at least three, or better, five days before a test.)

*Details of the individual oils, duration and quantities of treatment, and when and how to administer them, are all included in the *Aromatherapy Appendix II* on p. 301.

BACH FLOWER REMEDIES

Bach Flower remedies were developed by Dr. Edward Bach, a British bacteriologist and homeopathic physician. Dr. Bach first published a book about the remedies in 1931, which described how these flower remedies could improve a person's state of mind. Dr. Bach believed that a healthy state of mind is the key to maintaining good health and that if the mind is in a balanced state, the body will follow suit. He found that when he treated the personalities and feelings of his patients their physical distress could be alleviated as the natural healing potential in their bodies was unblocked and allowed to work once more.

The Bach remedies are flower essences prepared homeopathically. Bach discovered that the dew from each flower is charged with an essence (or energetic imprint of the flower's vibrational signature), and that these essences create an internal harmony that effectively treats physical problems and upsets by healing a person's psychological and emotional state.

These remedies work well on horses. When a horse is not responding to a treatment for a physical problem, I often try a Bach Flower remedy to see if the source of the problem is emotional. It is amazing how even one dose will improve the physical condition by first acting on the horse's mental state. For instance, I often suggest Bach Flower remedies to help with a sensitive horse's adjustment when he is moved to a new stable or to help a horse that lacks confidence from being abused by a former owner. In addition, Bach Flowers are often successful in improving the horse's response to any form of stress.

When using Bach Flowers, it is important to have an accurate understanding of your horse's mental state. Since you as the owner usually know your horse very well, you are in the best position to select a particular remedy or combination of remedies to improve that mental state. Because there are no ill effects if you pick the wrong one, Bach Flowers can be prescribed by the horse owner with little concern. However, if you have selected the proper remedy or combination of remedies, you will see positive results.

There are thirty-eight individual remedies, each corresponding to a specific negative emotional state of mind. For example, agrimony brings peace of mind to a restless animal, clematis helps inattention, rock rose calms a panicked horse. If more than one remedy seems to be called for, you can combine up to four remedies; however, in general, I find that the best results are achieved when only one or two remedies are used at once. There is also a *combination* available called Rescue Remedy. It is made up of five flower essences (impatiens, star of Bethlehem, cherry plum, rock rose, and clematis). This is frequently prescribed for stress and I have used it very successfully on horses that have suffered from extreme experiences such as trailer accidents, or trauma from fires or injuries. Since Rescue Remedy is a composite, do not combine this product with other remedies.

I have used Rescue Remedy for many years, both for myself and in my veterinary practice. The first time I had the opportunity to use Rescue Remedy for a serious personal injury was when I suffered a concussion after a fall from my horse, Charlie. On the way to the doctor, I took Rescue Remedy. Very quickly, my fuzzy vision cleared up, and I began to feel calmer. Within about fifteen to twenty minutes, the effect wore off so I continued to take additional doses until I got to the doctor. Each time, my vision would clear up and I would feel calmer again. When I have administered Rescue Remedy to animals in emergency situations I have always felt it was extremely helpful, but I had never observed such a dramatic reaction as the one I experienced when I was the patient. My response made me more aware that Bach Flowers work on a level so subtle that their effects often can be hard for a veterinarian or owner to observe. My personal experience made me appreciate Bach Flowers even more, and I was certainly grateful that I had

Rescue Remedy on hand that day for my own emergency.

On another occasion, when I was visiting a friend, her dog was kicked in the head by a horse. I felt helpless since I had no veterinary supplies with me. The dog went into shock, and the only thing I had with me to treat her was Rescue Remedy. She responded immediately. Her color and all of her vital signs returned to normal, and we could then safely transport her for further medical care.

The individual remedies come in small "stock" bottles. Only two or three drops of the remedy are mixed with water in a one-ounce dropper bottle and then given to the horse by syringe or on a sugar cube. If more than one remedy is needed, two or three drops of each remedy are mixed in the bottle.

Bach Flowers are a very useful adjunct to holistic therapy, opening the door to a whole new form of treatment. They are readily available at many health food stores, and a number of books are available describing their use. While these books refer to human use, an astute owner can correlate a horse's behavior and mental state to the descriptions in the book. You can also order Bach Flowers and books on this method through the mail from companies listed in Appendix VI.

How Bach Flowers Influence Behavior

Bach Flower remedies can have a great effect on behavior since their primary impact is on the emotions. These distilled extracts of flowers can be very useful tools when dealing with problems that stem from the horse's emotional center. Most health food stores that sell Bach Flowers also sell charts and books that describe the types of behavior most affected by each flower remedy. The books explain only how to use Bach Flowers for people, but the uses for horses are the same.

Focus on the most important or obvious emotional traits of your horse that need to be worked on and select one remedy (or a combination of remedies) that best suits your horse's needs. Although most sources say you can use up to five Bach Flowers at one time, I have found (as with using them for physical problems) that horses respond best to one or two Bach Flowers at a time when treating specific emotional problems.

My friend Sara has found Rescue Remedy invaluable for helping her with behavior. She buys horses off the racetrack, retrains them, and sells them as riding horses. When she started buying these Thoroughbreds, Sara experienced some problems when the horses first came to her farm. They had not seen other horses running free since their yearling days and certainly had not experienced turnout for a long time. They were overwhelmed by the sudden change in environment and, as a result, constantly jumped around their stalls and refused to eat. A few drops of Rescue Remedy in the water stopped their agitated behavior and started them eating.

Any time a horse has been stressed, Bach Flower remedies can help. When I moved my own horse, Charlie, to a new barn he did not adjust well. I gave him a combination of walnut and aspen, and his behavior calmed down right away. I told the manager at the barn to continue giving Charlie this Bach remedy until the bottle was used up. He thought the treatment was ridiculous, but carried it out anyway. Two weeks later the manager called me for some more medication, because when the bottle was used up Charlie's behavior began to deteriorate. After we had used one more bottle, Charlie adjusted to his new surroundings and did not require more of that particular combination of remedies.

*For full details about each individual Bach Flower remedy and how to administer, see the *Bach Flower Appendix III* on p. 311. I have also included specific suggestions under the individual listing of problems in the *Horse Ailments* section in Part Three of this book.

CHIROPRACTIC

Chiropractic is based on the concept that the skeletal system of the body must be in correct alignment and that a misalignment can negatively affect the organs and other systems of the body. When I was first introduced to chiropractic, I was very skeptical. Now, having done chiropractic adjustments on countless animals, I am convinced that more is affected than we realize when the bones are out of alignment. The most striking example of a correlation between the alignment of the bones and the immune system is viral infections. Viruses are difficult to treat, and in the past I had found that acupuncture and homeopathy produced the best results. Then, when I began adding chiropractic adjustments to my treatment regimen, I found that horses responded even more quickly and required less treatment overall.

Interestingly, most horses do not mind the chiropractic adjustments. Once they understand what is expected of them, they usually become helpful, bending their necks as if to show me the angle that assists the most. Many areas of the horse can be adjusted, including knees, shoulders, ribs, pelvis, hocks, and tails.

How do you know if your horse needs an adjustment? Most cases come to me for chiropractic only after other methods have failed. But there are better ways to see if your horse needs chiropractic treatment. Neck or cervical vertebrae out of adjustment can be diagnosed several different ways. One way is to run your hands down the horse's neck, feeling for any enlargements that are sore to the touch and present on one side but not the other. A second check system is to run your hand over the lumbar area of the horse's back. The lumbar area stretches from the last rib to the high point at the top of the croup or pelvis. If the horse dips his back away from your hand or shows other signs of discomfort, vertebrae may be out of adjustment somewhere in the spine. Since the lumbar area is unsupported by any other bony structure, any vertebrae out of adjustment cause tension in the spine, which, in turn, causes soreness. Once the spine is adjusted correctly, you should be able to run your hand down the lumbar area with no discomfort to the horse.

Other areas can be more difficult to assess. I am often called in on cases involving unexplained lameness. In many of these cases there is no swelling or heat. Sometimes extensive diagnostic procedures such as X-rays, ultrasound, and nerve blocks have been performed but have not provided a definite diagnosis. When I conduct a chiropractic examination, I usually find that one of the joints in the affected leg is not in its proper position. One or two chiropractic adjustments often correct the lameness.

After successfully treating a horse using chiropractic on a referral case I am often asked why the other veterinarian failed to recognize that the joint wasn't in proper position on the X-rays. I explain that because X-rays are two-dimensional and only taken at one angle, it is sometimes difficult to tell that a bone is misaligned when viewing the X-rays. The chiropractic diagnosis is arrived at by in-depth palpation (feeling) of the individual joints of the horse's affected leg. The range of motion for each joint is checked as well. During the exam the horse may react with pain to the palpation of the affected joint. This form of palpation is very precise and requires experience to pinpoint the exact location of a misalignment in a joint. Once the chiropractic adjustment is done, palpation of the area should not elicit any pain.

Another problem area that can be treated successfully with chiropractic is the rib. Ribs can rotate slightly, causing a great deal of discomfort. Signs that indicate a misalignment of the ribs include: objection to brushing, resistance to being girthed, shifting leg lameness, kicking when trailered, and difficulty bending to the affected side. Rib misalignment has usually gone undiagnosed because it is not recognized as a problem by most vets. However, having seen the results of successful chiropractic adjustments, many veterinarians are now aware of the problems caused by rib misalignments.

A horse used for cattle-roping competition was once presented to me after the equine hospitals at two universities were unable to produce a diagnosis for shifting leg lameness. The lameness was seen some days in the front legs and some days in the hind legs. After about 30 minutes in the trailer the horse would begin kicking non-stop, presumably because he was uncomfortable. The only problem I found was two ribs out of alignment. This was a big dun Quarter Horse from Texas, and, true to his heritage, he was a very tough horse. His ribs were huge and had a lot of scar tissue around them where his body had tried to heal itself. Enlisting the aid of the resident farrier, I was able to adjust the ribs into place. This adjustment was followed by another five days later. After each adjustment, I also treated the horse with acupuncture to help the ribs stay in position and heal properly. The ribs healed, and the horse returned to his peak performance level, with no further bouts of lameness.

I often have to explain to owners how chiropractic works. One woman wanted me to adjust only the area that an equine massage therapist had identified as being out of alignment. I told her that the entire skeletal system needed to be in balance for the adjustments to stay in place. For instance, I would not adjust a pelvis but leave the neck out of alignment because the horse would compensate for the neck area and probably put the pelvis out again in a short period of time. It turned out that this client thought equine chiropractors charged by the area and that it would be more expensive to have me adjust the horse's entire body. Once she realized that the whole horse needed to be checked, she asked me to proceed.

Some people ask me how it is possible for a person to adjust horses, given their massive size. I explain that the muscle, tendon, and ligament structure of a horse are extremely strong, and therefore most misalignments are only slight. The biomechanics of a horse require each part of the body to work with the others in a specific manner. Even a slight misalignment can cause a big problem when a thousand pounds of force is behind it. A veterinarian's knowledge of the skeletal structure of the horse allows her to make precise adjustments to ease the bone back into its proper location. Many horses that are competed regularly are given preventive chiropractic adjustments on a routine basis to ensure continued consistent performance.

Chiropractic and Behavior Problems

How does chiropractic influence your horse's behavior? When I first started adjusting horses I knew their attitudes would improve if they were more comfortable, but I was surprised by some of the major changes that I saw. Some horses are less tolerant of discomfort and pain than others, so the reaction to displaced vertebrae or other chiropractic problems will vary from horse to horse. In the past, a horse with advanced training who suddenly refused to perform would be punished. Today's trainers are increasingly aware, however, that a performance problem is often caused by a physical problem such as a displaced sacrum that causes pain during movement.

For example, when the first cervical vertebra has lost normal motion, the horse is in a great deal of distress. In addition to the physical pain, there is also an emotional pain because the horse is unable to turn his head properly to see what is happening around him and is therefore always on guard. Looking around constantly is a necessary behavior for a flight animal. When the horse is unable to turn his head without experiencing pain, he must turn his entire neck. In a survival situation the extra time needed to turn the entire neck instead of just the head could be the difference between escape and being caught by a predator. As I said earlier, even though domesticated horses are no longer required to escape predators, this instinct is still intact. We acknowledge this inherent instinct with comments such as, "He thinks there's a bear hiding there," when a horse spooks over nothing of consequence.

Once the first cervical vertebra is adjusted into the correct position, some horses show dramatic behavioral changes. Spooky horses often settle down once they realize that they can freely turn their head, and their performance can improve greatly.

A mare brought to me for a checkup was known for her ill temper. She was so difficult that no one wanted to even hold her. I found the main problem was her first cervical vertebra alignment. Once I talked to the mare and calmed her down, she allowed me to make the adjustment. This mare didn't even like to be touched, but after the adjustment she came over to me and put her head in my arms! The mare had been brought to me so she could be prepared for sale. She was thirteen years old and her performance as a barrel racer had deteriorated. Four months after the chiropractic adjustment, I learned from the owner (who had not sold her after all), that she won every competition she had entered. I rechecked the mare once more and continued to hear about her incredible success over the next two years. The horse is retired now, but what a difference that one adjustment made in her life.

A certification program in veterinary chiropractic is now available and many holistic veterinarians are adding this treatment modality to their practices. See Appendix VIII for information on the American Veterinary Chiropractic Association that lists certified chiropractors around the world.

HERBS

The use of medicinal herbs declined with the advent of modern medicine, even though the pharmaceutical industry began by using the harvest of nature's own vast and bountiful plant kingdom. In fact, many pharmaceutical drugs are still made from compounds of herbs, and others are synthetic versions of these compounds.

Unfortunately, pharmaceutical drugs are often used to the detriment of patients, both animal and human. Andrew Weil, M.D., who has done considerable research on natural medicine, says that: "Adverse drug reactions account for the lion's share of iatrogenic illness [illness brought on by medical treatment] so common that any dedicated patient is sure to experience one sooner or later. They can be as mild as nausea, hives, and drowsiness or as serious as permanent damage to organs and death." [3]

When the active component is extracted out of an herb, it is no longer in the state nature provided. Dr. Weil explains:

In their enthusiasm at isolating the active principles of drug plants, researchers of the last century made a serious mistake. They came to believe that all of a plant's desirable properties could be accounted for by a single compound, that it would always be better to conduct research and treat disease with the purified compound than with the whole plant. In this belief, they forgot the plants once they had the active principles out of them, called all the other principles "inactive," and advanced the notion that prescribing refined white powders was more scientific and up-to-date than using crude green plants.... Drug plants are always complex mixtures of chemicals, all of which contribute to the effect of the whole.... In general, isolated and refined drugs are much more toxic than their botanical sources. They also tend to produce effects of more rapid onset, greater intensity, and shorter duration." [4]

According to Dr. Weil, "Our problems stem directly from the decision of scientific medicine to value the refined white powder over the green plant." [5] However, Dr Weil does not totally condemn the use of pharmaceutical drugs. For emergency situations, he and I agree that the quick action of the isolated compound can be lifesaving. Dr. Weil says that he prescribes herbs for most conditions and only resorts to pharmaceutical drugs in about one case in forty.

Medicinal herbs are used to treat many health problems faced by horses, and they can also be a wonderful support for the immune system and a boost to vitality. As with drugs, the use of herbs must be carefully monitored because each horse responds differently.

Among the herbs commonly used for treating horses are yucca, Pau D'Arco, garlic, psyllium, kelp, goldenseal, dandelion, and aloe vera. Because the identification, drying, and preparation of herbs requires special knowledge, I recommend purchasing prepared herbs, and a number of companies sell high-quality herbs

3 Andrew Weil, M.D., Health and Healing, (Boston: Houghton Mifflin Company, second edition, 1988), p. 97.
4 Ibid., p. 98-99
5 Ibid., p. 101

that are organically grown. Organically grown herbs are always preferable since they are usually more effective for treatment.

In addition to herbs that are native to North America and Europe, there is also an upsurge in the use of Chinese herbs. I have also used Chinese patent medicines, which are herbal-based medications made in China, and find them indispensable for certain problems. Chinese herbal formulas have now been developed specifically for horses and are widely available but you should not experiment with medicinal herbs on your own. Ask your veterinarian to advise you about which Chinese herbs are beneficial for your horse. If you are interested in herbal medicine and have never been to a Chinese pharmacy, I suggest visiting one in the Chinatown area of a large city. The array of herbs and other items used for healing is fascinating.

Herbal mixes formulated to treat specific health problems are marketed by various companies. Currently, there are herbal products available for coughs, immune system stimulation, stomach ulcers, chronic colic problems, and a wide variety of other problems. Some of these products can be particularly effective in helping to treat respiratory disease, digestive disorders, and irritable mares. After consulting with your veterinarian, contact one of the herbal companies (Appendix VI) to see if it carries the herbal formula he or she recommends for your horse.

How Herbs Affect Behavior

Many herbs and combinations of herbs are now being marketed with specific claims that they will affect the behavior of horses. Each product must be evaluated on its own merit and tried individually. A large percentage of the products are for calming horses. There is no single best product when it comes to calming a horse, as each horse will respond differently depending on

what motivated him to get excited in the first place. Excitement can be caused by several different chemical reactions within the brain, so a herb that works well for one horse may have no effect on another.

Valerian root is one of the most widely used herbs for calming. It is available in powder form, and most horses like it in their grain or will eat it alone. The dosage needed to create a calming effect will vary from horse to horse. With some horses a tablespoon of valerian root is enough, while other horses will have to consume a cupful for the desired effect.

Red raspberry is another herb used to influence behavior. The leaves are given to mares with estrus problems and to help keep the disposition pleasant. This herb is very effective when properly used and is often tried after other hormonal therapies such as injections and implants fail.

Caution: *I have dealt with a number of cases where an inappropriate herb or herbal combination was fed to a horse and caused harm, so take care when using herbs. Consult a veterinarian or herbal specialist for help when necessary.*

*Specific herbs are recommended for individual health problems in the Horse Ailments section in Part Three of this book.

*A complete list of herbs and their properties, and descriptions on how to administer them, is in the *Herb Appendix IV* on p. 321.

NOTE: The American Horse Shows Association (AHSA) bans the use of herbal remedies in all competitions sanctioned by their organization.

HOMEOPATHY

Homeopathy is a system of medicine developed two centuries ago by Samuel Hahnemann, a highly respected German physician. It is based on the principle that "like cures like," which is also referred to as the "law of similars." A pioneer in medical research, Hahnemann found that a substance that produces a certain set of symptoms in a healthy person can cure a sick person manifesting those same symptoms. This was not a new theory. Many centuries earlier, Hippocrates wrote, "Through the like, disease is produced, and through the application of the like it is cured."

For instance, the homeopathic remedy allium cepa is made from red onions, which can make your eyes water when you cut them. If you have a cold and your symptoms include a runny nose, coughing, sneezing, and headache, allium cepa is the remedy that would probably be prescribed. A cold with a different set of symptoms would call for a different homeopathic remedy. If the lungs are involved, the patient has a sore throat, and the cough is productive, the homeopathic remedy silica would be used instead.

The homeopathic medicine itself is a very dilute medication (often in parts per million) that stimulates the body's defense systems, allowing the body to heal itself. Although homeopathics are absorbed through the mucus membranes in the mouth very quickly, their effects are often gradual, and it can take up to a few days before you notice any improvement. In some cases, however, dramatic changes occur within minutes, depending on the specific problem being treated.

To give you an example, while traveling to visit my mother, I was reminded of how quick and effective homeopathics can be sometimes. During the trip, I became increasingly ill with severe nausea and a headache. By the time I arrived, I was vomiting and had barely enough energy to hold up my aching head. My mother called a homeopathic doctor who discussed my symptoms with me on the phone and then prescribed a homeopathic remedy. Within twenty minutes after taking the homeopathic sepia, I was able to stand up, and within another five minutes my nausea disappeared. I was able to enjoy my visit with my mother with no recurrence of illness.

Usually though, a response to a homeopathic is more gradual when treating chronic conditions such as liver inflammation. In general, liver problems are challenging to treat with any form of medicine because the liver must function constantly to filter the blood of impurities and is not ever given a rest. Homeopathics, however, are often effective in treating the liver. When the treatment is successful, the horse gradually recovers to develop a renewed appetite, a happier attitude, and improved performance.

Another example of gradual improvement using homeopathics is in the treatment of a muscle or tendon inflammation. Arnica montana, a homeopathic remedy based on the Alpine flower arnica montana, is commonly given for these conditions. Arnica montana eases the pain, acting in a manner similar to anti-inflammatory medications.

Homeopathic remedies are diluted many times and "potentized" through a method of vigorous shaking between dilutions. This process is known as "succussing." The potencies of homeopathic remedies refer to how many times the medicine has been diluted and succussed. They usually range from the low potencies of 3C, 6X, 6C, 12X, 12C, 15X and 15C to higher potencies such as 200C or 1M. The difference between potencies of "x" (dilutions of 10), "c" (dilutions of 100), and "M" (dilutions of 1,000) is based on the dilution of the original tincture. For instance, a potency of x means one part of the medicine was mixed with nine parts of a dilutant. The dilutant can be liquid (water or alcohol) or powdered lactose (milk sugar). After the first dilution is made, the mixture is shaken (succussed). Then one part of that mixture is mixed with nine parts of the dilutant and is again succussed. This diluting and succussing (potentization) is done a total of six times for a 6x potency. If the potency is 6C, one part of the medicine has been mixed with 99 parts dilutant and succussed a total of six times. A fascinating phenomenon of homeopathy is that the more dilute the medicine becomes, the stronger its potency. Therefore, a 10C potency would be stronger than a 10x potency because it has been diluted ten times more.

Because homeopathic remedies are so dilute, they often contain no chemical residue of the original substance. Yet, as I have explained, the less of the original substance present, the higher the potency. It is this aspect of homeopathy that makes it so difficult for practitioners of allopathic medicine to accept. In their book, *Alternatives in Healing*, Simon Mills, M.S. and Steven J. Finando, Ph.D., explain it well:

After a dilution of 9x, however, molecular chemistry suggests that there is no longer likely to be any significant amount of the original substance left in the medicine, and, not surprisingly, this has caused skepticism about the ways the remedies work. Yet homeopaths have found, from repeated experience that many of these greater dilutions are in fact even more effective than lower dilutions....

Some scientific study is coming closer to understanding how potentization works. It is known that a substance leaves behind 'footprints' even after it has been greatly diluted. Paul Callinan, an Australian scientist, experimented by freezing remedy tinctures to -200 degrees C; they crystallized into 'snowflake' patterns that were different for each remedy. And the more these tinctures were diluted, the clearer their patterns became. Quantum physics tells us that physical substances leave behind energy fields, and in the end, it may be this that will explain potentization fully. [6]

Providing your veterinarian with a detailed history of the specific health problem is of great importance when treating with homeopathics, because prescribing is based on the law of similars. As mentioned earlier, the law of similars simply means that a remedy is prescribed because, in its original, undiluted form, it would produce symptoms similar to those being treated. Symptoms considered important to a homeopathic veterinarian go well beyond those an allopathic veterinarian would use in making a diagnosis or in prescribing medications. Consequently, a homeopathic veterinarian will ask you to keep detailed records of changes in your horse's behavior, habits, or attitudes.

I regularly prescribe homeopathic remedies and have found them useful for all facets of veterinary treatment. Horses respond well to homeopathics and seem to be even more responsive than dogs and cats. Homeopathics are versatile and can be an effective solution to many problems that are often thought to be untreatable. For instance, many horses will not eat well when taken to shows. The cause is usually stress that can be alleviated with homeopathics.

Homeopathics can also be used to treat inflammation, internal organ problems, and specific areas of the body such as the skin or hooves. As an example, for over a century, the homeopathic remedy heckla lava has proven to be effective in treating horses with navicular disease and ringbone. In the 1800s, when horses were first used on paved surfaces, navicular disease and ringbone were on the increase. (X-rays had not yet been invented, so at the time these diseases were diagnosed by dissection of the

---

6 *Simon Mills, M.A., and Steven J. Finando, Ph.D.,* Alternatives in Healing, *(New American Library/Plume, 1988) p. 27.*

hoof.) There were no drugs to help alleviate the symptoms, no surgeries, and limited special shoes (no pads like today), so horses used extensively in big cities with cobblestone streets suffered greatly. Hekla lava was found to reduce the symptoms and give the horses great relief. I find that its effect can be enhanced when it is combined with acupuncture and get great results—usually returning horses with navicular disease or ringbone to full work in sound condition.

Some homeopathic remedies can safely be given by an owner just as you would self-prescribe an aspirin for your own headache and there are a number of first-aid problems that respond well to homeopathics. Consequently, there are several homeopathics that you should have on hand around the barn, such as arnica for inflammation, hypericum for cuts, and magnesia phosphorica for muscle soreness. (For more on homeopathics to keep on hand, see *The Horse Owner's Health Care Kit for Home and Travel* on p. 163.) However, a homeopathic remedy for a complex problem such as kidney failure should be prescribed *only* by a holistic veterinarian because the symptoms must be carefully compiled and evaluated to determine the specific remedy to use.

HOMEOPATHY AND THE HORSE'S PERSONALITY

Homeopathics can be used to directly affect behavior when used "constitutionally." Although not many veterinarians are doing this yet, in this method of homeopathic treatment the veterinarian analyzes the horse's personality and treats the horse with the homeopathic that best fits that type of personality. Since horses are difficult to analyze in this way, the homeopathic must be selected with care. The right constitutional treatment will decrease the extremes of the personality. I have used this method most often in racehorses, especially with individuals who did

not handle the stress of racetrack life well and were not performing to their full potential. Once they were calmer in the barn, these horses were able to stay more sound and perform better.

*In case you do not have a homeopathic veterinarian to prescribe a remedy, I have given specific homeopathic remedies under each health problem in the Horse Ailments section in Part Three of this book. The homeopathics I have listed there are ones most often effective for those ailments. It is important to note, however, that a homeopathic veterinarian may choose a different remedy based on the unique set of symptoms your horse is exhibiting.

*For a complete list of homeopathic remedies and their properties most commonly used in treating horses, see the *Homeopathics Appendix V*, on p. 329.

HYDROGEN PEROXIDE

NOTE: The hydrogen peroxide used by holistic veterinarians is thirty-five percent food-grade hydrogen peroxide and available only to veterinarians who administer it. It is not the same as the hydrogen peroxide sold in a drugstore or chemist.

Hydrogen peroxide is a controversial form of treatment that is given orally or intravenously by a veterinarian. There are many different theories as to why hydrogen peroxide might be an effective treatment but the most common one is that it supplies additional oxygen to tissues and cells and that some viruses and cancer cells cannot survive in this hyper-oxygenated environment. Research on the use of hydrogen peroxide is ongoing and may provide greater understanding of how and when it can be an effective treatment.

Although the results to date have been inconsistent, treatment with hydrogen peroxide has produced some astounding success stories.

In one case, I used hydrogen peroxide as a last resort to treat a horse with cancer after exhausting every other form of treatment. This brood-mare had initially responded well to several other treatments but she eventually developed reactions to all of them so that treatment had been discontinued. The hydrogen peroxide was administered intravenously over a prescribed course of treatment, and the mare showed grad-ual improvement. Her weight returned to nor-mal, and her energy and appetite gradually came back. Occasionally over the next few months, when her condition declined a bit, hydrogen per-oxide was again administered. The mare has since had two foals and continues to do well.

Because so little is clearly understood about hydrogen peroxide treatment, I do not advise its use except by an experienced veterinarian. I use it mostly as a treatment of last resort and rarely as a primary treatment.

LASERS

Although many of the methods and tools of alternative medicine have been in use for thou-sands of years, holistic veterinarians incorporate the tools of modern technology into their prac-tice as well. One device that I have found indis-pensable is the laser (see fig. 3.12). Lasers, which range in size from penlights to large tabletop units, emit waves of light that are used to treat specific problems. I find that laser therapy gives the best results in horses when treating eye problems, or muscle and tendon injuries, and when used as an aid to the healing of wounds.

Lasers are used in one of two ways: either to stimulate acupuncture points or, at the site of an injury, to speed healing. Some holistic veteri-narians feel that the laser is less effective than acupuncture needles and, therefore, should not be used instead of traditional acupuncture. In my own experience, however, each technique has its place. Also, I often use laser therapy as a follow-up to acupuncture since my clients can learn to use a laser and perform the treatment on

their own horses. My preferences for when to use laser versus acupuncture treatment are based on the results I have observed in cases over the years. Many of my clients have their own lasers and know which problems respond to laser treatment and which do not. I also instruct them to call me for guidance on whether to use laser treatment when an injury occurs.

Acupuncture points can be stimulated easily with the laser. The smaller hand-held penlight lasers come in a variety of wavelengths and they are only slightly larger than a pen. These little lasers have limited effectiveness, but they work well for eye treatments and wound healing. Larger laser units sometimes come with human acupuncture charts and some manufacturers offer a course to teach individuals how to use the laser. You will need to consult an equine acupuncture text to use the laser on a horse. Laser units can also be leased for short periods if a specific case requires it. While each company's lasers vary, the large units are basically self-con-tained and a bit larger in size than a shoebox. Various attachments are available for the part of the laser that touches the horse.

Caution: *When the laser is used near the eye, it should be used only on the acupuncture points surrounding the eye and not directed on the eye itself. A penlight laser beam directed into a horse's eye can result in damage to the eye and may cause an aggressive response from the horse such as kicking. There are special lasers made for use directly on the eye and other del-icate tissues, but they require extensive training for proper use and are not commonly available for purchase by non-professionals.*

In certain cases the laser has been invaluable. For example, I was called to treat Penny, a horse with a serious puncture wound. The possibility of infection was of great concern. Even if I had felt pharmaceutical drugs were warranted,

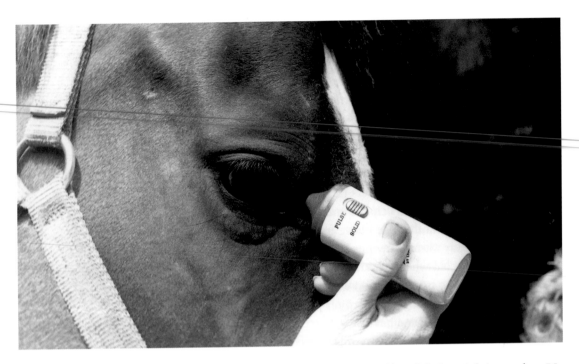

3.12 *Acupuncture points can be easily stimulated with lasers. This handheld penlight laser is being used on BL1 to encourage healing. Do be very cautious when using a laser near the eye; it should never be used directly on the eyeball itself. If a laser is directed on the eye and optic nerve, a horse will experience intense pain and as a result, react violently.*

Penny was allergic to most antibiotics and many other medications. I used the laser around the edges of her wound and on the acupuncture points associated with the immune system throughout the healing process and no infection developed. I have used the laser in this manner many times to stimulate healing when a horse is intolerant of antibiotics. It is a versatile aid in holistic treatment and, with continued research, we are finding many new uses for the laser in veterinary medicine.

NOTE: A list of acupuncture points and the areas they stimulate is in the *Acupuncture/Acupressure Appendix I*, on p. 291.

MAGNETIC THERAPY

Magnetic therapy is a healing method that has been in use for hundreds of years and presently there are more than 5,000 different magnetic-field therapy devices in use worldwide. In this therapy, magnets are applied to a part of the body in order to create a magnetic field that will increase circulation, oxygen utilization, and cell function in that area. Magnetic therapy is currently being used for treatment of fractures, wounds, degenerative diseases of the legs, circulatory deficiencies, strained ligaments, and treatment of joints. I use magnetic therapy frequently, particularly for sprains and strains. It's a good holistic alternative because it is both non-invasive and effective.

The use of magnet therapy in horses has increased dramatically in the last few years. A number of magnetic devices that are easy to use and comfortable are now made especially for horses. These include blanket magnets, hock wraps, leg or shin wraps, and hoof magnets (figs. 3.13 and 3.14).

touched around his hind legs, and his response was to jump around and threaten to kick. Neither disciplining him, nor positive-reinforcement training techniques improved his behavior. I had observed how much other horses enjoyed massage, so I thought it might help this problem if I could teach him that being touched on his body was a pleasant experience. After first massaging his back, I progressed to his hip area, then gradually down his legs. Although he was a little tense at first, he quickly relaxed, and let me work on the muscles of his hind legs. After a few more sessions I could groom and handle his hind legs easily.

There are many equine massage therapists who know specific massage techniques, but there is some debate concerning the qualifications necessary to act as a professional. The American Association of Equine Practitioners (AAEP) has a policy statement on massage which reads: "Massage is a technique in which the practitioner uses hands and body to manipulate soft tissue, thereby positively affecting the health and well-being of the animal. Massage should be performed by a graduate of an accredited massage school who has specialized training in equine anatomy, physiology, massage and veterinary ethics. The work should be done under the referral of a veterinarian." There are a number of accredited equine massage schools; however some offer a one-week training course —obviously not long enough to become a proficient equine massage therapist. Some states now have laws specifically concerning equine massage therapists, requiring that the therapist complete a human massage therapy course in addition to an equine massage therapy course before being able to be licensed to massage horses. Many states are considering adopting similar laws, so check with your state's licensing agency to obtain current information.

This is a confusing state of affairs. Check the qualifications of any equine massage therapist you are considering. Ask for a referral from your veterinarian, and speak to other individuals who may have already used that person's services. If you are still in doubt try to watch the massage therapist work on a horse. This will tell you if he or she is the right person for your horse. To prepare yourself for what to expect you may want to study the work of specialists in this field such as Jack Meagher (see below), who developed a trigger-point massage therapy which is a type of muscle massage. Another type of bodywork for horses is the TTouch, which was developed by Linda Tellington-Jones and is discussed in the next section.

However, massage isn't just for the trained professionals—you don't have to be trained in massage to do a bit of it on your own. As long as you are fairly gentle and don't try to do deep muscle massage, you can do some massage on your horse. (See figs. 3.15–3.20). I suggest you read *Physical Therapy and Massage for the Horse* by Jean-Marie Denoix and Jean-Pierre Pailloux (1996), or *Beating Muscle Injuries* by Jack Meagher (1985).

NUTRACEUTICALS

Nutraceuticals are food supplements that are believed to enhance the function and structure of a horse's body. They generally consist of naturally occurring substances found in the horse's body or a concentrated element found in the horse's natural diet. The U.S. government does not consider nutraceuticals to be drugs so they are not controlled by the U.S. Food and Drug Administration. Consumers should be aware of this. The manufacturers of these supplements represent an enormous industry and the information published by many of these companies can be confusing as well as misleading. (Remember, commercial manufacturers are interested in

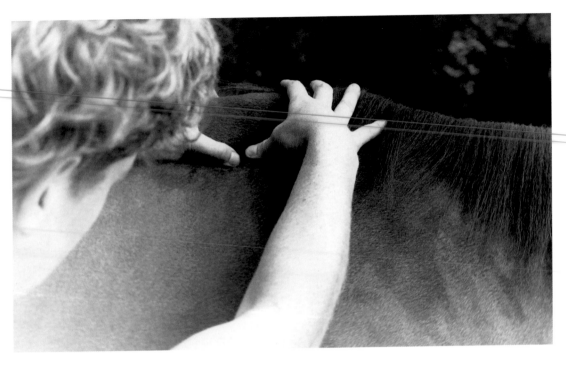

3.15 *A massage around the withers area helps to relieve tight, overworked muscles.*

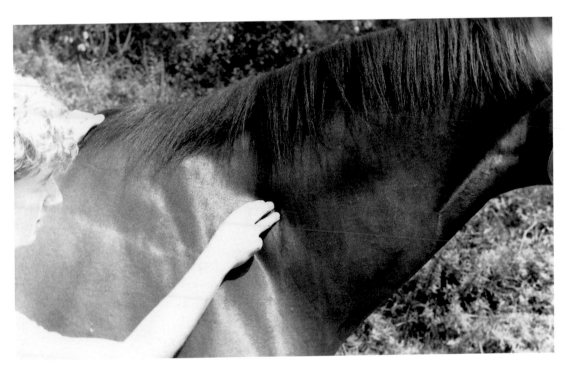

3.16 *The base of the neck is often tight. This area benefits greatly from a gentle massage.*

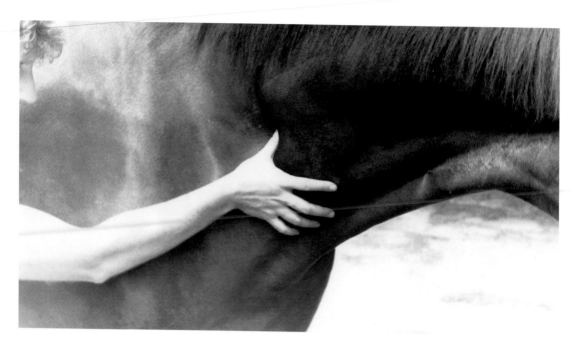

3.17 *Massaging the muscles along the cervical area enables a horse to stretch his neck downward with greater ease, which is a necessity for any working sport horse.*

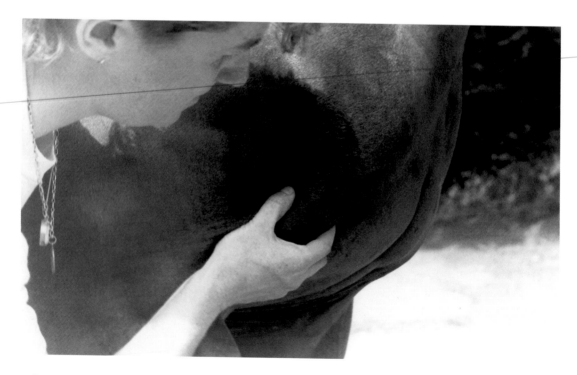

3.18 *A thorough massage of the biceps brachii muscle can help to increase a horse's range of shoulder motion and flex his elbow.*

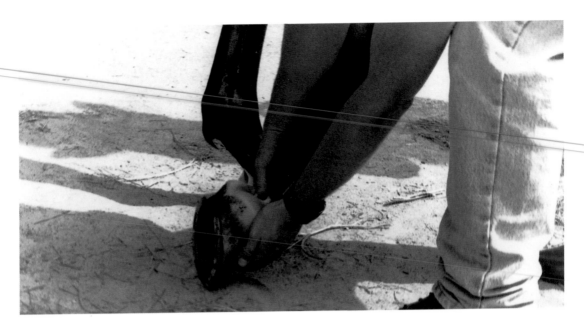

3.19 *When giving a horse a complete body massage, don't forget to include the muscles around the hoof. Flexing the foot, as you see here, relaxes the muscles over the back of the pastern for a more effective massage. Keep the hoof on the ground when you massage the front of the pastern area, and note that your thumb can be used to massage the heel at the same time.*

making money.) It's up to you as a horse owner to be vigilant and gather as much knowledge as possible about new products before adding them to your horse's diet. I discuss below some of the most common products, the reasons for feeding them, and any substantiated pros or cons related to their use. If you don't understand a product, consult your veterinarian before using it.

MSM (Methyl-sulfonyl-methane)

MSM is a naturally occurring sulfur compound found in all living bodies and in many raw fruits and vegetables. Since sulfur is a component in almost every cell in the body, it is a dietary requirement and it sometimes is not available in sufficient amounts to meet a horse's needs. Some of the highest concentrations of sulfur are found in the joints, skin, and hooves, so these areas need an even greater source of sulfur to maintain a healthy condition. Sulfur plays an active role in maintaining cell permeability, allowing nutrients and fluids to move in and out of cells, as well as allowing waste products and toxins to exit. It's used by the body in the production of insulin, which regulates the uptake of glucose by the cells. The cells then use glucose to produce energy. These two functions are essential to any horse but of even more importance to performance horses that have constant demands placed on their systems.

Sulfur is found in many of the horse's natural dietary sources; however its availability can be greatly diminished or destroyed by commercial processing. Cooking destroys sulfur, so any grains that are heated, such as extruded feeds (most senior feeds are processed this way), have no sulfur remaining in their final form. Storage also diminishes or destroys sulfur so any grain mix, or hay that is stored for any length of time, may have a greatly decreased supply or none at

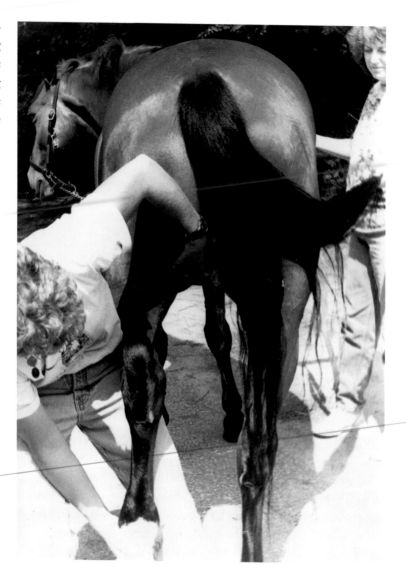

3.20 *Massaging the semimembranous muscle of the rear leg (the area under this practitioner's left hand) is very relaxing. Lifting the leg like this allows the muscle to relax thus making the massage more effective.*

all. But, even the sulfur in commercial MSM supplements evaporates quickly, so avoid premixing supplements with grain and allowing it to sit out over night because this may significantly reduce the amount of sulfur actually being fed.

Arthritic horses usually show the greatest improvement when fed MSM. This is because arthritis affects joints and joints require a high concentration of sulfur to function adequately. MSM can also help reduce scar formation, as it plays an active role in the structure of connective tissue involved in formation of scar tissue. In people, MSM has helped reduce allergic responses to inhalant and food allergens, though unfortunately, this has not been the case in most horses.

There have been no known side effects to feeding MSM and some new research has indicated that MSM may be useful in the treatment of digestive tract ulcers. It sticks to the surface of the gut tract, coats it, and protects tissues that have been damaged from ulcers or inflammation, thus allowing the tissue to heal. This coating action takes place down the entire digestive tract, so MSM can be helpful when treating small or large intestine ulceration, an increasing problem in the horse industry.

MSM is now available as a pure feed supplement—most often derived from kelp. It's a good choice as a feed additive for any performance horse. It is best fed to horses in this pure form. Follow the recommended dosage on whichever product you purchase since strengths of MSM sold over the counter vary.

Chondroitin

Chondroitin is one of the most popular feed additives on the equine market. It is a naturally occurring product that is derived from animal cartilage, mainly bovine (cows), porcine (pigs), fish, and marine mammals. Chondroitin is used by the body to synthesize glycosaminoglycans, one of the main building blocks required in the production of cartilage. When excessive cartilage damage has occurred the chondrocytes, cells responsible for synthesizing new cartilage, must have enough of these necessary building blocks available to build the new cartilage that is needed. Chondroitin also has an important role in neutralizing destructive enzymes found in joints. Levels of destructive enzymes increase in a joint when injury occurs, increasing cartilage breakdown. The addition of chondroitin to the diet helps reduce these enzymes.

Chondroitin products are available in powder and liquid form and vary in concentration and purity of ingredients. Chondroitin is a large molecule so it is unknown how much is actually absorbed as it is digested. The liquid products seem to produce a greater improvement in some horses, particularly in older ones, so it is possible that the liquid form facilitates absorption. There are so many products on the market, it is not possible to evaluate each one, and beware, price is not an indication that one product is better than another. Discuss the various products available with your veterinarian and other horse owners who use chondroitin products, and call the companies that manufacture the product for more information on an individual supplement.

As I noted above, most chondroitin is produced from bovine and porcine tracheas, which are readily available. Marine mammal sources, primarily whales, are not a good source of chondroitin for ecological reasons. Shark cartilage, the main fish source of chondroitin, contains only about 20 percent chondroitin by weight (many sharks are also endangered species so this source should not be encouraged). Most bovine- and porcine-based products contain 90 percent or higher purified chondroitin making them a better source.

Follow the dosage directions for whichever product you choose. Each product will differ depending on the concentration of pure chondroitin.

Glucosamine

Glucosamine is a substance naturally synthesized within the body from glucose and is paramount for the repair of compromised cartilage. If cartilage damage is extensive, the need for glucosamine is greater than the body can supply, so supplementing glucosamine can help meet this need. Glucosamine is one of the building blocks (see chondroitin for another building block) required by the chrondrocytes, the cells that form new cartilage.

There are three forms of glucosamine found in supplements: glucosamine sulfate, glucosamine hydrochloride, and NAG (N-acetyl glucosamine). The NAG form is expensive and not often used for equine products. The sulfate and hydrochloride forms are both broken down in the stomach allowing the glucosamine portion to be absorbed separately further down the digestive tract. Either form can be used in horses. The sulfate form is most commonly used, however the higher degree of purity and greater available glucosamine per unit weight found in the hydrochloride form has increased its use.

Glucosamines are usually obtained from crustaceans. When the shells are processed, they contain a high amount of glucosamine. Supplements containing glucosamine are available in a powder or liquid form. Like chondroitin, liquid glucosamine seems to produce a greater effect, especially in older horses. The addition of ascorbic acid (vitamin C) and manganese when supplementing glucosamine can aid in the absorption of glucosamine so look for products that contain these nutrients.

Glucosamine is also newly obtainable as an injectable. Although not commercially available as of this writing, it is chemically formulated by private laboratories and can be procured by veterinarians. The differences between the powder, liquid, and injectable forms are not really known. The injectable form usually given once a month may provide a horse's body with a greater supply of available glucosamine because oral supplements can be destroyed or lost during the digestive process. If injectable supplementation interests you, consult your veterinarian.

Remember, follow dosage instructions on the glucosamine product you select because each one may differ in purity and concentration.

Shark Cartilage

Shark cartilage is a controversial nutraceutical that is still being studied. The part of shark cartilage responsible for the medicinal effects attributed to it has yet to be identified. Arthritis and cancer, more specifically tumors, are the primary diseases thought to be helped by shark cartilage. Although recognized to contain chondroitin, a substance that provides one of the building blocks for cartilage repair as well as neutralizing cartilage–destroying enzymes, this does not seem to be the main action of shark cartilage. Its primary function appears to be the prevention of angiogenesis—the formation of new blood vessels. Blocking new blood vessel formation is helpful for the treatment of arthritis since the more blood vessels surrounding joints, the more inflammation will be seen to occur. The theory proposed is that inhibiting new blood vessels may reduce inflammation and prevent further degeneration of cartilage in joints. Studies conducted using shark cartilage have shown a decrease in swelling and pain and an increase in movement in joints affected with arthritis. So far, these studies have been conducted on dogs and people, not horses.

Angiogenesis is also an important factor in tumor development, so the blocking of this process can slow the growth, or cause a decrease in the size of a tumor. Results seem to vary depending on the type of cancer being treated. Amazingly, research suggests that shark cartilage does not interfere with blood vessel development in normal tissue.

The dosage for horses is not known. I would not recommend the use of this product until you have discussed it with your veterinarian. Since no studies have been performed on horses, its safety is unknown. There is also a decreasing population of sharks from which to obtain cartilage, making this a poor supplement choice both ecologically and monetarily. Furthermore, keep in mind that due to the short supply of raw product, many supplements claiming to be shark cartilage actually contain very little of the pure ingredient.

Caution: *There are contraindications for shark cartilage. Its use may interfere with, or delay, wound healing and it could prevent pregnancy from occurring. Recent surgical patients should not be fed shark cartilage until totally healed internally. Shark cartilage could also affect pregnancy and the blood vessels that support the embryo. These contraindications are important to note because the exact mechanism that blocks blood vessel formation is not yet understood.*

Colloidal Silver

Colloidal silver is a mineral supplement made up of small particles of silver electromagnetically charged and suspended in deionized water. The suspension is odorless and tasteless. Proponents of colloidal silver claim it is safe to use with no side effects; however there are no published reports of testing. In 1999, the FDA published a ruling on "over the counter" products containing colloidal silver stating that it is not recognized as safe and effective. The ruling further stated: "The indiscriminate use of colloidal silver solutions has resulted in cases of argyria, a permanent blue-gray discoloration of the skin and deep tissues." Unfortunately, there is no clear-cut answer concerning the toxic possibilities of silver.

What is known about silver products is that they can be effective against some bacteria, viruses, and fungi. When taken orally, silver accumulates in the body's tissues and does not leave, thus allowing a build up of the metal. There are also reports in the medical literature of neurological problems that developed after long-term use of oral silver products. However, colloidal silver is widely used to treat a huge variety of medical problems, usually when all other avenues have failed.

I reserve the use of colloidal silver for those cases that are nonresponsive to regular treatment, whether holistic or conventional. If the colloidal silver treatment is successful, I use it for as short a time as possible. My goal is to complete the treatment with colloidal silver in three weeks; however in severe cases treatment has continued for as long as three months. Most of the successful equine cases have involved treatment of bacterial infections when all antibiotics failed. These infections were usually in difficult locations such as tendon sheaths.

If you are considering treatment with colloidal silver, learn as much as possible first. Consult with a holistic veterinarian and then make an informed decision. Do not administer colloidal silver to horses suffering from liver problems since this organ must both filter and store ingested silver.

Coenzyme Q10

Coenzyme Q10 is also called ubiquinone. It plays an essential role in the proper transport and breakdown of fat into usable energy. However, when nutritional deficiencies occur or tissues need an increase of this important compound, a detrimental shortage can result. As the body ages the requirement for coenzyme Q10 increases as the natural levels in the body decrease. Although all the body's tissues suffer when coenzyme Q10 is deficient, the most metabolically active, or those needing energy greatest, suffer the most. The heart is the most sensitive to low levels of coenzyme Q10 and studies have shown that a deficiency is common when heart disease is present.

The use of coenzyme Q10 in horses has been minimal since the cost of a pure, good quality product can be prohibitive when used in horse-sized doses. Not enough research has been done to fully understand the extent of this supplement's usefulness; however its efficacy in treating heart disease is well documented in other species and is definitely worth consideration for use in horses. With today's performance horses, coenzyme Q10 may have an increasing role in aiding our search for ways to help maintain peak performance while avoiding tissue damage, structural weakening, and eventual breakdown.

The exact dosage for supplementing horses is not known. Usually, ten times the human dose is given.

TTEAM AND TTOUCH

TTEAM and TTouch are systems of animal training and healing developed by Linda Tellington-Jones which have proven to be phenomenally successful. Tellington-Jones studied the bodywork and movement system for people developed by Dr. Moshe Feldenkrais and adapted it for horses and other animals. His technique involves retraining the body to awaken brain cells, activate unused neural pathways, and release the bad-movement habits that have developed because of tension, pain, or fear.

The Feldenkrais system has two distinct parts—a series of movements or exercises called Awareness Through Movement and hands-on bodywork called The Feldenkrais Method of Functional Integration. In adapting Feldenkrais's work for animals, Tellington-Jones developed two comparable distinct parts to her system— the Tellington-Jones Equine Awareness Method, also referred to as TTEAM, which is a method of training, and the TTouch (Tellington Touch), a touch therapy.

The training method, TTEAM, has produced fabulous results for thousands of horse owners. I can attest to the wonderful help my horse Charlie and I received from TTEAM techniques used by Richard Lamb, a well-known eventing coach who uses TTEAM work as an adjunct to his regular training. I had decided to pursue riding Charlie even though he was young and very green. As our training proceeded, it was clear to me that his recent growth spurt to 17 hands had resulted in poor coordination. In short, he just wasn't quite sure where his legs were; nor did he feel comfortable about their range of motion.

To help Charlie become more aware of how he used his legs, Richard stayed on the ground while I rode Charlie through a series of obstacles. We started the training session by putting jump poles on the ground any which-way instead of in a row like cavaletti. Charlie had to carefully pick his way through them and, of course, he managed to hit every single pole. Then Richard did some awareness work on one leg at a time using a long white whip Tellington-Jones calls the "wand," and also did some TTouch work with Charlie. Charlie quickly learned to walk through the haphazard arrangement of poles without touching any of them.

In just one clinic Charlie showed great improvement, going from a clumsy youngster with a hollow back to a horse working with his head down and relaxed, his back round. He was halting with his hind legs engaged under him, and his balance improved. We worked with Richard several more times using the TTEAM approach. Each time, Charlie remembered the previous training, for which I am grateful. I have found his retention of this awareness quite amazing.

TTEAM encompasses a number of different exercises. At a TTEAM clinic, each horse is assessed first, and the instructor then decides which TTEAM exercises will be helpful for each horse. In addition to the TTEAM clinics, there are a number of videos and books available which allow you to work with the material on your own. (See figs. 3.21–3.23).

I frequently prescribe TTEAM exercises for horses. The one I suggest most often, "The Back Lift," helps sagging backs by strengthening the abdominal muscles. This exercise and many others may benefit your horse, so I suggest you check out the TTEAM videos and books and try to attend a TTEAM clinic. You and your horse will have a great time.

The second aspect to Tellington-Jones' work, the TTouches, is a hands-on therapy that you can learn to do yourself. The therapist's fingers make circular movements on the skin in specific areas in order to increase body awareness, circulation, and relaxation. This work has been credited with causing major changes in behavior and personality in animals, as well as faster healing of wounds, injuries, and stiffness. I have found that many horses truly enjoy the TTouches. In addition to the therapeutic benefits, I like the TTouch because owners develop a closer relationship to their horses through the one-on-one contact and seem to understand their horses better, including their physical limitations.

Tellington-Jones writes about her work with horses in three books, *An Introduction to the Tellington-Jones Equine Awareness Method* (1988); *Getting in TTouch: Understand and Evaluate Your Horse's Personality* (1995); and *Improve Your Horse's Well-Being: A Step-by-Step Guide to TTouch and TTEAM Training* (1999). You can obtain information on newsletters, upcoming clinics, list of practitioners in your area, or a catalog of videos, books, and equipment by contacting TTEAM at the addresses listed in Appendix VIII.

ANIMAL COMMUNICATORS

Although consulting an animal communicator may not seem at first to fit in a chapter on alternative treatments for horses, I'm including the information here because some people find this to be of great value helping them diagnose certain physical and behavioral problems of their horses.

There is a growing group of animal behaviorists who call themselves "animal communicators." They actually "talk to the animals" through a mental form of communication. Although many people are skeptical about such things, I have seen very positive and occasionally revealing results when animal communicators are consulted. They are consulted for various reasons. Some owners just want to understand their horses better, but most of the time an animal communicator is called upon to deal with a specific physical or behavior problem after repeated attempts to heal or correct it through more orthodox methods. For others it's just entertainment to hear what their horses have to say.

Many animal communicators do their work over the phone tuning in to your horse "long distance." I have seen numerous successful results, including solving undiagnosed health problems and finding lost pets. While there are many good animal communicators, it's important to be discerning when you are seeking this kind of help. After all, anyone can call himself an animal communicator, so it's important that you get referrals from people you know and trust and that you feel comfortable about the person you are consulting.

When consulting an animal communicator, remember that he is talking to an animal. You should try to look at your horse's perspective and expect to hear about things that are important to him, such as food or symptoms of illness. Horses, though generally positive, have a keen memory for negative experiences in the past. Sometimes, an owner can better understand and deal with problem behavior by learning from an animal communicator about the bad experience that started the behavior.

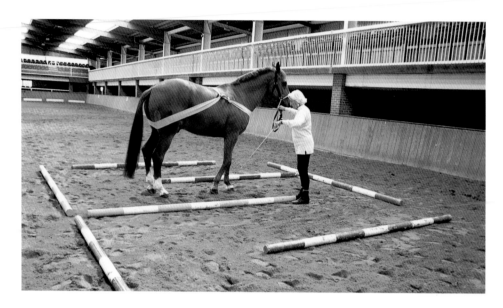

3.21 *Linda Tellington-Jones, founder of TTEAM (Tellington Touch Equine Awareness Method), leads a horse through a labyrinth.* NOTE: *The horse is wearing the Body Wrap; it gives him greater awareness of his whole body as he moves through the exercise. Improved coordination and balance result from this type of groundwork method.*

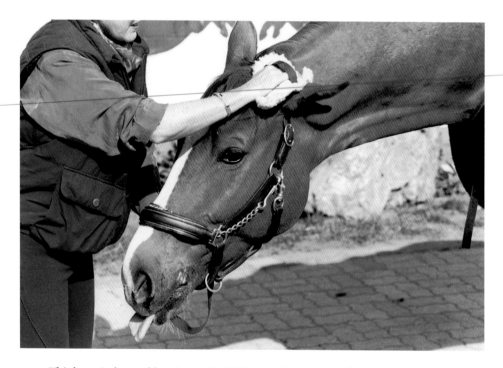

3.22 *This horse is thoroughly enjoying the Tellington Touch ear work. This TTouch is easy to do. Start at the base of the ear and stroke upward to the tip. A session of ear work will calm a nervous or frightened horse, reinvigorate a tired one, lower pulse and respiration rates, and alleviate pain and shock caused by injury or colic.* NOTE: *The sheepskin mitt often helps with horses that do not like their ears handled.*

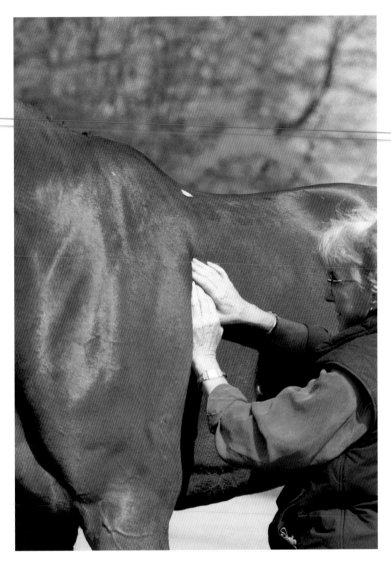

3.23 *Here, Linda Tellington-Jones works on a horse with the Lying Leopard TTouch. Hold your hand gently curved and use the area of your fingers and thumb from the tips to just below the knuckles together with the bottom of your palm to make contact on the skin. Push the skin one-and-a-quarter times clockwise around a half-inch (1.5 cm) diameter circle, slowly release, and move a short distance and repeat. This TTouch increases a sensitive horse's self-confidence, and soothes a horse with a nervous disposition.*

4 Conventional Veterinary Treatments

While I prefer alternative methods as the first option in treating horses, there is also a time and a place for conventional medicine. I am grateful that the options of pharmaceutical drugs and surgery are there when I need them. In emergency situations, drugs can literally save a life. In this chapter, I will give you an overview of the types of drugs commonly used in conventional veterinary practice.

ANTIBIOTICS

The antibiotic is one of the most commonly prescribed drugs and, unfortunately, also one of the most abused. Antibiotics are stressful to a horse's body because, in addition to killing the "bad" bacteria, they often kill many of the "good" bacteria that naturally inhabit the digestive system and aid in digestion. When the normal flora (bacteria) of the digestive system are gone, less desirable bacteria flourish and can cause digestion problems and/or gas. Problems with digestion are characterized by a change in the horse's attitude. Usually the horse is grumpy, and he may not enjoy being worked. The physical symptoms are often vague, such as a slightly loose stool, or discomfort when the girth is tightened. All of these signs in the horse may persist for a few weeks, and they generally indicate mild abdominal discomfort. Rarely does the discomfort progress to colic. Although the intended target of the antibiotic may be a specific area such as a puncture wound in the skin, remember that antibiotics spread throughout the body and may affect its overall bacterial balance. For example, when the antibiotic treatment kills off the normal skin bacteria that keeps the fungus on the skin in balance, the horse may develop a fungal infection on his skin. You may have noticed side effects yourself after taking antibiotics. For instance, when women take antibiotics, they sometimes develop vaginal yeast infections.

Antibiotics also cause stress on the liver, kidneys, and other organs that must filter these drugs. The immune system is forced to work

Calcium: A calcium supplement can be effective in some horses as a mild sedative. It seems particularly effective in Thoroughbreds. You can buy a calcium supplement for horses at the feed store. When administering it as a sedative rather than just a nutritional supplement, give the same dosage the label recommends for nutritional purposes. Or, as an alternative, you may choose to use homeopathic calcarea carbonica in a potency of 30C, given twice a day.

Caution: *Check with your veterinarian before adding calcium to your horse's diet; too much calcium may cause a dietary imbalance.*

PHARMACEUTICAL TRANQUILIZERS

Aceromazine maleate: One of the most well known pharmaceutical tranquilizers, this drug is also the one most often given to horses. Although relatively safe, it should not be used for horses that have neurological problems, heart problems, or respiratory difficulties. Acepromazine maleate is broken down in the liver, so it should also not be given to horses that have a history of liver problems. Its effects last from one to four hours, but can take up to 48 hours to subside in older horses. As with all drugs, it should be used with caution—if at all. It is available in injection form and several different sizes of tablets. If you have a large barn with many horses or if you trailer your horse long distances, it might be wise to ask your veterinarian how to administer acepromazine maleate in emergency situations and keep it on hand.

Xylazine hydrochloride: This drug acts as a tranquilizer and a muscle relaxant, also providing some analgesia (painkilling effect). It is broken down in the kidneys and liver, so it should not be used for horses with liver or kidney problems. As a general rule I recommend that it only be administered by a vet. Precautions should be taken when using xylazine hydrochloride since one of the side effects occasionally seen is a tendency to kick with the hind legs.

MUSCLE RELAXANTS

Muscle relaxants are used primarily for horses that are suffering muscle spasms or whose muscles are exhausted due to overexertion. The natural choices can be administered by the owner, but always with caution. If muscle spasms are severe, your horse should be treated by the veterinarian. I will discuss both natural and pharmaceutical choices.

Selenium and Vitamin E: These nutrients are used in cases in which a deficiency is present or where muscles have been exhausted from overwork or because they were out of shape. While not much research has been done on the use of selenium and vitamin E for horses, they have proved helpful for these problems. Commercial formulations that combine selenium and vitamin E are available for horses. The label will give information on the appropriate dosage for your horse.

Calcium: A calcium supplement specifically formulated for horses is beneficial in cases where the muscle is out of shape or overworked. However, calcium is more effective if used prior to the muscle exertion rather than after the problem exists. Give according to label directions.

Magnesia phosphorica (Tissue Salt no. 8): This homeopathically prepared remedy aids in relaxing muscles. Use a potency of 6C or 12C three times a day and administer according to the guidelines in the *Homeopathics Appendix V,* p. 329. If no relief is seen after one day's treatment, consider another option.

Arnica montana: This homeopathic remedy decreases inflammation in and around the muscle. Use a potency of 12X or 30X, or 6C to 30C, three times daily and administer according to the guidelines in the *Homeopathics Appendix V*, p. 329.

Methocarbamol: This pharmaceutical drug is available in both injectable form and tablets. It should be administered only under the supervision of a veterinarian.

ANESTHETICS

NOTE: Surgery is discussed later in this chapter; for additional information relevant to anesthetics, please see that section.

Anesthetics are a group of drugs people often fear, and to some extent this fear is warranted. There is always a certain risk involved in the use of anesthetics, and this risk must be respected. However, the advancement of pharmaceutical technology has provided us with a large variety of anesthetics that can be used more safely than ever before.

Because it is impossible to tell which horses will be sensitive or allergic to an anesthetic, great care is used when anesthesia is administered. Anesthesia must be detoxified by the body, which puts additional stress on the organ that is responsible (usually the liver or the kidneys), and the horse must be thoroughly evaluated with a laboratory work-up before anesthesia is administered. You can't just assume that your horse will tolerate anesthesia well.

Avoidance of anesthesia during old age is best. However, if the horse has an infected tooth that must be removed or needs other surgery, a safely administered anesthetic will be necessary. When delicate anesthesia must be administered to a very aged horse, I would suggest consulting a Board Certified Veterinary Surgeon (see *Surgery*, p. 66).

To be certain you have done as much as possible to ensure your horse's safety during anesthesia, follow your veterinarian's instructions carefully for pre-anesthetic care such as withholding water and/or hay. Don't be afraid to ask questions of your veterinarian to make you as comfortable as possible with the anesthesia procedure. Your peace of mind will be transferred to your horse, lessening his anxiety as well.

STEROIDS

Another category of pharmaceutical drugs that is greatly overused is corticosteroids, commonly known as "steroids." Steroids are synthetic drugs that are related to the adrenal hormone cortisone. This family of drugs is used primarily to treat dermatitis (skin problems), joint inflammation, and shock. They are prescribed as injections, pills, or topical creams. Steroids are considered by many to be a miracle drug because they can cause inflammations, skin disorders, and allergies to disappear almost overnight. Unfortunately, there are some dangers that accompany steroid use. Steroids work because they suppress disease. At the same time, however, they are toxic, create dependencies, and weaken the immune system by suppressing the functioning of the thymus, lymph nodes, and white blood cells.[1] Additionally, steroids suppress other body functions and can also lead to degenerative problems when injected in joints. Also, laminitis (founder) occasionally results from steroid use.

I am certainly not condemning the use of steroids entirely. What I am saying is that steroids are overused and are relied on in some cases when they could—and should—be avoided. The alternative to steroids can require a more complex form of diagnosis and treatment, which is often why some veterinarians opt to treat with steroids.

Sometimes, however, there is no choice other than to use steroids. For instance, if shock occurs during an illness or after a traumatic injury, steroids can literally save a horse's life. In

---

1 *Andrew Weil*, M.D., Health and Healing, *(Boston: Houghton Mifflin, 1988), p. 193*

other cases, symptoms can be very severe, such as difficulty breathing caused by an allergic response, and immediate treatment with steroids can alleviate these symptoms until other types of treatment can be employed.

A second family of steroids, known as anabolic steroids, has been associated with use by human athletes. Anabolic steroids cause an increase in muscle mass and are most often used in the horse industry for racehorses and horses shown in hand. Although the use of anabolic steroids is banned at horse shows in the United States, there are still those who use them either when they are not showing the horse or when they know drug testing will not be performed at a horse show. Like corticosteroids, anabolic steroids have a place in veterinary treatment, and can be helpful when treating certain cases. However, indiscriminate use of anabolic steroids can cause serious metabolic disorders, and they should not be used unless prescribed by your veterinarian.

The bottom line with steroid use is to be sure that there are no other alternatives because steroids can be very detrimental to your horse's health.

SURGERY

Much like human medicine, veterinary surgery has advanced to the point that it is no longer practical for a general veterinarian to do every type of surgery possible. Surgical techniques are changing and developing so quickly that it's almost impossible for a general veterinarian to keep up with all the latest advances. In addition, some surgeries require special equipment that can be very expensive. There are now veterinary specialists, called Board Certified Surgeons, who specialize in surgery. Like many veterinarians I do some types of surgery myself but refer more complicated cases to veterinary surgeons. If surgery is required, you will get state-of-the-art surgery from a specialist.

But let's take first things first and look at the question of whether a particular surgery is necessary. If surgery has been recommended for your horse and you're not comfortable with the idea, get a second opinion. Veterinary medicine is following the example provided by human medical practices, and second opinions are now commonplace. If your regular veterinarian has recommended a major surgical procedure that requires laying your horse down and using inhalant anesthesia, you may want to get a second opinion. If your veterinarian does not give you a referral, ask for a referral from the American Holistic Veterinary Medical Association (see Appendix VIII) or your local or state veterinary association.

Some of my clients seek second opinions for even the most routine procedures, and I encourage them to do so if they have any doubts. This concern shows how much they care for and value their horses. I would probably do the same thing in their place. As a matter of fact, I have done just that when I am not sure if there is a more advanced technique available for one of my own horses. Although I enjoy doing surgery and keep fairly current, another veterinarian may look at the case from a different perspective, which is sometimes valuable.

If your veterinarian recommends surgery, you should ask these questions before making the commitment:

1. Are there non-surgical alternatives that you can consider?
2. Will my horse safely tolerate this type of surgery?
3. Will this surgery completely repair the problem?

If the answers to these questions satisfy you, then you should consider proceeding with the surgery. If, however, they have raised more questions, talk it over with your veterinarian or get a second opinion. Any surgery carries with it some risks.

If major surgery is unavoidable here are some precautions that can be taken to help your horse through it:

1. Check that the veterinarian does laboratory tests to make sure that your horse's body is in shape for surgery. If the tests show abnormal values and the surgery must be performed anyway, at least the surgeon will be forewarned and prepared for possible complications.

2. In consultation with the surgeon, choose from the following homeopathic remedies to help your horse deal better with the surgery:

Ferrum phosphoricum (tissue salt no. 4) to support the oxygen-carrying capacity of the blood and strengthen the blood. Give 6x, 12x or 6c twice a day for three days prior to surgery and for one week following surgery.

Phosphorus 6c, 12c or 30c to help promote blood coagulation thereby reducing blood loss during surgery. Give three times a day the day before surgery, the day of surgery, and the day following surgery. Phosphorus may also be given by the surgeon during the operation if excessive bleeding is a problem. If severe blood loss occurs during surgery continue the medication for five days following surgery.

Carbo vegetabilis 6c, 12c or 30c twice a day, given one day before and two days after surgery to help prevent excessive gas formation and encourage normal intestinal tract motility.

VACCINATIONS AND NOSODES

Vaccinations have become a highly controversial subject for holistic veterinarians and owners who prefer a natural approach to their horse's care. Many veterinarians are beginning to realize just how detrimental some of the standard vaccinations are to the immune system. Have you ever noticed that your horse may seem less active and have a poor appetite after vaccinations? This lethargic period may continue for as long as two weeks and is particularly noticeable in older horses. Some older horses act as if they were suddenly affected with a case of generalized arthritis—a day or two following the vaccination their movement becomes stiff and painful.

A vaccine utilizes the bacteria or virus of a specific disease which has been altered through reproduction or killed so it is no longer active. The vaccine is given with the intent that it will help the body develop immunity to that particular disease. Dr. Richard Pitcairn, a veterinary specialist in immunology, explains the problems with vaccinations in his book, *Dr. Pitcairn's Complete Guide to Natural Health for Dogs and Cats.* Although Dr. Pitcairn's explanation refers to dogs, the same principle applies to horses. He says:

There is an implicit assumption among many people that vaccines are 100 percent effective. This belief can be so strong that a veterinarian may tell you, "Your dog can't have distemper (parvovirus, hepatitis, or whatever) because he was vaccinated for it. It must be something else." But one thing I learned from my studies in immunology is that vaccines are far from 100 percent effective. Obviously it is not just the injection of the vaccine that confers immunity; the response of the individual animal is the critical and necessary factor. Several things can interfere with the ideal body response (production of antibodies and immunity). These include vaccinating when the animal is too young, sick, weak, or malnourished; using the wrong route [e.g. the method of administration, such as in the muscle by injection or in the nose] or schedule of administration; and giving the vaccine to an animal with an immune system that has been depressed as a result of previous disease, inheritance or drug therapy.[2]

In some cases, the use of nosodes is a viable alternative to vaccinations. Nosodes are used to boost the immune system's response against a specific disease, usually one of the diseases that is vaccinated against. A nosode is similar to a homeopathic remedy because, like homeopathics, the active substance has been diluted many times yet is very effective in stimulating the immune system. Just like in regular vaccinations, the active substance in a nosode is the bacteria or virus of a specific disease; it is the homeopathic dilution and potentization that distinguishes nosodes from regular vaccines. Most veterinarians who practice homeopathy also use homeopathic nosodes.

Nosodes are sometimes used alone instead of a vaccination as a more natural type of immunization, but they can also be used as an adjunct to conventional vaccines. When used as an adjunct to conventional vaccines, nosodes help the body cope with the side effects of the vaccine. They are generally given once a month.

While nosodes can be very effective in some places, they may not always provide sufficient protection when used as a substitute for vaccines. In the southern United States, where strong strains of virulent viruses flourish in the hot, humid climate, I have not found nosodes to be strong enough to prevent some viruses. However, using the nosodes in addition to vaccinating strengthens the reactions of the immune system and decreases the side effects of the vaccines. Before I began using nosodes as an adjunct to vaccines, I found that some horses I vaccinated would come down with symptoms resembling a virus even though they had been vaccinated against it. When I started giving the nosodes as well, the problem diminished to the point that it rarely occurred. To decrease the side effects of vaccination, especially in older horses or horses that have previously had problems, I like to use nosodes following vaccination and then repeat the nosodes once a month until the next vaccination. (It is important to note that nosodes will not stop an allergic reaction to a vaccine.) Nosodes for horse vaccines are not commercially available. Most homeopathic veterinarians make their own.

You should discuss the issue of vaccines with your holistic veterinarian who will know the risks of specific diseases in your area and what your horse needs. When possible, it is best that vaccines be given separately so the immune system is not overburdened. Unfortunately, the current trend is to mix vaccines rather than separate them, because it is considered easier to give just one injection.

My own solution to the issue of vaccinations is to use them for the viruses that are prevalent and endanger a horse's health. I give individual vaccinations separately as often as possible, allowing at least one week between them, and then follow up with a nosode specifically for that vaccine.

Now, let's review some of the diseases for which horses are most often vaccinated.

Tetanus

A tetanus vaccination is usually recommended at least once a year. In areas where outbreaks of

---

2 *Richard H. Pitcairn, D.V.M., Ph.D., and Susan Hubble Pitcairn,* Dr. Pitcairn's Complete Guide to Natural Health for Dogs and Cats, *(Emmaus: Rodale Books, 1982), p. 250.*

the disease have occurred recently, twice a year is advisable. Tetanus lives in the soil and there is no season of the year in which it is more prevalent. The yearly vaccination for tetanus is called tetanus toxoid. It works by stimulating your horse's immune system to produce antibodies against the bacteria that produce tetanus. Although this protection is helpful, if the horse is exposed to a massive amount of tetanus bacteria, the body's immune system may not be able to respond quickly enough to prevent the illness. For that reason it is best to give an additional injection called a tetanus antitoxin when an injury occurs that has the potential to expose your horse to tetanus, such as a deep puncture wound or a gash covered with manure. It is best to give this antitoxin as soon as possible following an injury. But giving the antitoxin when you are aware of an injury is not a substitute for giving the regular tetanus toxoid injection, since it is not possible to discern which injuries might carry tetanus. Also, you may not notice every single injury your horse gets.

There is not a homeopathic nosode that generates enough of an immune response to protect your horse from this deadly disease, so vaccination for tetanus is a must.

Encephalomyelitis

I recommend vaccinating for encephalomyelitis about one month prior to the beginning of the mosquito season. This timing will help ensure an active immune system so your horse's protection is at its highest point when the mosquitoes that spread this disease become active. The main vaccine for encephalomyelitis covers the Eastern and Western forms of encephalomyelitis; however, in certain areas of the United States it is also recommended to vaccinate for Venezuelan encephalomyelitis, since outbreaks of this strain occasionally occur in South America, Central America, and Mexico. All forms of encephalo-myelitis are severely debilitating and often fatal. It is therefore highly recommended to vaccinate yearly against this disease.

There are currently no homeopathic nosodes or other natural preventives for encephalomyelitis.

Rhinopneumonitis

Rhinopneumonitis is caused by a virus known as the equine herpes virus, and it can manifest in the horse in three different forms. One form of this disease, called EHV4, causes mainly respiratory symptoms such as those seen with a cold; however, it can progress into a deadly case of bronchopneumonia in some horses. The second form, EHV1, causes abortions and, on rare occasions, a respiratory infection. The third form that is recognized is a neurological form considered an allergic type of reaction to an EHV1 infection. All of the forms of rhinopneumonitis have the potential for causing death—EHV1 can be deadly for the unborn foal, and the other two types can be deadly for the horse. This disease can be very contagious and is spread through the air, feed, or water, or through direct contact with an infected horse. Vaccination immunity or immunity from a natural infection is very short. Considering these facts, this disease cannot be ignored, particularly for horses such as race and show horses that are regularly in contact with other horses.

Constant vaccination for rhinopneumonitis is sometimes recommended, but vaccinating on a frequent basis can put a constant strain on the horse's immune system. Unfortunately, that means there is no clear-cut answer to the recommended frequency of vaccination for this disease. I prefer to not constantly vaccinate for the respiratory form of the disease but rather to allow the horse's own immune system to protect it. The veterinarian should assess the specific needs of each horse before making a decision on how often to vaccinate for rhinopneumonitis.

I have found homeopathic nosodes, combined with acupuncture to stimulate the immune system and a top nutritional program, to be effective in dealing with this disease. One option that is used by some holistic veterinarians is to vaccinate the horse only once for rhinopneumonitis to establish an immune system response to the disease and then to use homeopathic nosodes. Another choice is to never vaccinate for the disease and use only homeopathic nosodes to stimulate the immune system against the disease. There are also many choices in between these two options, such as vaccinating twice a year and using nosodes between vaccinations, or vaccinating once a year and using nosodes the rest of the year.

If you have a mare used for breeding purposes, it is best to consider your decision about vaccinating carefully since abortion can be caused if your mare contracts rhinopneumonitis. Vaccinating to prevent EHV1 is recommended during the fifth, seventh, and ninth months of pregnancy. The subtype 1P of the EHV1 virus is the most common in causing abortions, so the vaccine should contain this subtype.

Strangles

Strangles is a disease that is much feared because it can lead to a long illness or even death. Unfortunately there are problems with the injection form of vaccine for strangles. The vaccination often causes horses to feel or become ill and can result in a sore muscle or an abscess in the area where the injection is given. Older horses can suffer the most, sometimes feeling unwell for long periods of time following the vaccination. Because of the problems associated with this vaccine, it is not usually recommended unless your horse is going to a barn or show grounds where strangles is known to be

a problem. Before moving your horse to a new location, it is best to ask if strangles has been reported. If so, you should vaccinate against strangles at least two to three weeks prior to the move.

There is a new intranasal form of vaccine for strangles. It is squirted into the horse's nose. It is actually absorbed more quickly than the injectable vaccine, and also avoids the common side effects of injection for strangles—abscesses and/or extreme muscle soreness.

The bacteria that causes strangles can live in the soil for many years, so don't underestimate how serious this problem can be. In young horses, the lymph nodes under the throat are most often infected, but in older horses, internal abscesses can form which are extremely difficult to treat.

When a horse is allergic to the vaccine for strangles, it is best to keep his immune system at its peak by using acupuncture, high quality nutrition, and a homeopathic nosode. A homeopathic nosode can be used to stimulate the immune system in general to help protect against the disease if you choose not to vaccinate. The effectiveness of the specific nosode for strangles is unknown at this time.

Equine Influenza

Equine influenza is a viral infection which has symptoms similar to an upper respiratory infection, including coughing, fever, and nasal discharge. This disease can be spread by direct contact with a horse that has the infection or by aerosolized droplets containing the virus. Aerosol transmission occurs when an infected horse coughs, expelling droplets containing the virus into the air. These infected droplets are then inhaled by a horse nearby. Horses most at risk are the young and those who have a great deal of exposure to other horses.

There are two main types of equine influenza virus—A1 and A2—and many strains of the virus within these two main types. The A2 virus is thought to cause most influenza infections, as well as being the most severe form of influenza. Like most "flu" viruses, the equine influenza virus has mutated or changed its form since it was first discovered. Two of the most current strains of the A2 virus that are now available in vaccines, are Prague 56 and Kentucky 92. An influenza vaccine that does not include these strains will not protect your horse against the most current forms of influenza that have been identified.

Vaccinating for influenza virus may provide about six months of protection against the particular strains of virus covered by the vaccine. As most horse owners have experienced, however, there always seems to be a form of upper respiratory disease that horses get despite the vaccinations they receive.

I have treated many cases of upper respiratory illness caused by viruses. Horses who are maintained on top nutrition and kept in good physical condition are able to quickly recover from an influenza-type virus. I encourage owners to call in the veterinarian as soon as they notice the symptoms of any upper respiratory illness so it can be treated immediately with homeopathics, herbs, and acupuncture. Whether the illness is due to a bacterial infection or a virus, holistic treatment is usually very effective, especially if it is begun immediately. All cases must be monitored carefully, though, to be sure a bacterial infection does not get worse. Antibiotics may have to be prescribed, particularly for older, or already debilitated, horses.

Unfortunately, because many owners wait to see if veterinary care is really necessary for respiratory illness, I am often called to treat horses only after other home treatments have failed. Sometimes these horses have been sick for a month or more, and they run the risk of having permanent damage to their lungs, heart, or both.

Homeopathic veterinarians prepare their own nosodes for equine influenza.

Rabies

Although rabies is not common in horses, its consequences can be devastating. Therefore, vaccination against rabies is necessary for many horses in the United States, especially since the disease has become more widespread in recent years. Currently the vaccine is required annually for horses, but I hope a longer-term rabies vaccine for horses will be developed soon. The dog rabies vaccine is required only every two to three years, depending on where you live.

Rabies can be hard to detect since the symptoms are often not those typically associated with the disease. I have seen several cases—in horses, dogs, cats, and bats—and none of the animals exhibited the common symptoms of excessive salivation or trying to bite people or other animals. One case involved a racehorse that was being taken to his next race, which was one of the Triple Crown series for Quarter Horses. The horse was rearing up and falling over, experiencing muscle spasms, and colicking. I treated him for colic, stabilized him, and then sent him to a large clinic for observation. Unfortunately, the horse died three days later. Even the clinic was surprised when the diagnosis came back as rabies, since the only typical sign of that disease exhibited by the horse was muscle spasms.

There is currently not a holistic prevention or treatment for rabies. Vaccination is the best preventive, but I also recommend using a nosode along with it to help prevent any side effects to the immune system. Nosodes can be obtained from homeopathic veterinarians.

Equine Viral Arteritis

Equine viral arteritis is a disease that most commonly affects horses at racetracks. Although it is not as common as many other diseases for which horses are vaccinated, it can cause lost time in training. And, because it also causes abortion, this disease is of some concern to the breeding industry.

In addition to abortion, there are a variety of signs of equine viral arteritis, including nasal discharge, skin rash, eye irritation, and swelling of the legs. However, horses can be exposed to the disease and develop antibodies without ever showing any signs of illness. Stallions can act as carriers once they have been exposed to the disease and should be tested for it prior to the breeding season because they can transmit the virus to mares either during natural breeding or through fresh cooled or frozen semen. The virus is also transmitted through aerosol droplets exhaled by horses with the disease.

Equine viral arteritis can be kept to a minimum by isolating sick horses and testing breeding stallions to prevent its spread. There has been very little opportunity to treat it with holistic medicine, but supporting the immune system with acupuncture, minimizing stress, and maintaining a good level of nutrition are all helpful adjuncts to conventional treatments. Your veterinarian will manage the disease by treating the specific symptoms that develop.

If you wish to breed your mare to a stallion that is positive for equine viral arteritis, the mare should be vaccinated first. It takes about three weeks for an effective immune response to occur; then she can be safely bred without risk of abortion. Stallions can also be vaccinated to protect them from the virus.

Nosodes for equine viral arteritis are available from a homeopathic veterinarian.

Potomac Horse Fever

Potomac horse fever is caused by ehrlichia risticii, an organism found in the United States, primarily along the East Coast. Since the area of infection is limited, I advise not to vaccinate against this disease unless you plan to go to an area where it is prevalent.

Nosodes for Potomac horse fever are available from a homeopathic veterinarian.

Equine Rotavirus

Equine rotavirus occurs in foals from two to 160 days old, resulting in diarrhea. It can be mild and last for a few days or it can be explosive and severely dehydrating. Since this virus can affect the breeding industry, much research has been done to develop a vaccine to help control it. As of this writing, a vaccine has been made available to farms in Kentucky for testing, but it is not yet available for general use.

The best treatment for the new foal is preventive care of the broodmare. A foal is more likely to be healthy and able to withstand a viral illness such as equine rotavirus when the mare is eating a nutritious diet that contains the correct balance of vitamins and minerals.

X-RAYS (RADIOGRAPHS) AND RADIATION THERAPY

X-rays are sometimes necessary in the diagnostic process, but questions arise concerning the safety of the procedure. Each time your horse is X-rayed, he is exposed to radiation. No amount of radiation is good for him, so X-rays should not be done unless they are justified. Two to four X-rays at a time probably don't pose a threat to your horse's health, but you can practice preventive medicine by giving additional vitamin C following the procedure. Vitamin C helps the body cope with the radiation because it acts as an antioxidant. (See *Antioxidant Supplements* on p. 87). The dosage will vary depending on the size and weight of the horse, but 8 grams per 1,000 pounds (about 450 kgs) is the general range.

Radiation therapy, commonly used to treat various forms of cancer, is not a procedure I use or recommend. (For alternative treatments, see *Cancer* in the *Horse Ailments* section: Part Three of this book.) If an animal who has already undergone radiation therapy is presented to me, the therapy for over-exposure to radiation is more complex. I treat each case individually based on the type of radiation that was used. A combination of supplements and dietary changes can help the horse's body eliminate some of the harmful radioisotopes. It is important to design a specific treatment program for each horse based on that horse's needs. A blood work-up and thorough exam will help the veterinarian determine exactly what those needs are.

Part II

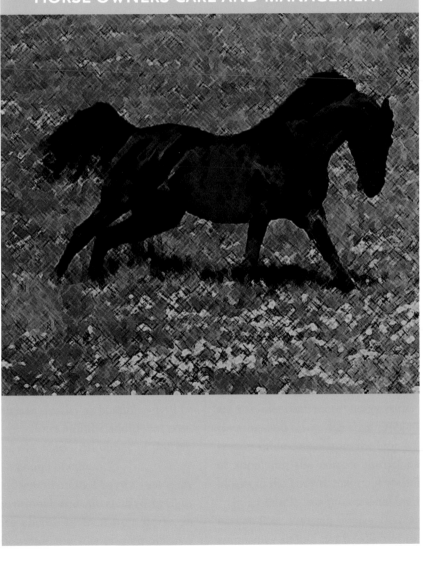

HORSE OWNERS CARE AND MANAGEMENT

The best way to see the reasonableness of removal of the "100% complete" claim is with an analogy, a human parallel. How many parents would take the advice of a pediatrician who placed a packaged food product on the exam table and told the parent that this is the only product they should feed the child day-in, day-out, for the child's lifetime, and further that they should be sure to not feed any other foods because that might unbalance the product? Even if the pediatrician gave assurances of nutrient analyses that exceeded required minimum levels, feeding trials, and even if the label guaranteed "100% complete and balanced," how many parents would accept such counsel? [1]

The federal regulatory agencies have led us to believe that bags of food are all that our horses will ever need. But, as Dr. Wysong points out in his article, to claim that any feed is "100% complete" would indicate that feed manufacturers know everything there is to know about animal nutrition. In fact, less is known about animal nutrition than human nutrition—and certainly no one in the scientific community is given credit for knowing with absolute certainty a human's nutritional needs. The study of human nutrition is ongoing, and from time to time medical researchers identify nutrients required by the body that were previously unknown. This is one of the reasons I feel a top quality diet that exceeds government nutritional standards for horses is needed to assure vibrant health.

Many veterinarians do not ask what you are feeding when they treat your horse. Like your own medical doctor, most of them have limited training in nutrition, so they do not focus on the link between health and diet. Fortunately, as scientific findings continue to conclusively prove this vital link, both medical doctors and veterinarians are becoming more aware the "we are what we eat." This old axiom is as true when it comes to our horse's health as it is for your own. Owners who appreciate this obvious connection between diet and health, are converting to better quality diets for their horses.

In my practice, questions concerning diet are a routine—and important—part of any exam, and I record the owner's responses on the patient's chart. Sometimes a change in diet is the only thing necessary to clear up a health problem. When the horse has been fed a low quality diet for a long period of time, however, it can be difficult to correlate an illness to any one cause. When a change in diet leads to an improvement in the condition, I know that I have probably identified the primary source of the problem. In any event, a review of the diet is an important step in the treatment of even the most advanced health problem.

I have seen dramatic examples of almost immediate results from a switch in diet. For instance, a 25-year-old mare in the barn where I kept my horse had a chronic cough. The cough was most severe in the late spring and summer and was therefore thought to be associated with plant allergies. All the measures that might help alleviate the cough were already being implemented, such as keeping the dust down and wetting her food. She was also being given antihistamines, which did not help. Since nothing else was helping with the cough, I suggested a change in the diet and recommended a high-quality extruded feed. Her owner agreed to try the feed, and within two weeks the mare's condition improved dramatically. Since the change in diet she has had only an occasional cough.

Every feed company wants you to believe it has the perfect feed for your horse, but no one

1 R.L. Wysong, D.V.M., "The Myth of the 100% Complete Manufactured Diet," Journal of the American Holistic Veterinary Medical Association, February-April, 1992, Vol.11, No. 1, p. 17.

knows exactly what a perfect feed is. Ideally, each horse should be individually analyzed for his own unique nutritional requirements, and a feed should then be formulated to meet that horse's needs. Nutritional needs vary from breed to breed and on the exercise requirements of the horse. A horse that is used for light trail rides will have different dietary needs from a racehorse that gallops daily. Many horse owners do not realize that all horses should not be fed the same diet, and I routinely encounter horses that are being fed a diet inappropriate to their needs.

There are so many variables to be considered when deciding on which feed will best fulfill your horse's needs that most horse owners are not sure where to start. You can find basic feeding guidelines in many books, and some feed companies now offer consultations with equine nutritionists at your farm or by telephone to help advise horse owners. Since the horse feed market is so competitive, you should be able to find a company that will answer your questions and help you work out a diet for your horse. Remember, however, that most feed companies will work out a diet using only feeds that they sell, which may not necessarily be what is best for your horse. So consider checking several different sources before making a final decision. It may also be helpful to discuss the alternatives with a veterinarian who is experienced in equine nutrition. If that isn't possible, consult a university veterinary school or an equine nutritional specialist. Your horse can only perform at his best if you feed him correctly. It is really worth the time and effort to check into different diets, both for the horse's health and to invest your money as wisely as possible.

GRAINS: MAKING THE BEST CHOICE FOR YOUR HORSE

Should you feed your horse assorted whole grains that you mix yourself or premixed sweet feeds or pellets (known as cubes or nuts in the UK)? Each of these options has a place in feed programs. First, the horse's preference must be considered: what will he eat? Many horses will not eat anything unless it is sweetened with molasses, so that may be the deciding factor. However, if your horse will eat either type of feed, then the question remains as to which is the best for him.

If you choose to feed whole grains, you should know the nutritional breakdown of the grains so that you can properly balance your horse's diet. This can be difficult, since nutritional breakdowns may not be available for individual bags of grain. You may have to use an average, because the breakdown can vary depending on how long the grain has been stored and where it was grown. The disparity can be significant because soil conditions differ from region to region, and the quality of the soil determines the quality of the grain. For instance, horses may need less grain to maintain their weight if they are fed a grain that was grown in the rich fertile soil of the midwestern United States rather than grain grown in the South where soil is less fertile. The additional problem of spoilage during storage must also be considered if you live in a climate that is hot and humid. So, when selecting the grains you will feed, it's best to investigate what types of grain are available on a consistent basis, where the grain is from, and what information is available concerning the grain's nutritional contents.

Premixed Feeds

Over the last several years, premixed commercial feed products have become both more varied and more specialized. It is now possible to buy feed formulated specifically for sport horses, pleasure horses, broodmares, and older horses, just to mention a few. In these premixed feeds, the carbohydrates, proteins, and fat are balanced to best meet the dietary requirements for the designated category of horse.

There are also premixed feeds in which the mineral content has been specifically balanced for feeding with certain types of hay. Horses, like humans, need calcium in their diets. If the ratio of phosphorus to calcium in the horse's diet is too high, the greater levels of phosphorus can interfere with the body's ability to absorb calcium. All grains are usually higher in phosphorus than calcium, and grass hay generally contains only small amounts of calcium. As a result, horses that are fed a diet consisting primarily of grain and grass hay sometimes develop calcium deficiencies. Vitamin-mineral supplements can provide an additional source of calcium, but the amount may not be sufficient to counterbalance the phosphorus in the diet. Determining the level of available calcium in your horse's diet is a complex process and not one that you should attempt on your own. If you suspect that your horse's diet is lacking in calcium, consult an equine nutritionist or feed one of the grain mixes formulated with the correct mineral balance for the type of hay you use.

Pelletized Grains

Pellets are so commonly fed to horses that owners often use them without stopping to consider whether they are the best choice. I strongly recommend feeding whole or premixed grains whenever possible, but there are admittedly some horses that seem to prefer pellets and reach their optimum weight and performance levels when the grain portion of their diet is pellets.

Pellets can also be a useful option when storage of feed is problematic. High heat and humidity can cause a breakdown of the essential vitamins and minerals in grains. Insects are also a problem when feed is stored on a long-term basis. Most grains—no matter how high in quality—contain insect larvae that will mature over time and begin to consume the grain. Often these problems can be minimized by storing grain for as short a time as possible. In some areas, however, the heat, humidity, and insects are so bad that the only solution is to convert the grain to pellet form in order to reduce its moisture content. This, in turn, reduces the rate of mold formation and allows for longer storage and safer feeding practices.

The extent to which a horse can utilize the nutrients in a pellet depends on two factors: the quality of grains used to make it and the type of pellet. It is critical that the grain be of high nutritional quality because the hot temperatures used in the manufacturing process result in some loss of nutrients. If you choose to feed pellets to your horse, you should first check the feed bag label to determine the grains that were used and the nutritional content of the pellets. You should only feed pellets for which the nutritional content was measured after the grain was pelletized; otherwise, you have no way of knowing how many nutrients were lost in the manufacturing process. If the label is not clear on this issue, check with the manufacturer.

Different types of pellets vary in moisture content and in the degree to which the grain is compressed during manufacturing. For the horse to get the most nutritional benefit from the pellets, they must easily absorb moisture and break down in his digestive tract. Although there are gastric secretions in the horse's system that assist in digesting food, they will not necessarily help to hydrate dry pellets. Before feeding any pellets, you should test them to see how well they absorb moisture and break down. Put a handful of pellets in a small bucket of water and monitor how long it takes for them to absorb the water. If they do not break down into a mushy consistency within 30 to 45 minutes, try another brand.

Finally, if you have a horse that does not drink much water, I advise against feeding pellets because they absorb water from the body as they break down and may leave the horse insufficiently hydrated.

PESTICIDES AND HERBICIDES ON FEEDS

There is growing concern about possible health risks to horses caused by pesticide and herbicide residues on feeds. Tolerance guidelines for pesticides have been established for humans, mainly with respect to carcinogenic risk. Testing for other possible effects to body systems, such as the immune system or pulmonary system, has not been done in horses, yet pesticides continue to be used on equine feeds. Nor have investigations been done on the possible synergistic or interactive effects of those chemicals in combination with each other or when they are combined with a medication or feed additive.

Occasionally, I have been called on to treat a horse that was experiencing digestive problems of a non-specific nature. The first place to start ruling out possible causes of a digestive problem is by testing the individual components of the horse's diet, either by conducting laboratory tests or by using applied kinesiology muscle testing (see Chapter Ten). Often I find that one or another component of the diet is not agreeing with the horse. I check the grain first, then the hay, then the supplements. If a feed or supplement appears to be the culprit, I recommend that the owner switch to an entirely different source or stop feeding that one part of the diet for at least five days to see if the digestive problem improves. You will be surprised if you start testing your horse's feed and supplements using muscle testing since it is common to occasionally find one ingredient or another that does not test well. Even if a horse is not noticeably experiencing digestive problems, the build-up of chemicals may cause a major reaction in the future.

Most horses digest oats well and I have never worked with any who were allergic to oats—although there must be one out there somewhere. So when testing indicates that a horse reacts poorly to oats, I usually suspect that the reaction is caused by a chemical residue on the oats rather than by the oats themselves. In every case I've seen involving oats, the horse has improved when fed oats from a different source.

On one occasion I was at a racetrack working in a barn where the majority of the horses had experienced poor workouts for several days. Some of these horses had races scheduled in the near future, and their laboratory blood work was normal, so some quick answers were needed. After muscle testing the horses, I concluded that a new load of timothy hay was not testing well for any of the affected horses. The hay had previously been checked for molds but not for chemicals. Apparently something on the hay was not agreeing with the horses and was causing them to perform poorly. The horses returned to their normal performance levels once they were no longer being fed the suspect hay.

FOOD ALLERGIES AND SENSITIVITIES

Food is often the culprit when a horse has a health problem such as hives, which is an allergic reaction. However, food allergies or sensitivities are not always so outwardly noticeable, and I frequently encounter horses with digestive upsets that have gone undiagnosed for long periods of time.

Digestive problems are often caused by foods that contain toxins in the form of molds, fungus, bacteria, or mycotoxins. Many of these contaminants cannot be seen with the naked eye, so don't inspect every bite of food your horse eats in the hope of identifying them. However, there are some signs that may indicate the presence of toxins in your horse's feed. Gradual weight loss, poor attitude, and a dull or bleached-out coat are some of the first signs that the body is struggling to deal with toxins. Hooves sometimes develop ridges or rings around them and can become dry. Although these are very general signs, they are sometimes significant if nothing else in the horse's environment has changed.

If you suspect there are toxins in your horse's food you can use muscle testing to determine which part of his ration is causing the problem (see Chapter Ten) or have the feed tested for various toxins at a laboratory. I use muscle testing first because it's quick and I've found it to be very accurate. Muscle testing can then be followed up with a laboratory test.

One feed that commonly causes an allergic reaction or sensitivity is corn (known as maize in the UK). The fat in corn is very susceptible to oxidation that can cause the corn to become rancid and lose over fifty percent of its nutrients, within three weeks after being cracked. The vitamin E in the corn also deteriorates very quickly and may need to be supplemented if corn is the main grain in the diet. In addition, mycotoxins found in corn are of growing concern, and they may be the problem when a horse reacts negatively to corn. There are corn-based feeds available that are free of mycotoxins, so check the feed label carefully. If you suspect a mycotoxin problem, have the grain analyzed at a laboratory, and, if necessary, switch to a feed that does not contain mycotoxins.

Crimped hay should also be avoided if the hay is from an area such as the midwestern United States where blister beetles are found. Blister beetles are very toxic to horses, causing kidney damage and eventually kidney failure. It takes only one-fourth of a blister beetle to cause serious illness in a horse. When the hay is harvested, it is processed in a manner that crimps or crushes the shaft of the hay. Any beetles in the hay are killed and baled right along with it. This is not a problem with regular non-crimped hay because even though blister beetles are sometimes baled along with the hay, they are still alive so they crawl out of the bales.

You should ask your supplier if the hay has been crimped, because it can be difficult to distinguish between crimped hay and regular hay. If you closely inspect it yourself, you may be able to detect crushed areas running down the length of the shaft, but often the crimper flattens or splits the hay shaft, making it difficult to tell if it has been crimped.

SELECTING THE RIGHT DIET FOR YOUR HORSE

Each horse has his own unique nutritional needs. In order to determine which feed most benefits your horse, you must weigh a number of variables. Here are some steps that you can take to help you shape the best diet to meet your horse's specific needs:

1. Find out what types of feed are available in your area. Will your feed company consider stocking new feeds?

2. Find out what grains are in the feed and in what proportion.

3. Once you have decided on some possible feeds, find out where each is grown. (Those grown in the northern and midwestern United States often have higher nutritional quality.)

4. Find out how fresh the feed is. You can get an idea of freshness by asking about the average storage time of the feed at the feed company.

5. Find out what vitamins and minerals are added to the feed and determine how they meet your horse's needs. I will discuss vitamins and minerals in more detail later in this chapter.

6. Check to be sure that the feed company excludes artificial fillers, binders, coloring

agents, and flavor enhancers.

7. Compare a number of available feeds. You may actually save money with a more expensive feed that is of higher quality because your horse will probably stay healthier.

8. Obtain samples of the feeds you are considering and use muscle testing to check your horse for any sensitivities to them.

9. If you have experienced feed problems in the past and have a very sensitive horse, you may want to send feed to a laboratory for testing to determine nutritional content and to check for toxins.

Be aware that companies sometimes change ingredients in their feeds. Or they may change management, and the new management may have lower standards. Keep ever vigilant; monitor your horse's coat, skin, and performance as indicators that the feed is continuously high in quality. Make it your business to check the ingredient list. You may also want to call or write to a feed company and ask for information on their standards and sources of ingredients. Remember both the specific types of ingredients and their quality affect the nutritional value of the final product.

To determine your horse's specific nutritional needs for protein, carbohydrates, and fats, consult your veterinarian or equine nutritionist. Or you can read up on the subject yourself. One excellent book is John Kohnke's *Feeding and Nutrition* (see Appendix VII). If the feed label does not list the exact percentages of protein, carbohydrates, and fats, or the exact contents of the feed, contact the company to obtain this information so you can make as intelligent a decision as possible.

The next step is to determine if the feed that you choose will actually work for your horse. Your horse's disposition might be a factor in deciding what types of grains to include in his ration. If he is the nervous or spirited type, do not feed oats as the main source of his grain. Excitable behavior is sometimes increased when oats are fed. Barley that has been soaked, steam rolled, or flaked is often a better choice for such horses.

Your horse may benefit from a diet in which part of the carbohydrates have been replaced with fats. This additional fat not only keeps the coat shiny, but it also gives the horse a more gradual and consistent source of energy since fat is broken down at a slower rate than carbohydrates. This type of diet helps to calm a nervous or temperamental horse by preventing him from experiencing a sudden rush of energy. High fat diets are also particularly useful for endurance horses who need a constant energy source to sustain long periods of exertion. Special feeds are available that provide a higher fat content in the diet; however, I prefer supplying some of the fat in the diet with an oil supplement. (See *Oils* in the next section, *Supplements to the Diet*).

SUPPLEMENTS TO THE DIET

Vitamins and Minerals

Many commercial horse feeds contain added vitamins and minerals designed to replace the nutrients that were destroyed in the processing of the feed, but you have no way of knowing the quality of these vitamins and minerals. I suggest feeding a grain that is as high in quality as possible in order to ensure that your horse gets all the vitamins and minerals he needs. In the southern United States, the soil is not rich enough to produce as high quality grain as that grown in the Midwest. Consequently, obtaining high quality feeds in the South is very challenging. Recently, I noticed that horses eating a particular grain brought in from the Midwest had substantially better coat condition and required less grain to support them. When I switched my own horse to this grain, the effect was the same. He was also happier and more cooperative after the switch.

Depending on the type and nutritional quality of grain available in your area, you may feel it's necessary to add some nutritional supplements to your horse's diet. Before you feed vitamin and mineral supplements to your horse, consult your veterinarian or equine nutritionist to determine the correct amounts. Over-supplementation can result in a diet that is too high in some vitamins, minerals, or other nutrients. For instance, if excessive amounts of B vitamins are fed, a horse may become excitable, highly energized, and unable to concentrate. A more dangerous example of over-supplementation is feeding too much calcium or phosphorus. Excessive amounts of either mineral can cause changes in the horse's bone formation, resulting in permanent damage.

Look for vitamin and mineral supplements that contain as many natural ingredients as possible and avoid additives based solely on chemicals. These synthetic versions of vitamins may not be absorbed as well by your horse. Also avoid supplements that contain corn, which is sometimes used as a filler and other times added to make the supplement more tasty. As discussed earlier, many horses are sensitive to corn, and it often carries mycotoxins. Remember we're trying to help our horses, not cause additional problems. If you're not familiar with supplements, start by comparing labels. You'll be surprised at the differences between brands.

Here are a couple of suggestions that can help ensure your horse utilizes the supplements to their full potential. Select a vitamin supplement and a separate mineral supplement because some minerals react chemically with vitamins, causing a reduction in the efficacy of the vitamins. New research also indicates that some

vitamins are more stable at a certain acid-alkaline balance (pH) and may lose potency if stored at a less ideal pH. Since most vitamins lose some of their potency during storage anyway, having the correct pH in the supplement may help decrease this problem. Supplement companies are now recognizing this and some are offering vitamins at the correct pH. Vitamins such as B1 and B6 are more stable at a pH of 2.5 to 3.0 while vitamins A, D, E, and B12 stabilize at a pH of 4.8 to 5.5. These are just a few of the vitamins that are pH sensitive.

In his book, *Feeding and Nutrition*, Dr. John Kohnke offers other warnings to heed when using supplements:

1. Avoid mixing supplements containing Vitamin E and Vitamin C into feeds containing supplements of iron or copper as these minerals can interact and destroy these vitamins.
2. Avoid storing damp feed [a feed mix that has had water added to it prior to feeding] with added minerals and vitamins (e.g. Vitamin E and iron) for more than 3-4 hours, as some of the vitamins may be destroyed by interaction with minerals in the moist environment.
3. Do not mix vitamin supplements directly into warm feeds (e.g. bran mashes, hot boiled barley or linseed) until they have cooled to room temperature. Mix in just prior to feeding.
4. Do not add mineral oils to the same feed as supplements containing Vitamins A, D and E as they will be absorbed into the oil and be less available to the horse.
5. Do not mix vitamins into feed containing alkaline electrolytes (particularly bicarbonate of soda) as some may be destroyed before the horse consumes

them, particularly in a damp feed [a feed that has had water added to it].

6. Do not rely on vitamin injections as the sole form of vitamin supplementation. Provide oral forms daily as a basic routine supplement, particularly to horses under stress of hard work and racing.

7. Do not mix calcium into pure bran mashes, as the calcium may be bound-up and made less available to the horse. In normal rations containing up to 10% bran, absorption of calcium will not be significantly reduced. [2]

Remember again to check all feeds, supplements, and medications for the quantities of vitamins and minerals present and to consult your veterinarian or equine nutritionist to be sure there is not too much of any one vitamin or mineral in your horse's diet. This is particularly important when supplementing with vitamin E and folic acid since the current treatment for equine protozoal myeloencephalitis includes a daily dose of these nutrients. While these nutrients are important, it is also vital that you do not inadvertently overdose them.

Oil Supplements

Extra virgin olive oil is an excellent oil supplement to increase the fat content in the diet. It is a naturally processed, cold-pressed oil that is well absorbed by the horse's digestive tract. Corn oil has long been used as an oil supplement, but many horses do not tolerate it—possibly because of the large number of chemicals used to process it. However, if you can find a non-chemically processed source, corn oil can be used. Like the grain, corn oil must be stored in a cool dry place so it doesn't become rancid or oxidized. If other oils are used as supplements they should be processed naturally, not chemically extracted. I prefer to keep fats from animal sources to a minimum since the horse's digestive tract is designed for vegetable-based fats.

Electrolytes

Electrolytes are mineral salts contained in body fluids that are composed mainly of sodium, potassium, and chloride, with lesser amounts of calcium, magnesium, and zinc. They are used in carrying out many body functions, particularly muscle contraction, and horses lose electrolytes when they sweat. A horse that sweats only lightly should not need added electrolytes because a healthy diet will provide sufficient elements to restore correct electrolyte balance. However, if a horse sweats excessively, too many electrolytes are lost in the process. When a horse is required to make great physical efforts in a short amount of time—such as running a race or galloping around a cross-country course—he will often require a quick replacement of electrolytes.

Caution: *An improper balance of electrolytes or a deficiency of electrolytes can be life threatening. Therefore, it is vital to provide extra electrolytes if your horse requires them. The need for electrolyte supplements varies according to the climate you live in, and the amount your horse sweats. If you are not used to giving them, and are concerned about your horse's electrolyte balance, discuss the procedures with your veterinarian.*

The veterinarian can take a blood sample and check the exact blood levels of the electrolytes before and after exercise. This step is rarely required but may be a good idea if your horse is experiencing symptoms such as tying-up, or exhaustion.

Electrolytes are available in commercial mixes that come with excellent dosage directions, or you can prepare a basic electrolyte mixture using salt and lite salt. Most commercial electrolyte mixes contain sodium, potassium,

---

2 *John Kohnke, B.V.S.c., R.D.A., Feeding and Nutrition, (Biribi Pacific, Rouse Hill, New South Wales, Australia, 1992), p. 187.*

and chloride. Some may also contain smaller amounts of magnesium, zinc, and calcium, but these minerals are often not included in electrolyte mixes because most horses get enough of them in their feed.

As an alternative to the commercial mixes, you can make your own electrolyte solution using the following recipe:

HOMEMADE ELECTROLYTE SOLUTION

3 parts sodium chloride (salt)

1 part potassium chloride (lite salt)

The daily dose of homemade electrolyte varies from one (14ml) to four tablespoons depending on the amount of exercise and the degree of sweating. Start with one tablespoon if your horse sweats a moderate amount and increase the amount when your horse sweats more. If you exercise your horse more strenuously than usual during a particular riding session, give him additional electrolytes that day. The best way to ensure that your horse ingests the correct amount of electrolytes is to add them to his feed, preferably at the evening meal so you can adjust the dose according to the day's activity level.

Alternatively you can add electrolytes to the water, but then you have to make sure the horse drinks the full bucket. Water containing electrolytes will taste different, so your horse may resist drinking it. Your horse should always have plenty of fresh water available, but this is especially important when you are giving him electrolytes.

Be careful not to exceed suggested dosages. If you stick to the dosages recommended you are not be in danger of causing an imbalance in your horse's system because any excess electrolytes inadvertently consumed will be flushed from his system when he drinks water.

Electrolytes are also available in a paste form. The paste electrolytes do not have to be combined with grain, so they can be given as soon as the horse has cooled down after excessive exertion.

Bacterial Supplements

Any horse that is on antibiotics (even injectable antibiotics) should be given additional beneficial bacteria in the form of acidophilus, lactobacillus, or one of the bacterial replacement products designed specifically for horses. (In the US, two of these are called Probiotic and Ration Plus and are available in feed stores.) This supplement should be given during, and for about a week after, antibiotic treatment. Antibiotics either kill the natural "friendly" bacteria in the digestive tract or significantly alter the balance of bacteria. If you have ever been prescribed an antibiotic, you may have suffered this side effect yourself and ended up with a stomach that hurt or was upset. (Many people take yogurt when they are on antibiotics because yogurt contains these same beneficial bacteria.) Horses are susceptible to the same side effects, but require even more friendly bacteria because of the type of digestive system they have. By adding beneficial bacteria to the horse's diet, you can speed up his recovery rate.

Acidophilus can also be helpful in the transition when a change is made in the horse's feed, since the new feed may cause different bacterial flora to flourish in the digestive tract. Feed it for about two weeks. Acidophilus and other forms of beneficial bacteria such as lactobacillus are available in capsules, powder, or liquid form in the refrigerator section of any natural foods store. If your horse is on antibiotics, either find a bacterial replacement product formulated specifically for horses or use three to five capsules a day of the products available from the natural foods store.

Yogurt can also be used; however it is not as bacterial specific as the products mentioned above made specifically for horses. If you choose to use yogurt, add one small container of the *plain* variety to the horse's feed once a day, or administer by syringe. Most horses like yogurt, though be aware that occasionally a horse will be sensitive to a dairy product such as this.

Digestive Enzymes

Digestive enzymes—protease, lipase, amylase, and disaccharidase—also help in the digestion process. These enzymes are substances produced within the body that break down the nutrients so they can be absorbed. But, when a horse is stressed by illness or other circumstance, his body may produce fewer enzymes. Supplementing the diet with additional enzymes will help the body to maintain a more constant supply of nutrients. The addition of digestive enzymes to the diet can also help older horses to maintain their health and weight since, with age, the body generally experiences a decrease in its own ability to produce enzymes. These enzymes, available in powdered form, are sold commercially under different product names, and can be obtained through a veterinarian.

Antioxidant Supplements

The discovery of free radicals may eventually be considered one of the most important breakthroughs in understanding the immune system and its ability to combat disease and degenerative conditions, including aging. Free radicals are highly volatile atoms that have at least one unpaired electron. This free electron causes a chemical reaction that leads to cellular damage when it becomes attached to another element. Free radicals can be extremely toxic. More than 30 years of research have proven that these overreactive molecules cause cellular damage. The cell damage from large numbers of free radicals has been linked to many degenerative diseases responsible for aging.

Stresses on the body cause high concentrations of free radicals that weaken the immune system. These stresses include chemicals in the food chain, polluted air and water, contamination by heavy metals such as mercury and lead, and exposure to radiation. Free radical activity in the body is also increased by excess amounts of fat in the diet, especially fats from rancid and heated oils. This is a special concern for horse owners because corn oil, which is commonly given to horses, becomes rancid very quickly, especially if it is stored in a barn. But free radicals are not all bad—the body actually requires minute amounts of them to remove a virus or bacteria from the body. It is high concentrations of free radicals that represent the challenge to your horse's health.

When the body is confronted with an overabundance of free radicals, it springs into action with its own free radical defense system composed of an array of body-produced enzymes called antioxidants, which are sometimes referred to as free radical scavengers. Free radicals become a problem when the body is unable to produce enough antioxidant enzymes on its own to combat high concentrations of these toxic invaders. While you can strengthen your horse's ability to deal with free radicals by selecting a high quality natural diet, you cannot totally avoid harmful amounts of free radicals from other sources such as pesticide residues on food and in water, air pollution, and heavy metal contaminants. Among their many other functions, beta-carotene and vitamins C and E are antioxidant nutrients because they play a supportive role in combating excess free radicals. Also helpful are specific antioxidant supplements such as blue-green algae or others made from whole food sources such as sprouted wheat that promote the antioxidant enzyme supply of the body. (See Appendix VI for product suppliers.)

Dr. Peter R. Rothschild and Zane Baranowski, C.N., explain the results of using antioxidant supplements:

Physicians and veterinarians utilizing whole food supersprout concentrates to improve the nutritional status of their patients report a long list of positive benefits that can only be related to an improved nutritional standard. These benefits include diminished joint pains and inflammation, more energy, better circulation, and, most importantly, significantly reduced recovery time after surgery or other types of convalescence after severe stress conditions such as physical trauma. Clearly, the degree to which a patient is well nourished does affect his ability to cope with stress. Apparently, whole food sprout concentrates supply the right nutrition for these circumstances. Due to the growing understanding of antioxidant enzymes, pharmaceutical companies are also pursuing the development of new compounds including [the antioxidant] SOD. These products, unlike whole food, contain isolated enzymes and could potentially create imbalances. Such new products will, of course, be regulated as drugs and require prescriptions. Fortunately, we have whole food "supersprout" concentrates at our disposal to naturally assist our body's maintenance of adequate antioxidant enzymes. [3]

As mentioned above, vitamin C is an excellent source of antioxidants—and less expensive than products such as blue-green algae or supersprout concentrates. Vitamin C supplements are available from many equine supply companies in a condensed powdered form. My favorite type of vitamin C is called Ester C which contains no preservatives, artificial flavors or color. It is less acidic and does not upset the horse's stomach when given in large amounts. I suggest five to eight grams per thousand pounds (about 450 kgs) of weight, although the dosage can be increased if the horse is injured. Another choice is to give your horse flavored 1,000 mg vitamin C tablets that are available at the health food store. They can be fed as a treat alone and are also readily eaten when mixed in the grain. There is also a number of other commercial antioxidant product available for horses. Check with your veterinarian or equine nutritionist for information on the latest products and see Appendix VI for suppliers.

Supplements for Hoof Growth

There are a number of products on the market that contain biotin (a vitamin) and methionine (a sulfur-containing amino acid) to assist in hoof growth. They work in tandem, so it is best when both of these nutrients are supplemented in the diet. However, they are helpful only if your horse has a deficiency of biotin and methionine. Since there is no way to accurately tell if your horse has a deficiency in these nutrients, you will have to feed the supplement to determine if it will have any beneficial effect. Hoof growth is very slow, so it can take four to six months to see results from feeding a biotin and methionine supplement. When giving hoof supplements, I also supplement the diet with acidophilus and digestive enzymes to assist with the digestion and utilization of these nutrients.

---

3 *Peter R. Rothschild, M.D., Ph.D. and Zane Baranowski, C.N.,* Free Radicals, Stress and Antioxidant Supplements, *(Honolulu: University Labs Press, 1990), p.4.*

Supplements to Calm a Horse

There are two natural supplements, thiamine and valerian root, commonly used to decrease nervous conditions in horses. You will have to experiment to see which works best for your horse.

Thiamin, also known as vitamin B1, can be fed on a continuous basis in the regular grain ration or given 20 to 30 minutes before riding. It is packaged for horses and available in feed stores, so check the label of any commercially available thiamine to determine the recommended dosage.

Valerian root is also an effective herbal calmer for horses. It can be used on its own, or you may want to try one of the commercially available herbal calming products for horses that contains it. Hilton Herbs makes several excellent products (see Appendix VI). In some cases, high doses of valerian are required. If you are interested in trying a product that contains valerian root, check the label for recommended dosage. If you want to try valerian root alone, you can purchase it in a health food store. Start with a dosage of one-half ounce (15 grams) a day in the feed or consult your holistic veterinarian about the dosage recommended for your horse. NOTE: Use of valerian root is banned at most horse shows and horse racing events.

Natural Laxatives

Bran and psyllium seed husks are the most common natural laxatives given to horses, but I do not recommend using bran as a daily laxative. My concern about the overuse of bran in horses' diets is twofold. First, bran contains some of the same elements that form enteroliths, which are stones that develop in the large intestine. They cause great discomfort and can block movement through the tract, resulting in continuous bouts of colic. Additionally, because bran is high in phosphorus, it is important that its use be balanced with sufficient calcium in the diet. Although horses should not be given bran on a daily basis, I have not found any problems with feeding my own horses a hot bran mash once a week as a treat. Most horses love bran mash and the change it provides in the regular feeding regimen.

Psyllium seed husks are often added to the diet to help remove sand and debris from the intestinal tract. They seem to be effective in helping to stimulate the intestinal tract, thus pushing fine particles out of it and diminishing the possibility of colic due to excessive sand ingestion. I always suggest adding psyllium to the diet when the horse is kept in a stall or a pasture where he might ingest sand when he eats. There are a number of products containing psyllium on the market, and they are all about the same. If you are uncertain whether your horse needs psyllium in his diet, ask your veterinarian. Be aware, however, that psyllium occasionally causes excessive gas formation due to the fermentation it can undergo in the digestive tract. If your horse has digestive problems or already suffers from excessive gas formation, do not use this product.

HOW MUCH TO FEED

Because of the differences in breeds, body types, and exercise levels, there is no general guideline on how much to feed. I suggest keeping track of all changes in the diet by creating a feeding record for each horse. Each time you make a change in the type or amount of feed or supplements, record the date and other pertinent information. This is much more accurate than trying to remember changes that were made months previously and can be very helpful, especially if the horse should develop a health problem.

If your horse needs to gain or lose weight, review the entry on *Weight Problems* on p. 288.

CHANGING TO A NEW FEED

When changing to a new feed, introduce the new feed gradually and monitor your horse closely for any reactions to the new diet. Start by replacing one-fourth of the ration with the new feed for five days. Then increase the new feed to one-half of the ration for five more days. After that, you can gradually phase out the old feed. Whenever a feed change is made, a different type of bacterial flora will flourish in the horse's digestive tract. This beneficial bacteria helps break down foods so the body can absorb the nutrients in them. They are present in many of the foods horses ingest and most horses receive a fairly consistent supply. However, a different feed may carry or support different types of bacterial growth, allowing one type of bacterium to flourish more than another. This upset in your horse's bacterial balance can sometimes cause a digestive problem such as colic. The possible negative side-effects of changing feeds can be minimized by adding an acidophilus or lactobacillus product to the diet during the transition and for a short period of time thereafter—about two weeks in all. (Refer to information on *Bacterial Supplements* on p. 86.)

NEED FOR FRESH WATER

Horses require a source of fresh water at all times. If water is not available, dehydration can occur faster than most people realize, particularly in hot weather. Water is not only a vital source of fluids but also contains essential minerals needed by the body.

Horses that regularly drink from impure sources of water such as ponds usually build a tolerance to most of the common bacteria found in the water. However, if serious disease-producing bacteria form in the water source, even these horses can become ill.

Mud puddles and algae-green ponds seem to attract horses to drink. I'm not sure why horses like that type of water. Perhaps it has an appealing taste. Although it usually causes no ill effects, I have treated cases of gastro-intestinal upset associated with contaminated water sources, so I advise caution when water sources are not known or appear questionable. If the water tank in your pasture is green and algae-filled, and your horse has suffered no ill effects from it, he probably will not have any problems in the future. That does not mean, however, that you should ignore this potential source of illness. Your horse's water tank should be cleaned and maintained regularly.

When presented with a questionable water source, such as a stream, it is best not to allow your horse to drink from it unless you are sure it is safe. Just because the water is clear, it does not mean that it is free from disease or pollution. If you are planning to trail ride in an area you don't know, try to obtain information about the water quality of ponds or streams in advance.

More and more, people are questioning the safety of their water supply, whether they have well water or depend on a municipal water system. If your horse lives in a stable that uses well water, the water quality should be checked periodically, especially if the surrounding area is used for farming or industrial activities. Much of our groundwater throughout the country has been affected by numerous contaminants that may be harmful to your horse, including fertilizers, herbicides, pesticides, insecticides, heavy metals such as lead and mercury, and other industrial wastes.

Despite the fact that municipal water authorities continually guarantee the safety of the water they provide, in recent years a number of cities have reported incidents of contaminated water causing hundreds of illnesses. Public confidence in water safety has eroded, and people concerned about the purity of their drinking water are choosing in greater numbers to install water filters on their home faucets or buy bottled water. Since bottled water is not an affordable alternative for horses, many people install filters in their main water systems to reduce contaminants.

Because water is such an important source of minerals for your horse, you should not use distilled water or water purified by a reverse-osmosis water-purification system. Both of these systems remove minerals from the water. If you want to install your own water purification system, you'll have some homework to do because several different types are available. An excellent assessment of these various devices can be found in the "Water" chapter of *Nontoxic, Natural and Earthwise* by Debra Lynn Dadd (see Appendix VII).

Some studies have indicated that an overly acidic pH of the water may cause minerals to be chemically bonded in the digestive tract and removed from the body. This issue has been a concern to owners of highly athletic horses such as racehorses who are looking for every advantage. They check the pH and adjust it to an alkaline state before giving it to their horses. The pH can easily be checked using litmus paper that is available in the drug store.

Whatever your choice of pure water, it should be changed daily, kept fresh in your horse's water trough or bucket, and available at all times. The container should be washed thoroughly on at least a weekly basis so algae, bacteria, and mineral deposits don't build up. In the summer, algae and bacteria are of greater concern so clean the water trough or bucket daily. In the winter, keep water free of ice. Electric water-heating devices and insulated buckets are available for use in cold climates. Though most people think of dehydration as a hot weather problem, a horse that doesn't drink enough can dehydrate in cold weather, too. Many horses don't like to drink cold water, so when the weather is extremely cold, offer lukewarm water at least twice a day.

TREAT FOODS

My own horse seems to live for his treat foods and truly enjoys having a variety to choose from. Treat foods run the gamut from sugar, carrots, and apples to commercial treats available in tack and feed stores. Treat foods should be just that—a special treat fed only once or twice a day. Commercially processed treat foods are not nutritionally balanced, and, like all treats, they should be given in small amounts so they don't interfere with, or take the place of, a balanced meal. Read the ingredient labels of processed treat foods carefully because some horses react to the artificial coloring, flavoring, or preservatives contained in many commercial treats. High amounts of sugar or molasses are also common in commercial treats and may cause some horses to become overly excitable shortly after being fed the treat.

As an alternative to commercial treats, you can feed carrots and apples, or make your own treats. Be sure the apples and carrots you give your horse are in good condition and not moldy or spoiled. I also strongly suggest that you cut the carrots into smaller pieces so that your horse cannot try to swallow them whole. You may say, "my horse always chews his carrots." My horse always chewed his too—until the one time when he didn't. The whole carrot became stuck in his esophagus (a condition known as "choke"), and he almost died. Choke requires immediate veterinary treatment, and it can be difficult to dislodge the food material. During the recuperation period, which can be lengthy, the horse cannot be in training. In my horse's case, it took two weeks for his throat to heal. If you want to make your own healthy treats, *The Original Book of Horse Treats* by June V. Evers contains recipes for a great variety of treats for horses. The recipes are fun and easy, and the horses love them. Additionally, you have the advantage of using fresh foods and controlling the ingredients you select.

Avoid human foods such as sandwiches, cookies, or hamburgers. (Believe me, people do feed hamburgers to horses, especially at horse shows). Although your horse might enjoy these foods, they are not good for him and can severely upset his digestive tract. Be careful feeding large amounts of anything your horse is not used to. Some of the worst colic cases I've seen have been caused by excessive consumption of human foods such as watermelon rind. Even if you have fed items like this to your horse in the past with no problems, remember there's always the first time.

FEEDING THE YOUNG HORSE

The foal's health is a reflection of the quality of the mother's milk. If the mother is on a high quality diet, you will be sure that the correct nutrients are present in the milk she is producing. While she is nursing her foal she will need more food in order to produce an adequate milk supply.

When the time comes to start giving grain to your young horse, you should use one of the commercially pre-mixed feeds designed specifically for youngsters. These feeds are formulated to provide an ideal balance of nutrients for this stage of life. If you stick to the recommended amounts of feed, your young horse should grow normally. You may also want to consult an expert in equine nutrition who can assist you in planning a diet that will provide the best nutrition for this important stage in your horse's development.

Sometimes people who own young horses that are being shown try to accelerate their growth and development by feeding a ration too high in carbohydrates, protein, and feed supple-

ments. Unfortunately, this kind of overfeeding often leads to problems with bone growth, including knees that won't straighten, and epiphisitis (a metabolic disease evidenced by enlargement of the limb joints). Although several factors can contribute to these problems, diet is one of the main factors, and it is the only one that can be controlled.

FEEDING THE OLDER HORSE

The older horse has different dietary needs as a result of a normal decrease in digestive efficiency. There is no specific age when this happens but there are some signs to look for that can help you recognize when your horse is starting to feel his age. Gradual weight loss is common and may be the first sign you notice that your horse has crossed the threshold into the "senior" years. While the weight loss may be attributed to a natural part of the aging process, you should always consult your veterinarian to rule out health problems that may be causing it, such as the condition of his teeth or the presence of parasites. Another sign of aging is a decrease in energy. Your horse may not seem to have as much stamina as he did in the past, even though his exercise program is the same. As a general rule, I consider a horse to be "older" when he turns 15. At this point, you should start to change the diet even if you haven't seen a difference in his weight and stamina.

Now available on the market are "extruded" feeds, which are ideal for older horses. This type of feed looks similar to breakfast cereal and is much easier for a horse to digest than whole grains of regular commercial mixes because it has been cooked in a process that gets rid of the (less-digestible) outer hulls of the grain. The energy content available from fat is often higher and more easily absorbed. There are several brands, each containing significantly different grains and energy sources. These extruded products have markedly different tastes and many horses prefer one over another, so you should experiment to see which one your horse likes best. You can ask your veterinarian which feed best fits your horse's nutritional needs.

Check the label on extruded feed to see if it contains beet pulp (called sugar beet in the UK). When fed alone, beet pulp must have water added since it expands greatly when exposed to water or saliva in the horse's mouth and can cause choke. According to the feed companies, the amount of beet pulp in extruded feed is so small that choke is not a problem, but my experience is different. If the feed you select contains beet pulp, be sure to take the precaution of wetting it down before feeding to avoid the potential for choke.

If an extruded product does not work for your horse, another feed choice that may increase the available energy in the ration is a pelleted feed. A ration with 12 to 14 percent protein content is usually suggested by equine nutritionists. When pellets are fed to older horses, they can be soaked in water to make eating and digestion easier, particularly if the horse no longer has teeth. Rolled or flaked barley is also a good energy source, particularly during cold weather. Some people suggest adding large amounts of oil to the ration for energy, but I don't advise it because too much oil sometimes causes digestive upset in older horses. Oil should be limited to between one-quarter and one-half cup (50 to 100ml) per feeding for the older horse.

SPECIAL DIETARY CONSIDERATIONS

Researchers are now coming to the conclusion that the genetic make-up of certain breeds dictates specific nutritional requirements. For example, in Europe, warmblood breeds are fed a diet with a calcium/phosphorus ratio different from that fed to horses in the United States. One of the reasons for this is that hay and grains grown in Europe generally have lower calcium content than those grown in the United States. When a warmblood is imported into the United States and given feed that has a different calcium/phosphorus ratio, his body may have difficulty adapting to the sudden change. Some experts believe that imported horses fare best with feeds that duplicate the calcium/phosphorus ratio fed to them in their native lands because the breeds have evolved to thrive on this particular mineral balance. Succeeding generations of horses in the United States might also be affected by this variance in the calcium/phosphorus ratio, but I am not aware of any research that shows how many generations it may take to adapt to the difference.

Some warmbloods—especially those from many of the former communist countries in eastern Europe—are descendants of very hardy stock accustomed to surviving on feed that is low in nutrients, and they may be particularly sensitive to changes in the type or amount of proteins in their diet. When fed either too much protein or protein from an animal source, these warmbloods may suffer a variety of ill effects, ranging from eye problems to immune system malfunctions such as overreactions to insect bites or to vaccinations and injections. New owners who import horses into the United States from Europe are often not familiar with the evolutionary history of these breeds, and they inadvertently feed a diet too high in protein. Proper dietary management can prevent most of the problems caused by excess nutrients.

TEETH

Teeth care starts with you as the owner. You should check at least once a week for any unusual changes in your horse's mouth. If your horse is not cooperative, you can at least feel the edges of his teeth on the outside of his head, checking

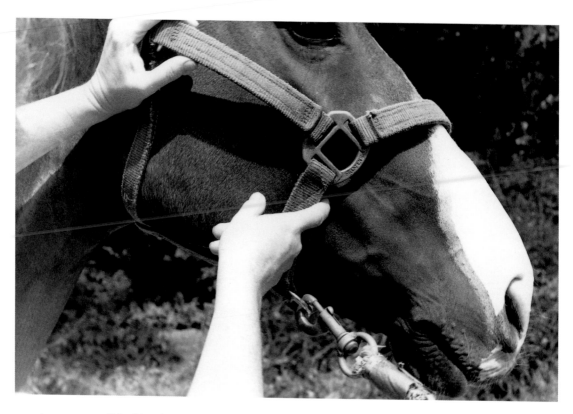

5.1 *An easy way of checking the outside upper edges of the molars for sharpness, is to run your fingers along the cheeks, noting any sensitive areas.*

for any excessive protrusions that differ from the other teeth and might be an indication of sharp edges or hooks forming (see figs. 5.1 to 5.3). Hooks are areas on the edges of the teeth that protrude and can become quite sharp, often causing abrasions to the adjacent soft tissues of the mouth. When this occurs, chewing is uncomfortable. Your horse may not be able to chew his grain thoroughly or it may drop out of his mouth. Either way, he is not getting the full nutritional benefit of the feed. So, not only does regular dental care save your horse from tooth problems, it can also prevent problems associated with poor nutrition.

Another problem that is commonly ignored is wolf teeth. These teeth are located on either side of your horse's mouth. (Not all horses have wolf teeth, so don't be concerned if you do not

see them in your horse's mouth.) It's a good idea to check the fit of the bit in your horse's mouth and see if it interferes with the wolf teeth. Slight discomfort can affect your horse's performance and responsiveness to the bit; ask your veterinarian to evaluate the wolf teeth and determine if they should be removed. The removal of wolf teeth is usually an easy, quick procedure performed by your veterinarian. If you have hesitated to have this done due to concern that it would cause pain to your horse, be assured that it is not a major operation. Many horses do not even require sedation.

Young horses can have problems as their permanent molars emerge. The baby teeth (deciduous teeth) appear as caps or covers over the permanent molars. These caps are gradually pushed up and fall off. Occasionally you may

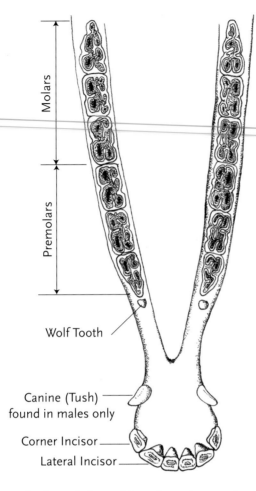

Molars

Premolars

Wolf Tooth

Canine (Tush)
found in males only

Corner Incisor

Lateral Incisor

5.2 *The upper dental arcade of a male horse. Mares do not have canine teeth—also known as tushes—shown here in the interdental space between the incisors and molars.*

even find them in your horse's feed bucket. Sometimes the caps are not shed and cause the horse to have an uneven bite. Your horse may exhibit difficulty in chewing or discomfort with the bit due to uneven pressure. Usually your veterinarian can easily pop these caps off without any pain to the horse.

As horses age, they gradually lose teeth and may require the occasional tooth pulled if it becomes infected. If your older horse has lost a few teeth, it's even more important to have his teeth checked regularly. Sometimes parts of a tooth may have remained in the horse's mouth, particularly if the tooth was broken. These remaining broken pieces can become infected due to a high bacterial content in the mouth. Infections of this nature allow bacteria access to the main blood circulation, which can result in infectious processes elsewhere in the body as well as overburdening the liver and stressing the immune system with constant stimulation.

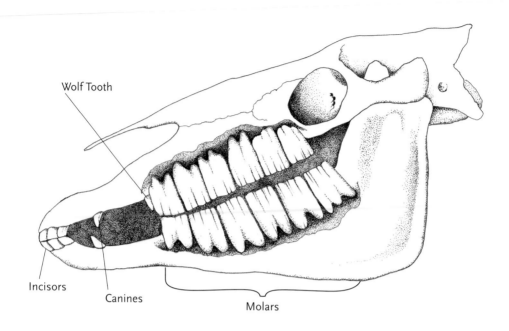

Wolf Tooth

Incisors

Canines

Molars

5.3 *A side view of an adult horse with a full complement of teeth.*

It's also wise to check your horse's gums regularly, particularly if he is kept on pasture or turned out daily. Some grasses produce awns or prickly coverings over their grain that can lodge in between teeth and in the gums. Thorns, sticks, and various other foreign objects can become stuck in the gums as well and result in an irritation or even an infection. Frequent checks can prevent this from becoming a problem.

6 Stable Management, Turnout, and Pasturing

STABLING

Stabling is often overlooked in terms of its significance in horse care. Your horse spends most of his time there and stable conditions can influence his overall state of being. It surprises me how many owners don't seem to realize how much a horse's surroundings affect him.

Some horses prefer a quiet setting and do not like a lot of activity around them. Others, like Charlie, love a constantly busy atmosphere and seem to thrive on new and interesting experiences. When I moved Charlie to a very busy stable with an indoor arena and 65 horses, some friends were concerned about how he would adjust to his new surroundings. After all, Charlie had been used to a small country barn with only ten other horses. He let us know right away by demonstrating a quiet, calm attitude despite all of the commotion in his new home. Not all horses adjust as easily to moving as Charlie did. Each horse has his own adjustment time when major moves are made.

To give you a different example, my Thoroughbred, Silver, had an insecure disposition. Once I realized this, I was able to adjust his environment accordingly. He preferred being in his box stall but was willing to go out to the pasture for brief periods of time with one older, quiet horse. Since he didn't really enjoy his time out, Silver liked having access to both his stall and a pasture, so he could return to his stall whenever he wanted. He did not like other horses—except his pasture buddy—and was happiest when kept in an area where no other horses could touch him.

I was once called to see a horse with a skin problem that had been treated and cleared up twice before but returned after a few weeks both times. After reviewing the entire case and eliminating any medical basis for the problem, I concluded that the horse was not happy in his stall. The excessive stress of living on the main aisle in a busy stable was too much for him. My diagnosis was confirmed when the horse went to a trainer who had a small, quiet stable in the country. After a week there, he came home with almost no signs of the skin problem. He was moved to an outside stall in a quiet corner of his home stable and has not had a problem with skin disorders since.

BEDDING

Bedding is required in all stalls, including those with rubber matting. In addition to the important function of absorbing moisture, bedding provides some cushion for the horse's legs and feet when he is standing in his stall for long periods. It also gives him a softer surface to lie down on and can serve as extra insulation during cold weather.

Straw

Years ago, straw was the bedding material used most often, and it is still the first choice for some horse owners. Since there is a lot of air trapped in its layers, straw seems to keep horses very warm. While straw makes a nice soft bed, it can be dusty, takes more time to clean out, and is heavy. By slightly dampening the straw, you can help to decrease the dust, but this is not advisable in the winter since your horse could get cold from lying on damp straw. Also, some horses like to eat straw and if it is over-consumed, it can cause colic.

Straw bedding can also carry fungal spores, which affect some horses. A horse with chronic respiratory problems such as heaves (*Chronic Obstructive Pulmonary Disease*, see p. 260) or a history of guttural pouch infections should not be bedded on straw. Long term exposure to high amounts of fungal spores accompanied by excessive dust can put a constant strain on a horse's respiratory and immune systems.

Wood Shavings and Sawdust

Wood shavings have replaced the use of straw in most places in the United States. Shavings are lightweight, easy to clean around, and they smell good. They are also easier to dispose of than straw. When the stall is cleaned out, the dirty shavings and manure can be used directly as fertilizer. Shavings are available in a variety of sizes ranging from large, thin, fluffy chips to sawdust. Most people prefer larger shavings because they are less dusty, but they may cost more.

Shavings are made from different types of wood. Some are made especially for use in horse stalls, while others are by-products from wood mills. It's important to know what is being used to make the shavings, since some horses can have sensitivity or allergic reactions to particular types of wood. It may only take a few minutes of exposure for a horse to develop a reaction, so don't use shavings until you have investigated their source, and do not take a chance if you suspect they are made from an undesirable type of wood. While allergic reactions vary, they can include hair loss, skin irritation, swollen legs, and even founder.

MOST COMMON TYPES OF WOOD SHAVINGS AND THEIR CHARACTERISTICS

Pine: Pine is the most desirable type of wood shaving since most horses don't react to pine. However, if the pine is too green, some sap may remain which irritates the horse's skin.

Cedar: Cedar is another wood that is popular. Although cedar smells good, it has high oil content which horses are sometimes sensitive to.

Oak Shavings: Oak is a good choice for shavings but is available only in areas where hard woods are milled.

Cont:

Black Walnut: Black walnut must not be used for bedding because it can be extremely toxic and even a short period of contact can cause disastrous results. Reactions can include hair loss, skin irritation, and even founder.

Cyprus: Another wood that is sometimes used in wood shavings in the southern United States is Cyprus. However, some horses are sensitive to Cyprus and react with skin irritations and swollen legs.

Maple: Maple, particularly red maple, can be toxic to horses and should not be used for shavings.

Black Cherry: Black cherry can also cause reactions and can be toxic if eaten.

A friend of mine learned the hard way how toxic wood shavings can be. He received a new load of shavings and used them right away. The shavings were from a new supplier and were by-products from a local mill. No instructions had been given to the mill concerning unacceptable woods and it turned out that the shavings contained a small amount of black walnut. Once in the stalls, it took less than 30 minutes for some of the horses to react to the shavings and then another hour to figure out what was happening. What do you do with an entire stable of horses that must be taken out of their stalls immediately? The horses were tied outside their stalls while the shavings were removed. Ten horses foundered, while several others developed fevers and difficulty breathing, and most went off their feed for several days. Three horses did not recover from the founder and had to be euthanized.

This nightmare could have been avoided if the mill had been informed about which wood shavings were unacceptable.

Though it is not preferable, sometimes sawdust is the only bedding product available. The problem with sawdust is that it is made up of very fine wood particles. The finer the particles, the dustier the stall. Every time your horse moves, he raises a bit of dust that he then inhales. Any type of dust should be kept to a minimum because, once inhaled, it can irritate the respiratory tract and make your horse more prone to infections.

Not only is the dust unhealthy for the horses, it's also unhealthy for you to breathe. Most sawdust and shavings, regardless of the size, contain some dust. To avoid inhaling this dust while moving shavings, you can wear a mask. This practice was started by people with allergies, but it has become very popular and is now commonplace in many stables. A surgical mask made of paper or the type of mask worn by house painters (available in a paint or hardware store) can filter the large dust particles and protect your lungs.

Another problem with both small shavings and sawdust is that the smaller the particles, the greater the chance that they will get into the horse's eyes and cause irritation. So, if you use sawdust or small shavings, check your horse's eyes frequently.

Shredded Newspaper

Shredded newspaper can be an inexpensive source of bedding material. Keep in mind, however, that some types of paper become very dusty when shredded, and the ink on the paper can cause some horses to have an allergic reaction. Fortunately, the increased use of soy-based ink has helped to decrease the reactions somewhat, but this is offset by the fact that many newspapers print some sections using colored inks that can be another source of allergic reactions. Your supplier of newspaper bedding probably uses recycled newspapers from many sources, so one batch may be fine while the next may include inks that cause problems.

Another problem with newspaper is that it tends to attract flies. I don't know why this happens, but it is a nuisance. Shredded newspaper also becomes clumped during processing and packaging, so it must be fluffed up when you put it in the stalls—unlike straw and shavings that the horses can move about. This means more work for you. On the other hand, newspaper is one of the best bedding for horses recovering from an accident, providing soft support that doesn't cling to wounds and is relatively free of pathogens.

Peat

Peat, which is available at nurseries and garden supply stores, is another type of bedding not often used these days. It provides cushioning support and gives good traction when the horse gets up. Peat is also very absorbent and keeps a horse dry. Consequently, peat works especially well for horses that lie down a great deal of the time, such as very ill horses, as long as they have no external wounds. In such situations, it is ideal to use peat as a base in the stall about six inches thick and then cover the peat with another six inches of shredded newspaper. The newspapers add a little more cushion to the bedding. The only drawback to peat is that it can become packed and heavy when you clean it out of the stall.

MAINTAINING THE BEDDING

People often ask me how deep the bedding should be. Remember that the bedding is your horse's mattress, so treat it as such. Horses are big, heavy animals and require adequate cushioning to be comfortable and prevent injury when lying down on a hard surface. If the bedding is not deep enough, you will notice abrasions or open sores on the front of your horse's fetlocks or on the sides of his hocks.

Rubber mats can help to decrease the amount of bedding needed. However, many people tend to skimp on bedding when rubber mats are in the stalls. Even with rubber mats, adequate bedding is required to provide cushioning and soak up the urine.

Some people like to clean stalls once a day, though I prefer twice a day if possible. You have to do what works into your schedule, but cleaning must be done at least on a daily basis since a build-up of manure and urine soaked bedding can be unhealthy for your horse. Bedding soaked with urine is wet and cold and is especially undesirable in the winter months. Also, if your barn is kept closed up during the winter, the ammonia given off by the urine builds up and can be irritating to the lungs and eyes of your horse. Excessive manure in the stalls also causes bacteria to thrive and get packed up into the hooves, leading to thrush.

If the bedding is on top of a really hard surface such as a concrete floor, it's best to provide as much cushion as possible by using the method known as "deep litter" bedding. This is accomplished by allowing the older, dirtier bedding containing no manure to pack down as a bottom layer anywhere from 12 to 20 inches (15 to 25cm) deep. The top layer of bedding should be removed once a week and all the wet spots should be dug out each time you clean the stall. Then, once a month or so, the lower layer must be removed and the process started all over again. However, remember that this is a guideline only and you will have to determine the frequency that's best for your situation. If your horse urinates excessively, the bottom-packed layer may have to be changed more often. The deep litter method is also not advised for use during the heat of the summer, especially in very humid locales.

WORMS AND WORMING

Intestinal parasites (worms) must be managed on an ongoing basis as part of your horse's routine health care. As shown in the illustration (fig. 6.1), *Lifecycle of Common Horse Worms*, there are many types of parasites. In this section, I will discuss the most common ones, as well as the basics of parasite control. As you will see, there are a number of factors that can influence both the types of wormer you should use and the schedule on which it should be given. It's important that you follow a parasite control program that is tailored to meet your horse's specific needs. Consult your veterinarian to determine the best parasite control program for your horse.

Strongyles

A form of roundworms that enters the horse through the intestine is strongyles, called redworms, or bloodworms. These can be large *(Strongyles vulgaris*, and *S. edentatus*, and *S. equinus)*, or small redworms (*S. triodontophorus* and *S. oesophagodontus*). They are destructive because of their migrations. The large strongyles can migrate to the main arteries supplying the hind legs, inflaming those arteries, or causing blockage called thrombi. On the way, the large strongyles can severely damage the walls of the intestines as they penetrate them as they exit and re-enter the gut. Their life cycle takes six months from eggs, to eggs found again in a fecal sample. *S. equinus*, as it exits the lower intestine (colon or cecum), creates nodules in the walls, then reaches the liver causing hemorrhage, damage, and scarring, returning after nine months to lay eggs in the intestine. *S. edentatus* also harms the liver, but has been found in the lungs, flank, and testicles as well, and has a ten-month cycle.

Small strongyles do not migrate through the body. They just form nodules in the intestinal wall and mature there over two to three months, damaging the wall and ingesting blood, sometimes causing anemia. Their cycle is three to four months.

S. westeri affects mostly foals and may penetrate the skin, be eaten, or ingested in mares' milk. Those that penetrate the skin mature in the lungs, are coughed up, and swallowed. They produce eggs in five to seven days after being swallowed. A heavy infection will produce diarrhea.

Ascarids

Ascarids *(Parascaris equorum)*, also often referred to as roundworms, are among the common intestinal parasites of foals. The various roundworms have similar lifecyles. Their eggs are passed in the manure onto the ground, where horses eat them with the little bits of sand and soil they ingest while grazing. Swallowed, the eggs travel down the digestive tract, while developing into larvae. The larvae can perforate the intestinal wall and migrate through the horse's body, eventually returning to the intestinal tract where, as adults, they lay eggs that are passed and start the cycle over again.

The worms can cause damage in several ways. As they migrate, they can poke holes, harming the liver, heart, and lungs; as adult worms they can damage the intestinal wall and rob nutrition from the body.

Bots

Another type of damaging stomach parasite is the bot that come from eggs laid by bot flies on the horse's legs and face. Once in the stomach, these eggs hatch and the larvae attach to the stomach or small intestine wall, causing damage. The larvae can also hatch before reaching the stomach and penetrate the mucous mem-

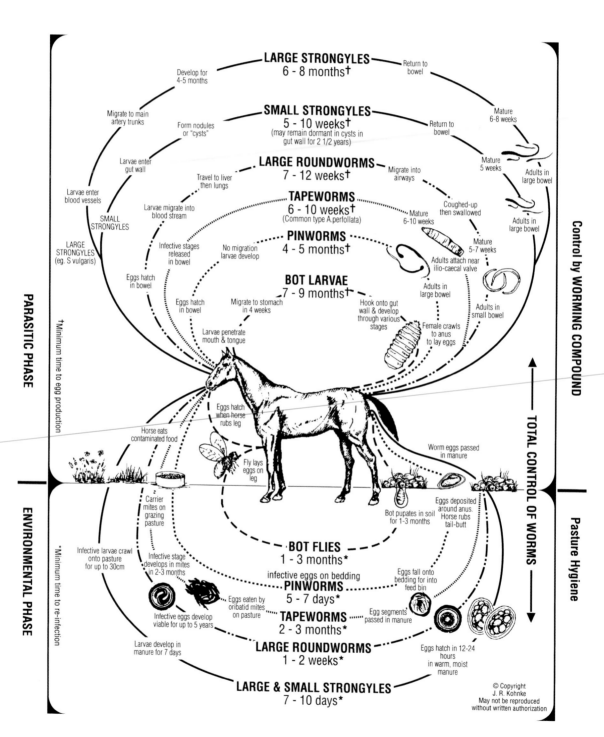

6.1. *The lifecycles of common horse parasites.*

branes of the mouth or get into areas around the molar teeth. It is difficult to get rid of these parasites and only certain wormers are effective against them. Ivermectin is a wormer that is effective against bots as well as other parasites. A wormer called Quest with the active ingredient moxidectin is made by Fort Dodge and available at feed stores. It kills bots as well as the other parasites that affect horses. The bot fly season starts when warm weather begins, usually early summer, and ends when the flies are killed as the temperature goes below freezing. In most areas of the United States worming for bots twice a year is recommended—usually in July and after the first frost in the autumn.

Tapeworms

The tapeworm is another parasite that may infect your horse. Check with your veterinarian to find out if tapeworms are a problem in your area and what product is most effective in treating them. Tapeworms are tough to eliminate and I have found homeopathics ineffective when worming for them.

Pinworms

Pinworms *(Oxyuris equi)* are mainly a problem in foals, although they are found occasionally in adult horses. These worms do not migrate through the digestive tract; instead the eggs hatch following ingestion and the larvae remain in the intestines where they compete for nutrients. After four to five months, the mature female makes her way to the horse's anus where she breaks apart and releases her eggs. The eggs are sticky and adhere to the anus and surrounding area. They irritate and cause the horse to itch, so tail rubbing and tail hair loss are the main signs of pinworm infestation.

The horse's parasite load is dependent on the quantity of eggs in the soil. Sandy soil provides the best conditions for propagation of the eggs.

The quantity of eggs also varies depending on the density of the horse population and the effectiveness of the parasite control program. When many horses are confined to a relatively small space, the number of parasites becomes condensed in that space, increasing the probability that a horse will pick up some parasites. Parasite eggs are tough and can live through most major weather extremes, therefore the passage of time does not improve a pasture once it has become saturated with parasite eggs.

When a pasture or paddock becomes saturated with parasite eggs, the best way to handle the area is to not use it for horses. Unfortunately, this is not always possible. Sometimes we have no other choice but to use a parasite-laden area. For example, in the southern United States, where my practice is located, there are some areas at older horse farms that have a very high parasite load, but there is not enough pasture land available to graze horses elsewhere. The southern climate allows parasites to flourish year round and many areas have nice sandy soil that is ideal for parasites. To help manage the horses in a parasite-laden area such as this, an intensive parasite control program is necessary.

If you are unfamiliar with the level of parasitic infestation in your area, take a fecal sample to your veterinarian and have a count made of the number of parasite eggs present. If you have a few fecal tests done at various times between worming, you will get an idea of the build-up of parasites which help you determine how frequently to worm your horse. In most areas, once every month or two is sufficient.

It's important to rotate the wormers you use. My personal preference is to worm with the same wormer twice then rotate to a different type. Usually rotating among three different families of drugs is effective. Check the label of each wormer to be sure that the main active drug (either the family name for the drug or the generic name) is different on each of the three. Some of the drugs used in effective wormers have a benzimidazole base or are from that family. Other families of effective wormers are pyrantel, febantel, and ivermectin.

Daily wormers are also available, but there are questions about their safety. However, for some horses that have suffered extensive internal parasite damage, I recommend using them. While most horses can tolerate a small number of parasites, there are horses with a history of poor parasite control who react to even a few parasites with recurring colic or diarrhea. For these horses a daily wormer seems the only effective alternative.

Do not rely on old folk remedies to worm your horse. Most do not work well and can cause severe reactions. Many herbal remedies for worming rely on herbs that cause an increase of intestinal contractions that dislodge the worms and force them out the intestinal tract. This is not an effective method for worming and it can cause great distress to the horse. It is particularly dangerous when large infestations are present, since increased contractions can result in intestinal rupture. Tobacco was once a remedy thought to be good for worming horses. However, it is not very effective either since only a few of the parasites are killed.

Newer on the market are combinations of homeopathics marketed as wormers. As with other products used as wormers one way to monitor effectiveness is by fecal counts. Some homeopathics work well and cause the body to expel the parasite. Other homeopathic wormers cause a temporary sterilization of the parasites so no eggs are expelled in the feces; however, the parasites are still present. Because of this even fecal counts can be misleading when you are monitoring these wormers for effectiveness. As a rule I do not recommend using homeopathic or herbal wormers.

INSECT CONTROL

Flies seem to come with horses. They are attracted to the horses themselves as well as to the manure and can be difficult to control. Every summer brings a renewed challenge to control flies in the stable area, pasture, and while riding. My horse Silver was very thin-skinned and sensitive, so flies were a constant annoyance to him. I particularly dreaded the large biting flies, such as deer flies, since Silver would go into a bucking frenzy to avoid being bitten. This was not a fun experience!

So what's the answer? Of course, keeping the horse's environment as clean as possible helps, but that's only part of the answer. Most horse owners turn to chemical insect repellents, feeling there is no other viable alternative. However, in addition to the health concerns associated with chemical insect repellents, they are not totally effective. Sunlight causes chemical change that leads to loss of efficacy, and repellent often gets covered by dust from the ring or the trail. Buying stronger repellents doesn't work because a horse's skin can only tolerate a certain strength of chemicals. If the chemicals are too strong, the skin will be irritated or, worse, burned. Chemical insect repellents can also cause serious allergic reactions for both owners and horses.

Since repellents are effective for only a short period of time, may be environmentally harmful, and could be unhealthy for both you and your horse, why use them? The best alternative is to make your horse less appealing to flies with a natural fly spray. There are several homemade fly sprays that work well and many new non-toxic commercially prepared fly sprays are now available on the market. They may not be quite as effective as chemical repellents, but they often do the trick without any harmful side effects. Here's one that you can tailor to your own needs, since some people prefer certain ingredients over others.

HOMEMADE FLY SPRAY

In a standard one-quart or one-liter spray bottle, mix the following ingredients:

2 cups or 400ml Avon Skin-So-Soft or 1/4 to 1/2 teaspoon oil of myrrh

2 cups or 400ml water

1/2 cup or 150ml cider vinegar

1/4 teaspoon oil of citronella

Shake before every use.

If you don't like an oily base, use the oil of myrrh instead of the Skin-So-Soft. Some people are sensitive to citronella, which smells like citrus. Citronella is not an essential ingredient, so either you can eliminate it completely or the amount can be reduced if it seems too strong to you. Most horses tolerate the ingredients in this mix very well, and some riders use it on themselves before riding to ward off biting insects as well as flies. Mosquitoes can be ferocious to riders as well as horses, so it is useful to have a safe repellent that both you and your horse can use.

Another safe and natural alternative is a dietary one. Some horses attract fewer flies when they are fed cider vinegar because the vinegar makes their skin less desirable to insects. Feeding cider vinegar not only changes the pH of the top layer of the skin, it also changes the pH throughout the skin layers. While effective, this method is slow—it can take months to work its way through all the skin layers and change the pH balance. If you want to try feeding cider vinegar, start four to six months in advance of fly season or your horse's worst itching season.

Not all horses like cider vinegar in their feed at first, but if started in very small amounts they often learn to tolerate it. It takes a little experimentation to determine the amount that will work for your horse. On average, a 1,000-pound (about 450 kgs) horse will require about one cup of vinegar daily to help repel flies. I do not recommend trying cider vinegar if your horse has sensitive digestion or has had other health problems. If you have any doubts about feeding it to your horse, check with your veterinarian first.

Controlling Flies in the Stable

Now let's explore the insect control options available for stable areas. The most well-known—but not the best choice—is an automatic spray system, which is usually set on a timer and sprays out insecticide at set intervals. One major drawback to these systems is that the spray is inhaled by any horses or people in the immediate vicinity. Depending on the content of the spray, it can be irritating to the nasal passages and lungs and can be easily absorbed into the body through mucus membranes like those in the nose. Some people just notice a mild irritation of the nose or eyes. (People who wear contact lenses are particularly susceptible to irritation.) Others have more serious allergic reactions such as headaches, nausea, sneezing, or breathing problems.

If people who are only occasionally in the barn can have these reactions, it's clear that a horse that lives under or near an insecticide spray system most of the time may suffer health problems too. Unfortunately, the signs of toxicity from these insecticides may not be easily detected. Internal changes can occur, and negative effects on the body systems may take years to show up. You need only read the cautions on a container of insecticide to see the potential danger to both humans and animals. What we do know is that insecticides can be harmful to the body, so it's best to keep exposure to a minimum.

Despite their potential harm to horses and humans, automatic spray systems are only marginally effective in controlling insects. Since they are set on the ceiling, the spray mostly affects flying insects in the area closest to the spray jets. Fly breeding areas in manure and dirty cracks and crevices are left pretty much untouched because much of the spray is vaporized and dissipated before it reaches the ground. The concentration of insecticide that does reach the ground is so small that it is not very effective in killing insects at that level.

I recommend that you use other fly control methods for the stable that are less toxic. They include fly traps, strips, and baits. *Fly traps* are containers that are filled with a substance which attracts flies. Once inside, the flies are either trapped or killed by the substance. These traps are hung around the barn but should be kept well out of a horse's reach. *Fly strips* are sticky strips that flies cannot escape once they land on them. These strips are hung from the ceiling and should also be out of the horse's reach since they could cause illness if the horse eats them. Both fly traps and fly strips are non-toxic and can be helpful in your fly control program. *Fly baits* come in powder, pellet, or granular form and are sprinkled on the floor of the barn or any other area that attracts flies. Although most baits are labeled as non-toxic to pets and children, they should be used with extreme caution and only when absolutely necessary. Some fly baits have a taste that can be attractive to animals as well as flies, and they can be lethal when consumed in even small amounts. I suggest using fly bait only in certain circumstances, such as sprinkling it on the collected manure if it is not possible to remove it from the barn area immediately.

One natural way to repel flies from an area is to hang a plastic bag with holes in it filled with chopped onions. Replace the onions every two to three days. This method can be extremely effective in eliminating flying insects. One bag covers an area about 12 by 12 feet.

Another very safe way to control flies is through the use of fly traps that you place outside around your whole stable/barn area. These are small metal containers that you fill and refill with a foul-smelling liquid (foul to humans, anyway) which attracts flies. They enter the trap and cannot get out. This system backed up with a monthly spreading (by hand) of beneficial nematodes that eat fly larvae on all manure piles, is most effective (see Appendix VI).

Yet another method that I am less sure about is sold in feed stores and through catalogs. It is known as the "feed-through system," in which a product containing a certain chemical is fed to horses and excreted in their manure. The manure of a horse treated with this chemical does not allow flies to reproduce. This product is only effective if it is being fed to all the horses and other livestock in the area and if the flies are also controlled in the stable area by other means. It is designed to not break down or alter its form in the horse's digestive tract, but I have not been around enough horses using it to determine its safety and efficacy. I would not feed this product to my own horses until its safety has been proven.

While these methods will all help in fly control, there are stable management procedures that should be implemented as well in order to cut down on the fly problem. Here are some suggestions:

1. Clean stalls and paddocks as often as possible. Manure attracts flies and gives them a place to breed.

2. Keep the stable area swept clean, free of debris, trash, and manure.

3. Do not keep manure near the stable area. If you are loading manure onto a wagon or manure spreader, move it away from the stable as soon as it is loaded. If that is not possible, sprinkle it with fly bait but be very careful to only sprinkle manure when it is out of reach of dogs because the fly bait may be toxic to them.

4. Keep trash cans covered.

5. Keep grain bins covered.

6. Keep water buckets and water devices clean so they are free of algae, grain, and hay.

7. Clean around grain buckets or feed areas at least twice a week.

8. Use fans aimed into stalls and the stable aisle to keep the air moving. The airflow from the fans makes it difficult for flies to fly around and discourages them from entering the area. Be sure that the fans are placed where horses cannot reach them, and do not leave them running overnight.

Controlling Flies in the Pasture

Controlling flies in the pasture is difficult but very important for your horse's well-being. Repellents that are sprayed or wiped on do not stay effective for long due to breakdown by the sun, heat evaporation, or horses rolling in the dirt and coating themselves with dust or mud. Fly masks and bonnets which have been around for some time protect the horse's eyes and/or ears and you can now purchase fly boots, and fly strips to protect the horse's legs, too. These prevent excessive stomping which causes leg injuries. For very sensitive horses you can also buy a fly sheet that protects the whole body, like a blanket does. (If you use a mask, make sure it's loose enough to slip off if it gets caught on something in the pasture.)

One method that is successful to a degree in repelling flies from around the eyes and ears is to apply one of the special fly repellents in ointment form made for horses. The advantage to ointments is that they are thick and sticky so they stay on longer. They also soften wounds or irritated areas. Be careful not to get the ointment in the eye or the ear canal, but apply it liberally over the entire top part of the ear and to areas on the sides and under the eye. (Do not put it over the eye, since it could run into the eye.)

Another method that has been used to keep flies away from a horse's head in the pasture is to use cattle ear tags that contain insecticide and attach them to a ring at the bottom of a halter that is left on the horse in the pasture. It is important to use a leather halter or a halter designed to break away if it gets caught on anything in the pasture. (In general, horses should not be turned out in nylon halters). These tags have been found to be very effective if they are replaced regularly. Make sure that your horse is not sensitive to the insecticide in the tags before turning him out into the pasture by putting the tags on the halter while he's in the stall or a paddock so you can monitor his reaction.

If you have ever seen the damage that flies can do to the ends of ears or the infections caused and spread by flies in a pasture situation, it's easy to understand the need to repel them with whatever means possible.

STABLE AND PASTURE HYGIENE

It is important to keep feed and water clean and free from insects and dirt. Feed your horse in a washable container that can be removed easily from the stall and cleaned. The water bucket should also be removed and scrubbed on a regular basis or, if it's an automatic water dispenser, it should be disassembled and cleaned. Routine cleaning will eliminate one more possible source of disease.

Feed and water buckets should be cleaned every two to three days, so a quick rinse with water and scrubbing with a stiff brush will take care of any accumulated debris. If a more thorough cleaning is required, use hot water and a mild cleansing agent, but be sure it is one that will not be toxic to your horse. Avoid cleaning agents that contain bleach, detergents, or pine-based oils, but if you must use them, be sure to rinse thoroughly. You should also be aware of chemicals in cleaning products that could also be toxic.

If your water buckets seem to grow algae quickly, it's a good idea to set them in the sun for an hour or so when not in use to help kill the algae that might be growing in tiny, hard-to-reach places. Most algae will not tolerate direct sunlight well. Remember, too, that your horse will probably drop saliva and feed into the buckets as he eats and drinks which could encourage growth of bacteria—another reason to clean buckets often.

If the water is kept in a large tank in the pasture, investigate the ways to help control bacteria and algae specific to your area. The methods of doing this vary according to climate so a local county agent or extension office will be helpful in giving you ideas. Keeping goldfish in the tank is an easy way to control algae, but you need to monitor the fish occasionally for illness and to determine if they need more food than the algae is supplying. One of the ways you can tell if a goldfish is ill by a sign of fungus that looks like white cotton on the fish's scales. If there is not much algae you will need to add fish food.

When watering your horses in a pasture using large water tanks, keep a check on the level to be sure the horses are drinking. Sometimes a problem can arise that deters horses from drinking but no one notices until they show signs of dehydration or colic. The horses might avoid the water because it tastes bad due to the growth of an unpleasant algae or bacteria. Or the horses could be upset by the invasion of a snapping turtle or water snake. This type of problem most commonly occurs when using watering tanks with flotation devices that automatically refill the tank with water. Since the water source doesn't have to be filled by anyone, the fact that horses are not drinking can go undetected for a period of time. So check regularly to make sure that horses are drinking from such a water tank.

In cold climates water will freeze hard in the tank. Heaters are available for the larger tanks, and work well. Where you have no supply of electricity you can use insulated buckets, or install small water tanks insulated with foam. These should allow you to break the ice to make a hole. Be sure to do this at least twice daily—depending on the temperature. If you see your horse eating snow this is a sure sign that he is not getting enough water. A horse can never get hydrated enough this way—snow is no substitute for fresh water.

TURNOUT

When horses are kept in stalls, they should be turned out daily if at all possible. Even a short free period in a larger open space will help your horse feel better. Turnout helps increase the circulation, particularly in the legs, and allows the horse to get rid of some of his excess energy. It also gives a horse the chance to roll. Rolling is a natural, healthy act that most horses enjoy.

If your horse has not been turned out on grass recently and you plan to start turning him out on a grass pasture, do so gradually, since the grass can upset his digestion. Start with a short period of time—about twenty minutes if the grass is green or thirty minutes if it's dry winter grass. Then gradually increase the time over a two-week period.

Do not leave a blanket on your horse when turned out unless someone is there to monitor him periodically to make sure the blanket doesn't become tangled in his legs or on a fence.

KEEPING YOUR HORSE OUTSIDE

Many horses live in a pasture year-round and do very well. Even in extremely cold environments, a horse can adapt and live comfortably outside as long as the feed is adequate. This means that the grass must be maintained and you will have to feed hay in the winter if you live in an extremely cold climate. If you are the person responsible for maintaining the pasture, you can get tips on proper pasture care from your local county or extension agent or an agricultural specialist.

It is also important that you determine how many horses your pasture can accommodate based on factors such as its size, location, and the type and amount of grass it contains. If the pasture is overpopulated, the horses may eat all of the grass so quickly that it does not have time to regenerate, eventually resulting in a "pasture" that is bare of grass. Your local agricultural experts also can help you figure out the right number of horses for your pasture space.

If the pasture grass is high in nutrients, your horse may not require much, if any, extra grain. I suggest having the grass tested in a laboratory so you know what nutrients are being provided and whether any missing nutrients must be supplemented. If you are not supplementing his diet with grain and your horse is being exercised a lot, his weight will help you determine if extra grain is required. If a weight loss is noticeable, start giving grain to your horse regularly.

Horses should have access to some type of permanent shelter if they are kept outside all the time. The best option is a three-sided shed that can protect a horse from wind, rain, and sun. If possible, build the shelter on high ground in order to provide good drainage, and not too close to large trees that could topple in a storm.

When horses are kept continuously outside, they may develop a condition commonly called rain rot. There are a variety of lay terms for this condition which results when moisture is trapped under the hair and fungus or bacteria grow on the skin, causing patches of hair to fall out. (See *Fungal Infections* under *Skin Problems* in the *Horse Ailments* section, Part Three.) Horses kept in a pasture should be monitored for this condition regularly so it can be treated promptly if it develops. The hooves also require monitoring for both excessive dryness and excessive moisture. Too much moisture can result in a hoof infection called thrush, or in extremely soft hooves. (See *Hoof Problems* in *Horse Ailments*, Part Three.)

Your horse may have more chances to hurt himself when he's in a pasture all the time, so be sure to check his entire body frequently for any small cuts or other injuries that require treatment.

7 Grooming

Regular grooming is just as important for your horse's well-being as regular exercise. If you do not groom your horse properly, his coat, hooves, mane, or tail will eventually show the results of your neglect. At minimum, your horse will be uncomfortable, which, of course, will affect his performance. Over time, prolonged neglect of good grooming can lead to more serious health problems such as skin or hoof infections.

Since not all grooming tasks need to be performed on a daily basis, it's best to keep a schedule on a calendar or in your appointment book to aid you in remembering when certain routines need to be done. I find that keeping a written schedule is particularly helpful with the grooming tasks I don't like to do such as sheath cleaning (something I'll cover later in this chapter), since it can be easy to forget about them for months. Some barn or stable managers keep calendars posted so that you can write down when your horse is due for certain grooming procedures.

BATHING

We all like to see our horses clean and beautiful, but since horses enjoy pursuits such as rolling in the mud and dirt, we are often disappointed! You may have noticed, however, that even when your horse has rolled in dirt or has not been brushed consistently, his coat still maintains a glossy shine. Horses in good health usually have shiny coats—even gray horses, although theirs are less obvious. A horse's coat is kept shiny by the natural oils from the skin that coat the hair.

Some horses' coats do not seem as shiny after a bath with shampoo. This is because the natural oil in the hair has been washed off, and it will require some brushing to recoat the hair. The degree to which the oil is removed depends on the type of shampoo. Some shampoos are more efficient than others at stripping oil from hair and should be avoided. Your goal is to keep as much oil as possible in the hair while cleaning off any dirty areas or stains.

Use a shampoo that is non-detergent, if at all possible. Detergent ingredients are great for er this by accident when they add a new supplement to the diet for other reasons and notice improvements in the condition of the mane and tail. For example, hoof supplements, which often contain biotin and methionine in addition to other nutrients, frequently bring about improvements in the mane and tail as well. Most of the time it's difficult to determine which ingredient is working since all of the ingredients are combined in the supplements and cannot be separated out. An alternative to the trial-and-error method of supplementation is to have your veterinarian perform a blood analysis, including the electrolytes, to see if any deficiencies are present.

Testing the hair itself—hair analysis—is sometimes used to diagnose skin problems. Hair analysis shows concentrations of specific nutrients, such as proteins or metals. However, the reliability of this hair analysis is questionable. I have seen hair analysis results that show differing concentrations of nutrients in the mane and in the tail of the same horse. These differences indicate to me that hair analysis may not accurately reflect systemic nutritional deficiencies and is not therefore a reliable diagnostic tool.

HOOF CARE

Let's review the basic daily hoof care for any horse. First, clean the feet thoroughly with a hoof pick and check for any foreign objects such as small rocks or sticks that might be stuck in the hoof. This cleaning also serves to allow air into the underside of the hoof, an important step in helping to prevent thrush, which is an infection around the frog. (If you suspect thrush, it's important to begin treating it as soon as possible. See *Thrush* under *Hoof Problems* in the *Horse Ailments* section, Part Three.)

The hoof should also be checked thoroughly for signs of excessive moisture or dryness, sensitivity to the hoof pick, bad odor, cracks, or injuries. Make a special point to check the coronary band, which is the top area of the hoof nearest the skin. This very sensitive area must be healthy to ensure good hoof growth.

Check the shoes for individual loose nails, an overall loose shoe, or a "sprung" shoe. To check for a loose shoe, you can pull the shoe from side to side while you have the leg lifted up or listen to the horse walk on a road or cement surface. A loose shoe will make a clanging sound when that hoof strikes the ground instead of the clear sharp sound that the other shoes will make. A sprung shoe is one that has been bent. You must check for a sprung shoe by looking at the back of the foot while you have the foot lifted. Also look at the heel of the hoof and make sure the shoe is level. A sprung shoe will have one side slightly bent away from the foot and may cause your horse to be slightly unbalanced when he walks. Sprung shoes are not always loose when they first occur, so you may not hear them when the horse is walked on a paved surface.

In addition to the basic routines detailed above, some horses may have special hoof care needs. Let's take a look at some of them.

Hoof Conditioners

If your horse has dry or cracked feet, you may need to add a conditioning treatment to your regular hoof-care regimen. Several types of hoof conditioners are generally available: lanolin-based creams, gel-like products, and oils. Opinions vary as to which conditioners do the best job, but I prefer the lanolin-based creams. Both gel and oil hoof products are petroleum-based and can clog the skin around the coronary band, so if you use one of them, avoid getting the product on this area.

In most cases, daily application of hoof conditioners is not necessary. It is usually sufficient to apply the conditioner about once every three days, being sure to coat the top and bottom of the hoof. If hooves have been blackened or dyed for a horse show, use the product recommended by the dye manufacturer to take off as much dye as possible after the show. (Even clear dye should be removed because all dyes dry out the hoof.) Once the dye is removed, wash the hoof, let it dry, and then apply some conditioner. You may find that you need to apply more conditioner the next day if the hoof is still dry.

Some horses develop dry or cracked feet because they live in a dry environment, and others are just naturally more prone to having dry feet. In either case, a hoof conditioner may help to alleviate the problem. Occasionally, however, dry hooves can be caused by other factors, such as a fungal infection, a dietary deficiency, or a systemic illness. If your horse has a dry hoof problem that is severe or persistent or one that does not respond to treatment with conditioners, you should consult your farrier or veterinarian to make sure the dryness is not a symptom of a more serious condition.

Hoof Tougheners

Dry, hard, rocky ground, such as is found in the southwest United States, can be punishing to tender feet, particularly those that have been recently re-shod or trimmed. In addition, some horses just seem to be more sensitive on the soles of their feet than others, regardless of the terrain. Toughening up the bottoms of the hooves can make horses with sensitive feet more comfortable and decrease their incidence of stone bruises.

The commercial product I have found most effective for toughening hooves is one called Tuff Stuff commonly available in horse supply stores and catalogs. Iodine tincture is an old remedy sometimes used for this purpose, but I don't recommend it because it dries the hooves out more than it toughens them. Venice turpentine and Reducine are also commonly used to toughen hooves. Although most horses do not experience any ill effects when these products are used on their feet, you should consult with your veterinarian before trying them.

Remember to apply any hoof-toughening product to the bottom of the hooves only. If you are using Reducine (a blistering product that can be used on hooves), be especially careful not to get it on the horse's skin because it is a blister and may irritate the skin. Watch for excessive drying, and do not over-treat with any hoof toughener. An application every two or three days should be sufficient to achieve the desired results.

THE SHEATH AND ITS CLEANING

The sheath is the soft structure between the horse's hind legs from which he extends and contracts his penis. There is a space up inside the sheath that can collect dirt, sand, and other debris. If too much dirt and debris become trapped inside the sheath, the horse may show signs of discomfort such as becoming uncooperative when being ridden.

The covered area surrounding the end of the penis must be cleaned also because debris can accumulate there as well. The debris in this area sometimes becomes hard and compact forming into an oblong mass. Because of its shape and texture, this mass of debris is often referred to as a "bean."

It always amazes me how many people own geldings and don't know about this important grooming procedure. Cleaning of the penile sheath must be done at least every six months—and sometimes more often. Since the sheath is located between the hind legs, you have to be careful. Some horses object to this procedure and may try to kick. It's a good idea to observe someone else performing the cleaning before you try it yourself the first time.

If your horse doesn't like you handling his sheath area, I suggest you begin your approach by stroking and scratching his belly. Reward tolerant behavior with praise or treats and gradually work your way nearer to the sheath area. This procedure may take weeks to accomplish, but often helps get you closer to your goal of cleaning the sheath. Even with this gentle, positive association method, your horse may still decline to drop his penis, or have you clean inside his sheath. If you are uncomfortable with your horse's reaction, consult your veterinarian for guidance and discuss sedating him. A tranquilizer usually causes a horse to drop his penis and the cleaning procedure can be accomplished much more quickly and safely. If necessary, most veterinarians will perform this service for you if your horse is difficult to handle.

A mild shampoo or special cleanser can be used to clean the sheath and the end of the penis. Dilute any shampoo with water before starting. It's important not to use a harsh soap, shampoo, or detergent that could irritate the sheath. There are products available in tack shops, equine-supply stores, and catalogs that are specifically made for this purpose. These sheath-cleaning formulas break up and clean out the debris more easily than regular soap and water, making them the best choice for this task. The material that comes out of the sheath is frequently smelly and unpleasant, so it's a good idea to wear rubber gloves. After cleaning the area, it's most important to thoroughly rinse it to prevent irritation from the soap or cleanser.

CLIPPING

There are generally two reasons to clip a horse—either as a basic grooming routine for general neatness or when the coat becomes too thick or heavy. Since space doesn't allow me to give a complete guide, I'll concentrate mainly on the pros and cons and a few things to think about when clipping your horse.

When deciding what to clip, you should consider your horse's needs first. If you're not going to a show, you may just need some basic clean-up clipping. This usually includes the bridle path, whiskers around the muzzle, hair under the jaw, the fetlocks, and possibly the long hairs that are located on top of the hooves. Years ago bridle paths were not clipped because it was believed that the mane under the bridle allowed for some ventilation and greater comfort for the horse around his ears. Although there are still some horsemen who feel this way, clipping of the bridle path is routine nowadays. The length of the bridle path can vary depending on the standards established by specific breed associations or the traditions of the discipline in which you compete. There is an excellent book, *Grooming to Win* by Susan Harris, that I suggest you consult for specific details.

There are several other parts of the head that some people clip, such as the ears. As a general rule, I do not recommend trimming all of the hair out of the ears because it protects the ears from both dirt and insects. Horses with especially hairy ears can be made to look neater by trimming the edges of the ears and trimming back any hair that sticks out of the ear. This leaves the internal hair to protect the ear. In the past, horses that competed in certain disciplines, such as hunters and jumpers, routinely had the internal hair clipped from their ears. I have been pleased to note recently that many competitors have begun to refrain from clipping their horses' internal ear hair.

Eyebrows and eyelashes act as antennae, alerting the horse to objects that are too close to the eye. If they are not there, there is a greater chance of your horse hitting his eye on an object and injuring it. Therefore, I suggest that you don't trim either the eyebrows or the eyelashes.

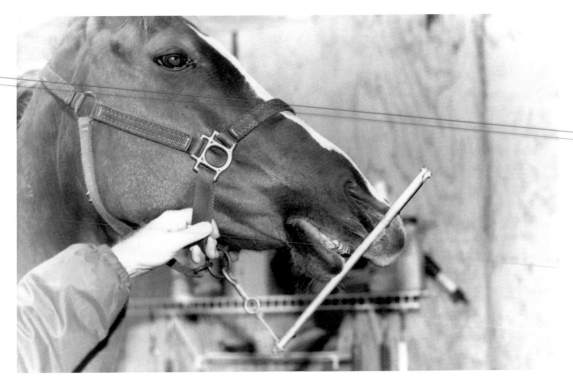

7.1 *There are various types of twitches used to restrain horses, but this humane twitch is the least severe, and will serve the purpose under most circumstances.*

If it is absolutely necessary to do so for show standards, trim them to no less than half their normal length.

If your horse grows a long or very dense coat during the winter, it may be difficult or even impossible for him to thoroughly cool and dry out after exercise. It is very important that he be completely dry when you return him to his stall, or else he may become chilled, which can have serious consequences.

One solution to this problem is to body clip your horse. Body clipping, which requires large, powerful clippers with very sharp blades, can be done in a variety of styles depending on the needs of the individual horse. If you are not sure how much of your horse's coat should be clipped, ask your trainer or veterinarian for advice. Body clipping is not a job for amateurs. If you have not body clipped a horse before, hire

an experienced person to do it for you so you can see how it's done.

Remember that if you body clip your horse, you are removing his natural protection against cold weather conditions, so he must be blanketed appropriately throughout the winter.

Controlling the horse is often a challenge, particularly when trimming ears. If you're like me, you are usually alone when performing these tasks, and don't have that much-needed extra hand to assist you in holding your horse still which is very helpful for this chore.

If needed, there are a couple of methods of control that might work for you but the first thing I suggest is to spend time getting your horse used to the clippers. I first introduce them after every exercise session, turn them on, and hold them near the horse. When the noise no longer upsets him, I touch him with the clippers, rubbing them over his body so he can feel the vibration and hear the change in noise as they move. Once your horse has accepted the clippers, try clipping a small area. Remember that the clippers will make a different noise when hair is actually cut and the horse might be startled.

I usually give the horse all the time he needs to become accustomed to the clippers. This might be one or two days or two weeks. It took my horse Charlie a week to accept the clippers and another week to not jump around when his hair was cut. Now it's "old hat" to him. However, if it's been a while since he's been clipped, I repeat the introduction procedure to make sure he remembers what's expected of him. If you're in a hurry and rush into clipping when you haven't done it in a while your horse may react badly and a lot of training may be ruined. A quiet, easy clipping session is your goal so remember to take your time.

Despite your best efforts, your horse may be one that just won't accept the clippers. He will require restraint and may respond well to a twitch. There are several types of twitches that help owners and veterinarians perform many tasks over a horse's objections. A humane twitch is one that is all metal; it is slipped over the horse's nose and has a cord attached which is tightened around metal handles and snapped on to the halter (fig. 7.1). This type of twitch

enables you to twitch your horse and perform the procedures on your own without help.

There are other types of twitches that have a rope or chain that loops over the horse's nose and is twisted until it is tight. These twitches are more severe and therefore less humane, and I prefer to avoid them unless no other method is effective on an individual horse. Another drawback to these twitches is that most of them require someone to hold the twitch in place as long as it is on the horse. Consequently, you cannot use one for clipping unless you have a helper available to hold the twitch.

A twitch is all that is needed to restrain most horses for clipping. But there are some who require a tranquilizer. The use of a pharmaceutical tranquilizer should be a last resort and certainly not used as a substitution for taking the time to train an inexperienced, frightened horse. One tranquilizer that is effective when clipping is detomidine (sold under the trade name Dormosodan). It is called the "remembering" drug by some horsemen, due to the fact that, once used, horses seem to remember that they submitted to the clipping procedure and don't require the tranquilizer again. If your horse requires sedation, check with your veterinarian for guidance. And remember, a tranquilizer must be administered before starting any procedure since once the horse becomes excited or upset many tranquilizers are not effective at all.

8 Tack and Equipment

PROPER FITTING TACK

Many horses are presented to me with health problems that stem from improperly fitted tack. Let's look at some areas of concern.

The Bridle

Fortunately, horse owners are becoming more aware of the importance of using a bridle that fits properly around the bone structure of the horse's head and thus provides maximum comfort for the horse. Bridles are available in a vast number of styles, which vary according to the requirements of different riding disciplines. For instance, the style of bridles used for Western pleasure riding is quite different from those used for upper-level dressage. The basic components of the bridle are the same; however, regardless of the style, and the same criteria for proper fit apply to all types of bridles.

The parts of the bridle to check for proper fit are the browband, the headpiece or crownpiece, the noseband (if there is one), and the cheekpieces, or side pieces (figs. 8.1–8.6). Here is what you should look for:

The browband must be long enough to fit comfortably around the horse's ears and to allow the cheekpieces to lie flat against the sides of the head, positioned under the cheekbones. If the browband is too short or is adjusted too high, it can pinch the bottom of the horse's ears.

The headpiece, or crownpiece, that goes over the horse's poll, just behind the ears, should lay flat against his head. If you are using a noseband, it should be secured to the headpiece by running it through the ends of the browband in order to prevent it from moving excessively in the poll area. Horses usually sweat a lot behind the ears, so an ill-fitting headpiece can cause chafing and raw spots.

The noseband—also called a cavesson—should be adjusted so that it is snug enough to be effective but still allows the horse adequate room to breathe. Remember that he must be able to breathe properly not only when standing still while being fitted, but also during strenuous exercise. I find that the "flash" and "drop" types of nosebands commonly used in dressage are often adjusted too tightly.

As mentioned above, the cheekpieces of the bridle should lay flat against the sides of the horse's head. Check to be sure that the attachment to the bit is comfortable and is also laying flat so that no area of the horse's face is being rubbed.

If you are not sure whether a particular bridle fits your horse properly, have a trainer or other experienced horseperson check it for you. Before using a new bridle, you should also clean it thoroughly. New bridles are sometimes coated with wax or oil to protect the leather, and some horses have bad reactions to these preservative substances.

The Bit

The question of which bit to use is one that every horseperson faces. Usually we base the decision on a combination of factors including what will control the horse best, what is allowed in the discipline in which we ride, and what we have on hand. There seem to be constant changes as to which bits are fashionable to use. At one point, the fashion in Western riding was high curb bits with copper mouthpieces and rollers that allowed the horse to play with the bit. (When all of the horses at a show played with their bits in the ring, the resulting cacophony sounded like a symphony orchestra tuning their instruments!)

Many different types of metals and various combinations of metals have been used to make both English and Western bits. Most bits are made of steel, silver, copper, alloy, rubber, nylon, or plastic. (Silver bits have some silver in them but are actually made of a combination of metals.) All metal bits wear better than bits made of rubber, nylon, and plastic, which can be chewed by the horse no matter how hard the material, but these types are often used short-term—with young or green horses—as a more sensitive training bit. (NOTE: These should be monitored

for chew marks that can cause sharp edges). Silver, copper, and some alloy bits can cause a reaction in the horse's mouth that makes him salivate and increases play with the bit, while steel bits do not have this effect.

Before choosing a bit, it is important to evaluate the inside of your horse's mouth. The shape of the palate (the hard area on the inside top of the mouth) can vary from horse to horse. The palate is usually flat or has a slight arch, but occasionally a horse's palate will have a high arch. The shape of the palate may influence your choice of bit for your horse. Palates that are flat and closer to the tongue will be less tolerant of bits that put pressure against this area such as a bit with a curb or port. Sometimes even the joint of a simple snaffle can push against a flat palate and cause discomfort. A double-jointed snaffle may work better with a flat or low palate because its flat, thin, middle piece will fit comfortably against the palate. A horse with a noticeable arch in his palate is usually comfortable in a wider variety of bits. You may find, however, that bits with curbs or ports are not as effective on such horses because the high arch diminishes the amount of pressure felt on the palate.

The bar—the lower inside of the mouth where the bit makes contact—should be checked for any abnormalities. If you are unsure about what a normal mouth looks like, compare several horses or ask your veterinarian to explain. The bars should be a healthy pink color and smooth. You may find that your horse has scars or anatomical abnormalities here. If so, you should select a bit that does not interfere or is more comfortable in this area.

A nice Thoroughbred mare named Jenny is one of my regular patients. Her owner was having problems controlling Jenny when she galloped over a cross-country course. I evaluated the mare's performance and explained that

Jenny, a former racehorse, was equating the cross-country course with the races. The start box on the course reminded her of the starting gate on the track, and she loved all the excitement associated with racing.

The bits that had been tried—everything from a strong curb to a gag—had been completely ineffective, and Jenny's owner was at her wit's end. When I examined the bits, I noticed that all of them allowed Jenny to do the one thing that she had been trained to do when racing—lean into the bit. An examination of her mouth revealed a rather high arch to her palate and normal bars. It was no wonder the curb bit had not phased her. In fact, it had only provided an even better straight piece for her to bite down on.

I suggested trying a double-twisted snaffle, a harsh bit by any standard, and having Jenny schooled by a professional trainer with a very light hand. This bit would not give Jenny the even pressure to pull against, and used properly it might get her attention. The trainer rode her in this bit, and eventually the owner was able to switch back to a lighter bit once Jenny realized that the cross-country course was not a racetrack. Sometimes knowledge of a bit of anatomy and insight into a horse's background can assist us in finding answers to our training problems.

The Saddle

Up until recently, saddles were designed and purchased primarily with the rider's comfort in mind. Only slight attention was given to which saddle was best for the horse. Each horse is shaped differently, and a saddle that fits one horse perfectly may be completely inappropriate for another. An incorrectly fitted saddle can be very uncomfortable for the horse and can cause physical problems such as chronic back pain. Extreme discomfort may also lead to behavioral problems because the horse is unable to perform without experiencing pain.

It is important to find a saddle that is comfortable for you as a rider as well, so that you are able to ride safely and to the best of your ability without interfering with your horse's balance. You should start, however, by selecting saddles that fit your horse well. After you have found several saddles that are right for your horse, the next step is to decide which one suits you best. There is a wide array of saddles available for just about every discipline now, so you should be able to find one that is a good match for both you and your horse. The process of choosing the right saddle may require significant time and effort on your part, but in the long run, it will be worth the effort. Let's discuss some things to consider when evaluating whether a saddle fits your horse properly.

EVALUATING SADDLE FIT

The tree is the basic frame on which the saddle is constructed. The width of the tree varies somewhat among different types and models of saddles. Some saddle models can be purchased in several tree sizes (usually narrow, medium, or wide and extra wide) designed to accommodate the builds of different horses. The basic shape of the tree, and how the saddle is constructed on top of that tree, are the components that make one brand of saddle different from another.

To evaluate how well a saddle fits, place it on your horse's back without a saddle pad. You can check the fit more precisely. First look at the saddle from a side view and note the center of balance of the saddle, or where you will have your weight centered when you are sitting in the saddle. This point should be in the center of the saddle's seat and be level whether the saddle is English or Western. It is the most crucial aspect in evaluating saddle fit. (See figs. 8.7–8.10).

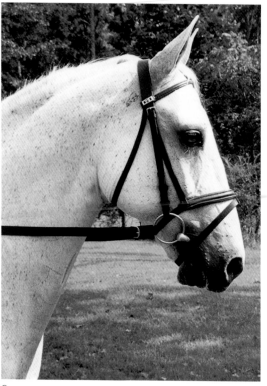

8.1

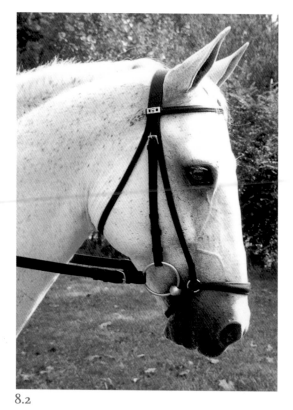

8.2

8.1–8.6 All of these bridles and bits fit well, achieving both effectiveness and comfort.

8.1 A loose-ring snaffle bit and a flash noseband.

8.2 A loose-ring snaffle and a dropped noseband.

8.3 A double bridle made up of a bridoon snaffle, curb bit, and regular noseband.

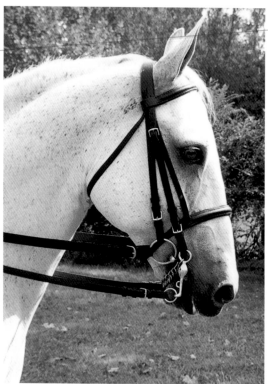

8.3

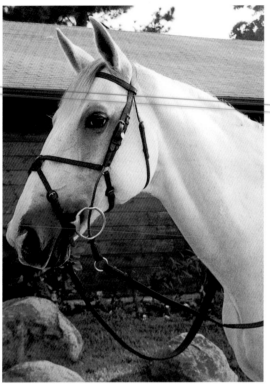

8.4

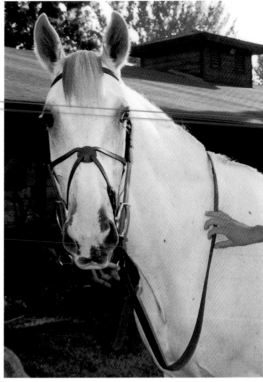

8.5

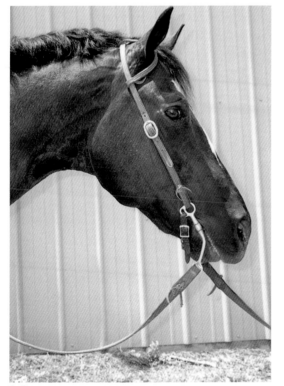

8.6

8.4 *An eggbutt gag snaffle with a figure-eight noseband fitted correctly, side view.*

8.5 *The figure-eight noseband fitted correctly, front view.*

8.6 *A Western training snaffle with curb chain in a one-ear headstall.*

If this center of balance in the saddle is not level then the tree may be too wide or too narrow. The front of the saddle should not be higher than the back. If the front of the saddle appears higher than the back, the tree is too narrow and does not fit down properly on the horse's shoulders. Instead, it will pinch his shoulders, put pressure on his withers, and cause the rider's balance to be thrown backward. If the front of the saddle is low and close to the horse's back, the tree is too wide and will cause the rider's balance to be pitched forward. In either case, the saddle will be uncomfortable for the horse.

You should also check the places where the saddle actually touches the horse's back to make sure that all areas on the underside of the saddle will evenly support the weight of the rider. Slide your hand under the saddle, first in front, then under the middle, and lastly under the rear area. Each of these areas should fully touch the horse's back. Another way to test the evenness of a saddle before you buy it is to apply some baby powder to the horse's back and then put the saddle on over the powder. Press down evenly on the saddle and then carefully remove it from the horse. When you check the underside of the saddle, the pattern of the powder should be consistent on both sides of the saddle.

You can check the evenness of a saddle you already own by examining the sweating pattern on your horse's back after exercise. If there are dry spots under the saddle, or the sweating pattern is not the same on both sides of the horse, the saddle does not fit properly.

CORRECTING FOR PROPER FIT

Perhaps you already own a saddle that suits you well, but you suspect that it doesn't fit your horse properly. What can you do to make the saddle more comfortable for your horse so that you can still keep using it?

You can evaluate the fit of the saddle yourself by following the steps outlined above, but I suggest that you contact someone who has some expertise in saddle fitting to check the saddle for you as well. It may be a challenge to find a saddle-fitting expert in your area, but it's worthwhile to do so. Ask your veterinarian or local tack shop for recommendations or check with trainers or horse clubs and organizations. You can also search the Internet for saddle fitters.

Once you locate an expert, he will first check the saddle's tree to make sure it isn't crooked or broken and then check to see how it fits the horse. If the tree does not fit properly, there is usually little that can be done to correct the problem, although some English saddles are made with trees that can be adjusted.

With an English saddle, the saddle fitter will then check the panels to make sure the padding is not uneven or broken down. Various materials are used for padding inside the panels, but under constant use, all of them will eventually break down and lose their concussion-absorbing properties. Re-stuffing of the padding material may be necessary as frequently as once a year, so the panels should be checked regularly.

Western saddles do not have adjustable trees, and most new ones are designed to be an exact fit on the horse's back, requiring only a light, regular Navaho-type saddle blanket underneath. If the tree of a new Western saddle is too wide, using extra saddle pads sometimes helps improve the fit. Beware: the extra pads can also cause the saddle to roll and move excessively. If a Western saddle tree is too narrow, it should not be used on your horse; adding extra pads under a saddle that is too narrow will only make it fit tighter and pinch around the withers.

If you are thinking about buying a used Western saddle, be aware that many older ones were actually designed to be used with one or two thick saddle pads. This is a factor that you should take into consideration when fitting a used Western saddle to your horse.

Finally, remember that although Western saddles are not padded in the same way that English saddles are, they will sometimes require reflocking with sheepskin on the underside in order to help cushion the saddle.

COMPUTERIZED SADDLE FITTING

There are now systems available that evaluate saddle fit by using computers that measure the evenness of pressure over the horse's back under the saddle. These systems are extremely expensive and are usually owned by saddle-fitting specialists. They can be helpful in assessing the fit of a saddle as well as determining whether particular pads improve or interfere with the way the saddle fits.

Saddle Blankets and Pads

People ask me more questions about saddle blankets and pads than about saddles. In recent years there have been so many changes in what goes under a saddle that it's been difficult to keep up with them all. Sometimes I'm asked about a pad that I haven't even heard of. I always investigate the usefulness of a pad before I recommend its use to a client.

Most people use pads to help increase the comfort of the horse and to keep the saddle clean. Pads have also become popular as a cheaper way to try to fix saddle-fitting problems instead of buying a new saddle. As mentioned earlier however, pads may not provide a solution. Your horse will be the best judge, telling you if the pad you are using is doing the job. If your horse's back is sore, make sure he doesn't need a chiropractic adjustment first. Then investigate the saddle fit and finally, the pad. Prolonged back soreness should always be checked by a veterinarian.

Different styles of pads are used for various types of riding. For instance, dressage riders favor square, quilted cotton pads, hunt seat riders often use fleece pads in the shape of the saddle, and Western-pleasure show riders prefer a woven Navaho-type blanket. Sometimes, two or three different types of pads are used at the same time with Western saddles. And for all types of saddles, there are therapeutic pads made of a high concussion absorption material that make a saddle more comfortable for the horse, as well as special materials to cover pads to help dissipate heat from the horse's back and absorb sweat.

Pads designed specifically to improve saddle fit really don't work and are no longer much in use. For example, pads designed to lift the back or front of the saddle are ineffective and only compound the problem of incorrect saddle fit.

There are several questions to answer before using a pad or blanket:

1. Will this pad fit under my saddle?
2. Does this pad interfere with the balance of my saddle in any way?
3. Is this pad easy to keep clean?
4. Will this pad be comfortable, not too hot, and soak up sweat if it is next to the horse's skin?

If these questions can be answered to your satisfaction, consider the special purpose of the pad and whether it will work. Many manufacturers rely on the testimony of satisfied users in advertising their products, but I don't consider this sufficient evidence that the pad will work for me. Just because it worked for someone else's horse does not mean it will work for yours. No two horses' backs are alike, just as no two saddles—even if the same model—are exactly the same. You should assess your own horse's needs and make your choice based on this knowledge.

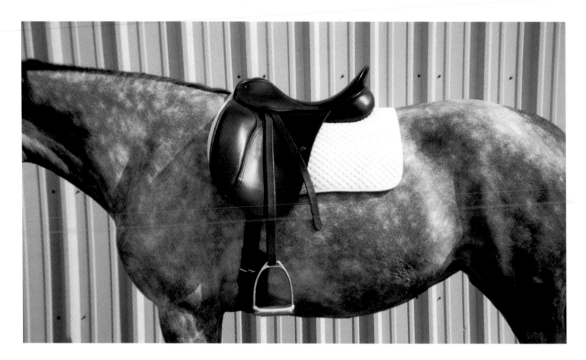

8.7 *A dressage saddle that fits very well. note that the center of the seat is flat, the panel sits evenly on the pad, and the stirrup leather falls in a perfectly straight line from stirrup bar to stirrup.*

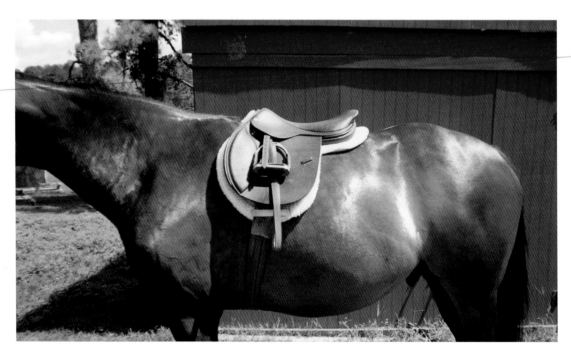

8.8 *This close contact saddle fits this horse. The girth is in a good position and the pad is just the right size for the saddle and has been correctly pulled up off the withers so it matches the arch of the pommel, not causing any friction.*

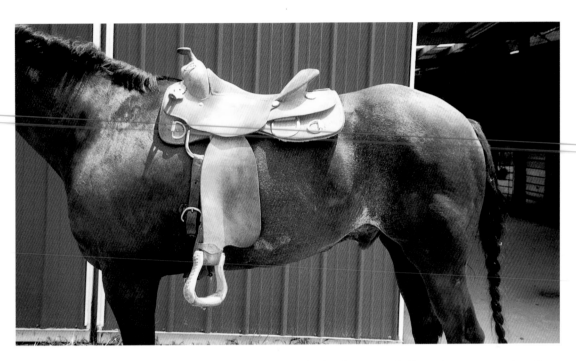

8.9 *This Western stock saddle sits correctly on this horse's back. The pommel allows clearance over the withers and fits down on the shoulders without pinching, and the lowest point of the saddle is where the rider's center of balance will rest.*

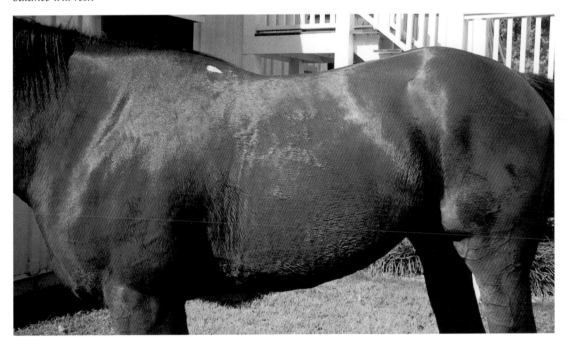

8.10 *When a saddle does not fit properly, a horse can be left with scars that often turn the affected area's hair white. This horse suffered because of a saddle that put too much pressure on his withers.*

Let's review some of the different types of saddle pads on the market today.

FOAM PADS

Foam pads are made of foam rubber. Some come with covers, while others are just bare foam. They provide some concussion absorption, but the amount varies with the density of the foam. Although this type of pad can work well, when foam is used constantly it tends to break down quickly and loses its concussion-absorption ability. If you use a foam pad, replace it every four to six months to maintain the highest level of concussion absorption possible.

HIGH-DENSITY FOAM PADS

High-density foam pads have appeared on the market during the last few years and have become very popular. The shock absorption provided by these pads is excellent, and they are more effective than regular foam pads. Having experimented with them myself, I can say that these pads work well and seem to make the horses very comfortable. However, as with regular foam pads, their concussion-absorption ability breaks down within six months to a year. So check your pad regularly for signs of breakdown, such as thin areas, and replace it when you find them.

GEL PADS

Gel pads are filled with various types of soft substances that have the ability to move around inside a liner. The gel substances used are designed to decrease concussion. When a computer saddle-fitting system is used to measure how much pressure is distributed by these pads, they do not test well. In some pads the gel tends to move out of the area of highest pressure over time. Consequently, not enough gel is left in that area to provide adequate concussion absorption. A newer type of gel pad now on the market is made with thicker gel that stays in place under pressure. The results of using these pads have been promising. Be aware that some gel pads can build up excessive heat under them causing irritated skin. They sometimes even burn the skin slightly so watch for this problem in the summer months.

POLYURETHANE PADS

Another newcomer to the pad market, the polyurethane pad, has proved to be effective. All of the owners I know who have tried them have found that their horses perform better when these pads are used. The only drawback to polyurethane pads is the heat generated under them during hot weather. Some people have remarked about the weight of the pad and it does seem rather heavy when compared to light-weight foam. The horses seemed unfazed, however, so it does not seem to be a concern.

The breakdown properties of this type of pad vary according to the density of the polyurethane and how often it is used, but the wear time seems to be longer for foam pads. As with all other pads, I recommend regular checking for thin or worn areas.

SHEEPSKIN PADS

The sheepskin pad is best used when only one pad is needed and it works especially well with horses that have allergies. Sheepskin is usually not the answer for a tender or sensitive back since it offers little concussion absorption. Nevertheless, a sheepskin pad can be very useful, particularly when you need a pad that is comfortable, cool, and moves well with the horse. With proper care a good sheepskin pad can last for years. (The sheepskin pads available today are not all cured by the same method so follow the cleaning directions that come with the pad.)

FLEECE PADS

A synthetic copy of a sheepskin pad, fleece pads have the advantage of being easily washed and always looking clean. The level of concussion absorption will vary from pad to pad according to what the pad is made of. Some of these are back-to-back synthetic fleece, while others have a layer of foam rubber in the middle.

Synthetic fleece itself has very little concussion absorption, and because there are different materials used in making it, it's not possible to say when a pad will need to be replaced. If the pad shows signs of wear and looks matted, it's definitely time to replace it. Occasionally a horse will show a sensitivity or allergic response to the synthetic material used to make the fleece, so monitor your horse's back if you use a fleece pad, particularly in hot weather.

QUILTED PADS

Quilted pads are made of cotton or a cotton blend and are filled with either foam or synthetic batting. They are one of the most popular types of pads. Quilted pads come in square shapes or saddle shapes and can be used with other types of pads—for example, under a foam pad. If you are using a quilted pad alone it is important that the saddle fits correctly since they do not provide any help in absorbing concussion. These pads are easy to wash and dry quickly.

NAVAHO BLANKETS

The Navaho horse blankets used today are similar to those traditionally made by Navaho Indians in the southwestern United States. These extremely popular blankets are made of wool or cotton and absorb sweat well. Because they are made of natural fibers, these blankets usually breathe well and help to keep the back cool during exercise. Be aware that there are imitation Navaho blankets that look like the real thing but are made of synthetic materials rather than wool or cotton. These synthetic Navaho blankets can cause the same problems as fleece pads.

FELT PADS

The felt pad is inexpensive, comfortable for the horse, and rarely causes a sore back or irritates the skin. The concussion-absorption capacity of felt pads is minimal when compared to that of high-density foam pads, but there is some air space between the layers of felt, so the pad is usually cooler than a high-density foam pad, and it does absorb some sweat from the back. Felt pads are difficult to clean so can be used over the top of a regular blanket such as a Navaho, but of course you do lose the sweat-absorption property of the felt. These pads can be used with both Western and English saddles, but are more commonly used with Western ones.

BANDAGING FOR EXERCISE

I will discuss bandaging for stable use in Chapter Ten. Here I'm going to address bandaging for exercise.

We see horses exercised in bandages or boots so often that you might assume it's proper always to use them when exercising your horse. However, I do not advise using bandages of any type unless they are needed for a specific reason. The less you do to cover your horse's legs, the better. Anytime you apply a bandage to a horse's leg you could alter the pressure on the tendons and potentially cause a problem. Of course none of us want to do this, but the fact is I see far too many tendon injuries that are the result of improper bandaging.

The two basic reasons for using bandages are to support the leg and to protect it. If protection is needed, boots are an alternative to bandages. I will discuss boots later, but first, let's consider the type of bandages that are available and the intended use for each of them.

Polo Bandages

Polo bandages are probably the most common bandages used on horses. They are widely used during regular exercise to help protect horses from injuring their legs if they "interfere" (accidentally kick themselves) while in motion. Polo bandages are made of synthetic material that is thick, soft, and fluffy. These bandages provide protection to the legs from impact, but contrary to what many people believe, they do not provide support to the tendons. In fact, if incorrectly applied, even a soft polo bandage can actually cause a tendon injury. Polo bandages can also be dangerous if they are not tight enough. During exercise, they can slip down and get stepped on by the horse. Polo bandages, like any other bandage, should be applied at a slight angle, not straight around the horse's leg. (See figs. 8.11–8.13).

Most polo bandages are made with Velcro fasteners and for regular exercise this works well. Be sure that when you have finished applying the bandage the Velcro closure is located on the outside of the leg. (I learned this lesson the hard way when a horse I was riding hit the Velcro closure on the inside of his hind leg with his opposite hind hoof. The whole bandage came loose and got tangled in his back legs, nearly causing a fall.)

If you are using polo bandages with Velcro for vigorous activities such as galloping or jumping, the bandages must also be secured with tape or large safety pins so there is no chance they will come loose. If you decide to use tape, you can choose masking tape, adhesive tape, or duct tape. It must be applied in a barber pole fashion around the bandage so there is no possibility of constricting the tendons. My personal favorite is duct tape that has been split in half and wound around the length of the bandage. While some people might consider this much taping to be overly cautious, anyone who has ever seen a horse step on a bandage and flip or fall over at a gallop would disagree. At most racetracks where bandages are used at gallop speed, safety pins are mandatory for all bandaged horses.

Track Bandages

Track bandages that are applied the same way as polo bandages are made of knit cotton or synthetic fabric. These bandages are thinner and have less stretch than polo bandages so provide more support to a horse who needs tendon support when they are correctly wrapped. However, because they can be tightened and have a limited stretch, they have greater potential to do harm if incorrectly put on. As a general rule I do not recommend daily use—a horse should have strong enough tendons for regular exercise without this sort of support unless he is being brought back to work after a tendon injury, or beginning a rigorous exercise program involving galloping, for instance, when they can be used until the horse's tendons get stronger.

If the stretch in a track bandage becomes too loose, a wash usually will tighten the bandage back up so it can be used again. If washing it no longer tightens it, it's time to replace the wrap. I recommend using track bandages made of cotton because cotton has more stretch and will provide more support. Also, there are horses that develop a skin reaction to synthetic fibers, particularly when mixed with the sweat that occurs under the bandage, so cotton is usually the better choice. Occasionally, it may be appropriate to choose a fiber other than cotton, such as elastic or a blend containing elastic, if your horse has an old injury in need of special protection. These kinds of bandages should always be removed right after exercise so circulation returns to normal. They are not suitable for trail riding or any prolonged period of work.

Most track wraps now come with Velcro fasteners at the end, but every once in a while I still see an old set of bandages with ties that are wrapped around the horse's leg and tied to secure

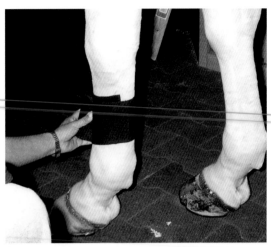

8.11

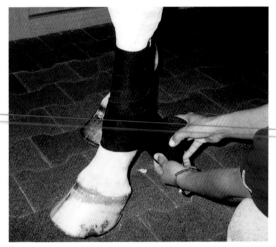

8.12

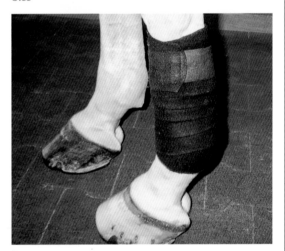

8.13

8.11–8.13 Polo bandages offer good lower leg protection during work sessions and are easy to apply once you get the knack. Begin by placing the end of the wrap on the side of the cannon bone and making one circuit of the leg so that when the wrap comes back around it holds the end in place. Continue around the cannon, first working down the leg to just below the fetlock joint. It's best to wrap at a slight angle because this will help prevent slippage. Only pull the wrap tight around the front of the cannon bone, and not at the back over the tendons. Once you've reached the bottom of the fetlock, start back up until you have wrapped to just below the knee. End your wrap near the top of the cannon and on the outside of the leg. If your bandage is long (as in these photos), first wrap up to just below the knee, then down to the bottom of the fetlock joint, and back up again.

the bandage. I do not advise using bandages with ties. If you have some, I suggest replacing the ties with Velcro pieces or just using pins. The ties can cause a constriction if they are secured too tightly, but they are otherwise notorious for coming loose.

Do not use track bandages if you are unsure how to put them on properly. The angle at which they are applied to the leg and the degree of tightness both have a great impact on the effectiveness of the bandages, and secondly, if misapplied, they can cause injuries. The most common injury I see is due to the uneven pressure of the bandage on the tendons which results in damage to the tendon sheath and possibly an injury to the tendon itself—even a bowed tendon.

BOOTS

So many different kinds of boots are available that it's hard to keep up with all the new styles and which types are best for what. A quick and convenient way to review what is currently available is to look at the many tack and supply catalogs that display them. Boots, like polo bandages, are used to protect a horse's legs from injury but they provide no tendon support unless specifically designed to do so. They are available in a variety of materials ranging from synthetics to leather and are used over polo bandages in certain more rigorous horse sports as a fashion choice, and because they are hardy, shed water quickly, easy to clean, and buckle quickly.

If your horse just needs some basic protection for the cannon bone and fetlock while being exercised, the neoprene splint boot with Velcro closures is a good choice. (These are known as brushing boots in the UK.) They are easy to put on and keep clean and seem very comfortable for most horses. Be aware, however, that some horses have been known to have allergic skin reactions to neoprene. Otherwise, their biggest drawback is that they can be very warm because the neoprene material does not breathe. They also do not shed water well and might become heavy and uncomfortable when they get soaked. Be very careful using boots that use a strap under the fetlock. These can cause great harm if not put on properly.

Plastic boots are a better choice if you are going to be riding through water because they do not hold it. Like the neoprene, however, they can become warm over a long period of time. Leather boots, some lined with sheepskin, are also used for protection and are seen often on hunters and jumpers. Leather is the best choice if your horse has sensitive skin, since many sensitive horses are less likely to be allergic to natural materials.

Newer on the market are boots designed to provide some type of support to the tendons. Most of these boots have a portion that is under the fetlock and extends up the cannon bone to just below the knee. There has been controversy concerning the use of these boots since some injuries have occurred while they were being used. Studies in the past have indicated that any uneven pressure on the tendons can cause injury so, depending on its design, the potential for injury exists if the boot isn't put on properly. The leg conformation of each horse will be a little different as will the proper application of a support boot. However, support boots can be very helpful to many horses when used correctly.

The other problem I have noticed when support boots are being used is that the rider sometimes forgets the horse had been injured. For instance, if boots are being used because a tendon was sore and needed support and the horse works much better when the boots are on, there is a tendency for some riders to get carried away and overwork the horse. In other words, there is potential for abuse—however unintentional—and this may be the source of some of the problems reported with support boots. Remember, the faster the gait the more pressure on the tendons, so it is essential to have even pressure over the tendons when boots or bandages are being used.

As with bandages, if you have not used support boots before, have an experienced person demonstrate the proper position to put them on the leg. Clean the boots after each use; sweat can build up on them and irritate the skin as well as providing a good place for bacteria to grow.

I find it interesting to watch horses at racetracks and note what is used on their legs. Many top trainers, understanding the potential for injury from using boots (or bandages) incorrectly, do not use anything at all on the horse's legs when galloping them. When I am examining a horse, I make it a point to ask what is used on the horse's legs during exercise, particularly when I'm working on racehorses. I've noticed that a growing number of trainers are using bandages or boots only when the horse needs protection from interfering or has been injured previously.

9 Exercise and Conditioning

CONDITIONING YOUR HORSE

Understanding your horse's exercise and fitness needs is important, whether you are preparing him for competition or just riding for pleasure. Knowing your horse's basic fitness level, how long he should exercise, and what types of exercise he can perform will make your riding time safer and more productive for both you and your horse.

Even if your horse is only ridden occasionally and just for pleasure, you should be attentive to the correct amount and type of exercise he will tolerate. I use the word "tolerate" because of the way horses respond to continued exercise when they are tired. Many become resistant or uncooperative; they are not as careful in their use of the body because their muscles are fatigued and their attention span may be wandering.

Unfortunately, fitness is an area that is often overlooked by horse owners. I frequently see a lack of fitness in my patients—surprisingly, sometimes even in top-level competition horses.

This problem often manifests with back problems, which constitute a large proportion of the cases I am called to treat.

Just like people, horses need a comprehensive exercise program to achieve the correct level of fitness. Most exercise programs do not feature enough diversity to achieve all-around fitness in part because of the ongoing loss of riding areas. A large number of horse owners are faced with the problem of trying to maintain an exercise program but having nowhere to ride. Many of today's stables are land-locked or completely surrounded by other farms or subdivisions, making it difficult to ride off the property. It is a very big challenge to keep a horse fit without enough land to ride on and there is no simple answer to this problem. Each owner must tailor an exercise program to accommodate his or her particular situation.

First, evaluate your horse as an athlete. What is his current condition and how long do you have before he must be fit? If you have ever had to get your horse fit for a competition before, you will have some idea of how long it will take to achieve the desired fitness level. Many horses that have been maintained at a high level of fitness for a long period of time in the past can be returned to a fit condition in less time. For example, racehorses—whose cardiovascular, respiratory, and muscular systems have been developed to full capacity—generally become fit a little faster than the average Thoroughbred who has never been conditioned. The respiratory development of a racehorse alone can aid him in the conditioning process.

Some breeds, such as the Arabian, seem to have a natural capability for fitness and endurance and therefore have been very successful as competitive endurance horses. Check into the requirements of any competitive sport you are considering and also research which breeds are used the most for that sport. Sometimes breeds are favored because of tradition, but more often some horse breeds predominate because they have exceptional abilities that help them to excel at a particular sport. Nevertheless, there are always exceptions or exceptional horses who are successful at a sport regardless of their breed. The Quarter Horse stallion Rugged Lark has not only been shown successfully in Quarter Horse shows in many different divisions, but he is an accomplished dressage horse as well. Another exceptional horse that defied the rules was Stroller, a large pony, who represented Great Britain in the 1968 Olympics. Despite his diminutive size, he won a silver medal in show jumping. Another small horse that successfully competed in world-class competitions was the Connemara-cross, Seldom Seen. This little horse won national dressage championships in the United States and did well in Europe showing against some of the best horses at grand-prix level. Although Connemaras are known for their athletic ability, it was a significant feat for a smaller horse to be so successful against larger horses that were bred specifically for dressage competition.

Now, let's review some of the components of a good exercise program.

THE CARDIOVASCULAR COMPONENT

The cardiovascular system includes the heart, the circulatory system, and the various components of the blood. Too complicated you say? Actually it's not all that complicated. You can learn to monitor your horse's heart rate with a little training. All you will need is a stethoscope and some practice using it. Ask your veterinarian to assist you in learning how to use your stethoscope and where to listen to your horse's heart (fig. 9.1).

The horse's normal resting heart rate ranges from 35 to 45 beats per minute, and each horse will have his own specific resting heart rate within this range. If you listen to your horse's heart rate daily for five days you should be able to determine what his average resting heart rate is. If your horse has a heart rate above the normal range, consult your veterinarian and have a thorough diagnostic work-up done. It is unusual to have a low resting heart rate. If your horse has a heart rate in the lower range, it usually indicates that the heart is large and has a high stroke volume or amount of blood that is pumped during each beat.

Knowing your horse's resting heart rate will assist you in monitoring his progress with the conditioning process. Also, because the heart rate will sometimes be elevated during an illness or other stress, the ability to determine the resting heart rate will help you evaluate your horse's condition if you suspect a health problem.

Take your horse's resting heart rate before he has done any exercise. Be sure he is calm and standing still, not moving or eating. That's why it is called the resting heart rate. During exercise, the heart rate can increase to a range of 215 to 250 beats per minute. As your horse's fitness level rises, his heart will work more efficiently, so the increase in heart rate may not be as high, and it will return to a resting rate more quickly. If it takes your horse a long time to return to his resting heart rate after exercise—say longer than 20 minutes—then you should have your veterinarian check him.

If you are planning to start an intensive conditioning program, consider asking your veterinarian to perform routine blood work to evaluate your horse's present status first. A CBC (complete blood count) and chemistry profile should be included to determine that the horse is in the best possible shape to start the conditioning program. (It is especially advisable to do a blood test on Quarter Horses because of a certain genetic condition called hyperkalemia that is potentially fatal when the horse is stressed. If you are thinking about competing a Quarter Horse, ask your vet, or contact the American Quarter Horse Association to obtain more information about hyperkalemia).

If any levels of the blood work are out of balance, your veterinarian can advise you on how to correct them. It's also a good idea to monitor the blood work throughout your horse's conditioning process, particularly if he has not been in an intense conditioning program before. Advances in technology have made it increasingly quick and easy to perform blood work-ups and there are now portable units available so some blood chemistry tests can be performed right at the farm.

THE RESPIRATORY SYSTEM

It is important that you have a basic understanding of the respiratory system so you can safely condition your horse. There are several different parts of this system where problems can occur during the conditioning process, so we'll discuss each of them.

Horses have a respiratory system similar to yours, with lungs, bronchi, a trachea, a pharynx, larynx, and nasal passages. Since the respiratory system provides oxygen to the horse's body, it is of vital importance to the horse when exercising.

When starting a fitness program you should know what your horse's respiration level should be during various activities. Watch your horse's flank for each complete breath—the inhalation and exhalation. Respiration is measured in breaths taken per minute. You can practice on yourself first by timing how many breaths you take in a minute. Use a watch that can measure in seconds and time the respirations for fifteen seconds. Then multiply by four to get your respirations per minute. A single respiration is when your horse breathes in and expands his chest and then breathes out and relaxes his chest. When you are counting, use the expansion part of the respiration as one breath.

RESPIRATION RATE	
GAIT	BREATHS PER MINUTE
Rest	20
Walk	50
Trot	80
Canter	100
Gallop	130

Average respiratory rates for horses weighing 1000 lb. (approx. 450 kgs).

The respiratory rates I have given above are only averages, and the rates for individual horses will vary. If your horse exceeds this range by a large margin, it is an indication that he is not in condition and needs an exercise program to improve his respiratory fitness.

When they are exercised some horses make noise, others have a chronic cough or nasal discharge, and some just seem to struggle to breathe. If your horse has any of these problems when exercising, do not ignore it. Discuss the

9.1 The correct location to listen to your horse's heart with a stethoscope. If you cannot hear his heart in this location, move the stethoscope further toward his chest.

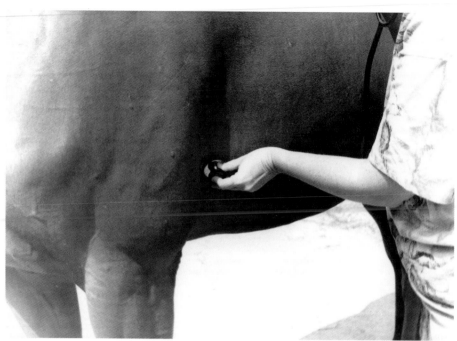

symptoms with your veterinarian. There are many possible causes, some of which can be easily treated. Otherwise the condition could worsen. (For more information on possible causes see *Respiratory Problems* in the *Horse Ailments* section, Part Three.)

THE WARM-UP

Some warming-up can be done even before you tack up your horse and begin riding. Start with some good stretching exercises which I think are most helpful and important.

These stretches will get you started. Follow them up with under-saddle stretches before starting riding. The classical stretches under saddle—used by dressage riders—encourage the horse to perform in a "long and low" type of body frame. This type of stretch rounds the horse's back up and stretches the back muscles, as well as developing balance and helping the horse learn to relax and carry himself. If you are not familiar with this type of stretching, you can find it detailed in many books on modern dres-

sage techniques, or you can watch dressage riders as they warm up. You might also consider taking a dressage lesson to assist you in learning this technique. Start the exercises at a walk, and when you are comfortable, try doing them at the trot. Five minutes of this exercise while going both directions should be sufficient—two to three minutes each way. I also suggest using this stretch as a break during your regular exercise program to relax and rebalance your horse.

Another excellent exercise to incorporate in your warm-up is working on hills. This is beneficial to horses in all disciplines. Start slowly, even if your horse is used to regular exercise, since hill work uses different muscles than he normally might use. It's best to start at a walk on a hill that is not too steep. Be sure your horse is on the bit, but not over-flexed. His head flexion should remain slightly in front of the vertical. If your horse's head is in the correct position, he will engage, warm up, and strengthen the muscles he uses most when ridden. This is also

STRETCHING EXERCISES

1. Using a treat such as a carrot, entice your horse to stretch his head to his side. Stand at his shoulder so he stretches around you. Stretch both sides (fig. 9.2, p. 138).

2. Entice your horse to follow the treat between his front legs. This not only stretches the neck area but raises the back as well (fig. 9.3, p. 138).

3. Lift the horse's front leg as if you were going to clean his feet by taking the hoof in one hand and steadying the knee with the other. Slowly move the leg below the knee in small circles. Start with 10 circles and gradually increase to 20 circles (fig. 9.4, p. 139).

4. Still holding the leg up, put both your hands under the knee and gently lift the leg in front of the horse so the knee is moving toward the chin. Five repetitions of this stretch should be adequate (fig. 9.5, p. 139).

5. Next, placing one hand under the cannon bone and the other on the hoof bring the leg slowly in front of the horse. Begin with the leg in a low position near the ground and do this stretch once. As your horse becomes more flexible, bring the leg a little higher (fig. 9.6, p. 142).

6. Move to the horse's hindquarters and bring his hind leg forward making sure to hold the cannon bone with one hand, and the hoof with the other. If your horse is resistant, it is likely that he is lacking flexibility. Do not force the leg to come further than is comfortable. When he becomes more limber, you can gradually ask for more extension. Do this stretch once each session (fig. 9.7, p. 142).

7. Life the hind leg as if you were going to clean the hoof and gradually extend the leg behind the horse. Keep it low to the ground at first. This is the same movement a horse performs by himself when first stretching after lying down. As you and your horse become more comfortable doing this stretch, you can gently raise his leg just as he does on his own. Be careful since some horses are less trustworthy than others and if nervous, or touchy, may kick (fig. 9.8, p. 143).

8. If your horse is comfortable having his tail handled, the tail stretch is a good exercise. However, it is only advised for the most dependable horses, since some horses will not tolerate it. Hold the hair at the tip of the tail, and stand directly behind the horse at the farthest extension of the tail. The tail's angle should be level with the horse's croup or the angle from the top of the hip to the base of the tail. Put your weight against the tail, but do not pull. Your horse should pull again you. Hold this stretch for one to two minutes. Stop if your horse shows any signs of discomfort. Don't take the chance of being kicked. If you are concerned, place a bale of hay behind your horse's hind legs while you stretch his tail.

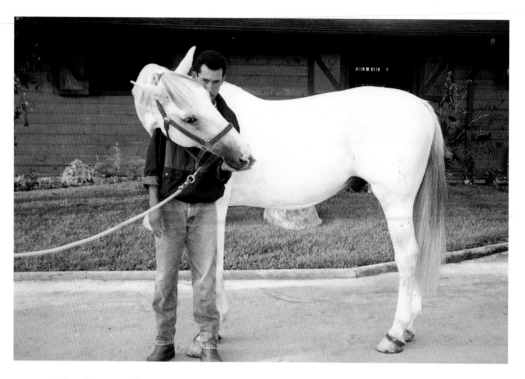

9.2–9.8 Stretching exercises. (Text p. 137)
9.2 Neck stretch.

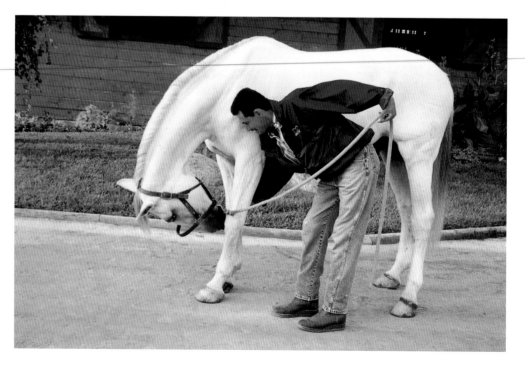

9.3 Topline stretch.

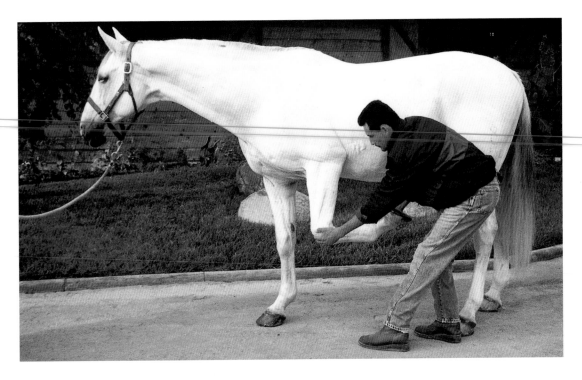

9.4 *Lower leg circles.*

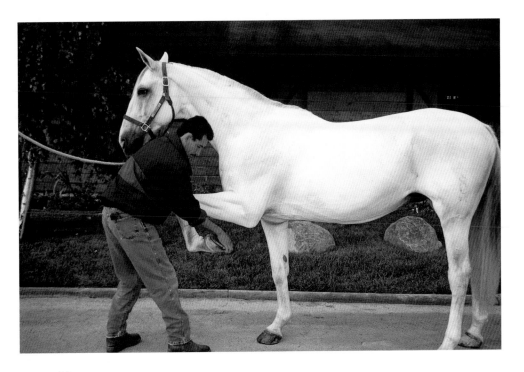

9.5 *Leg lift.*

an excellent way to strengthen the muscles that support the stifles.

If you are just starting your horse on a conditioning program, walk him up and down the hill no more than three times. If the only hill available is very steep or extremely long, decrease the number of repetitions. You will have to monitor your horse's breathing while doing the hill work. If it increases greatly after one or two times up the hill, then stop. Individual horses will vary as to how long they should be worked on a hill. It is important to monitor your horse's progress. Start with hill work every other day at a walk, both up and down. Then, after two weeks (or sooner if you think your horse is ready), proceed to trot up the hill, still keeping your horse's head in the flexed position slightly in front of the vertical. Continue to walk, not trot, down the hill. Once your horse becomes stronger he will enjoy this exercise, and you can use it as part of your regular warm-up two to three times a week.

Another way to use a hill for stretching is to go across the side of the hill, so one side of your horse is higher than the other. Use a hill with a gradual incline, not an extremely steep one. Start the exercise at the walk and go about 500 yards; then reverse and walk with the other side on the high side of the hill. This stretch lets the shoulders, chest, and hip area really move, freeing them and giving your horse a little extra stride. Working across the side of the hill can also be performed at the trot, but I don't recommend proceeding to the trot until the walk stretching at an incline is firmly established and has been performed daily for at least one week.

Once the stretching is completed, you can proceed to other exercises that will help your horse with bending. Start at a walk on circles that are at least twenty meters wide. If they are smaller than twenty meters, too much stress will be put on the spine before the muscles are warmed up enough to allow a proper bending motion. Of course, any horse can be forced to bend in smaller circles during warm-up, but this can be harmful as it can stress the spine and cause the muscles to bunch up. Since we're trying to avoid muscles that are bunched up, be sure to keep your exercises straight or in large circles at first. Ten minutes at the walk is optimum to allow the tendons, muscles, and joints to increase circulation and prepare the horse to move into a faster gait with maximum flexibility. Ten minutes of trot can then follow the walk work. Be sure to allow a few periods of walk during the trot work, especially if your horse is out of condition. The canter or lope can then be performed. Five minutes of canter on a twenty-meter circle in each direction is usually sufficient.

LONGEING

Longeing is also used as a warm-up, especially with young or overly energetic horses. Be sure to start at the walk, if possible. I know with some horses it is difficult to begin walking; but try to stay at the walk for five to ten minutes. The walk should be forward and active, not slow and lazy, in order to warm up the muscles, tendons, and ligaments. Then proceed to the trot for five minutes and then the canter for five minutes. Your horse will get more out of the longe work if side reins are used. Side reins help the horse use his body more effectively, keep him balanced, and decrease his ability to misbehave. If you are unfamiliar with the use of side reins while longeing, consult a professional horse trainer.

Caution: *If your horse has a hock or stifle problem, it's best not to longe him, since longeing puts pressure on those joints and may aggravate his condition.*

REMEDIES FOR STIFFNESS

If your horse has a problem such as arthritis in some of his joints, he may be especially stiff at the beginning of the exercise period. There are several options that will help decrease your horse's discomfort. First is the technique called moxibustion, used over a joint area prior to riding. Moxibustion will help to increase the circulation and warm up the area. It takes only a few minutes and is very effective. I frequently teach owners how to use it. (For details on how to perform *indirect moxibustion*, see Chapter Three.)

Another option is to use arnica to decrease inflammation. Arnica can be applied directly on a problem area as a liniment (called arnica lotion) or given internally in homeopathic form. Or you can use BHI Traumeel, an ointment that contains arnica as well as other ingredients. (BHI Traumeel is available in most health food stores.)

If the exercise is going to be very strenuous, such as jumping or galloping, I suggest using dimethyl sulfoxide, commonly known as DMSO. This product can be very effective in warming up a joint if it is applied prior to exercise. Make sure the joint area is very clean before you apply DMSO. Because DMSO is absorbed quickly through the skin, you should use an applicator or wear latex or rubber gloves so you don't absorb any through your hands. If other products or medications are on the skin before DMSO is applied, it will also carry them across the skin barrier and into the tissue. So do not apply DMSO over other products unless that is your intention. I have known several people who applied DMSO on a leg that had been sweated the night before. The medication used to sweat the leg had not been completely cleaned off prior to the use of DMSO, and the horses became ill because the remaining sweat medication was carried into the horse's body.

The only medication that I intentionally apply under DMSO is arnica lotion. The DMSO assists in carrying the arnica into the tissues and has been very effective over tendons, muscles, and joint areas. I don't recommend using DMSO on a regular basis particularly if applications are repeated daily. We don't fully understand all of the effects of DMSO, so it should always be used in moderation. It can cause a burning sensation so some horses do not like it being applied. Since they can readily identify it by its strong garlicky odor, they may react strongly, so be cautious.

Counter-irritants readily available in drug stores and chemists have been used on the joints to help warm them prior to exercise. Counter-irritants produce heat in the area where applied by causing irritation to the skin. For this reason, I don't recommend them. Also, if used repeatedly, these products destroy the top layers of skin becoming counter-productive.

THE COOL-DOWN

The cool-down includes time both under saddle and after dismounting. There are many ways of cooling down a horse after exercise. The first step I recommend is walking at least five minutes before dismounting. This will allow your horse to decrease his respirations and relax his muscles.

Once you dismount, loosen the girth and lift the saddle slightly to allow a little air under the saddle blankets or pad for a brief moment. This starts the cooling process and allows the hot air trapped under the saddle to escape without significantly cooling the back; in other words, it makes cooling down a more gradual process. This should be done right after dismounting.

Cold Weather

Next, the horse can be led over to the area where the saddle and other tack are removed. If it is extremely cold (below 20 degrees Fahrenheit or

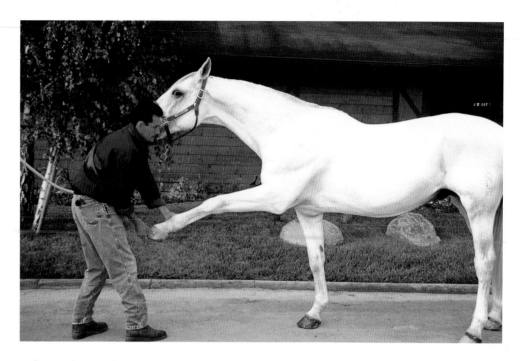

9.6 *Front leg stretch.*

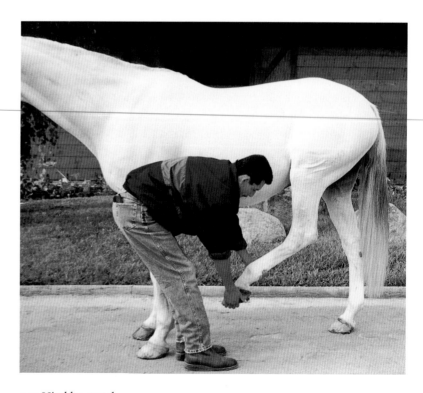

9.7 *Hind leg stretch.*

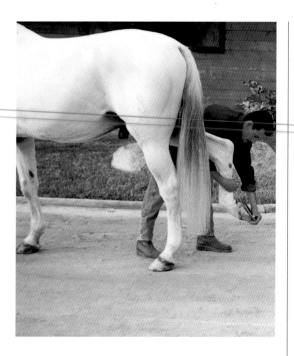

9.8 Hind leg extension stretch.

minus 5 Celsius), and the horse is very hot, it's best to hand walk the horse around for another five minutes with the saddle on to avoid a sudden loss of heat over the back and possible muscle tightening. (In extreme cold throw a cooler over the horse and the saddle as well.) Remember, your horse is not going to go into a nice warm house like you are after the ride, so be careful that he doesn't get chilled since it may be difficult to get him warm again.

Once the saddle is off, put on a cooler or anti-sweat sheet to keep your horse warm and allow for a gradual cooling off. Even if your horse is soaking wet with sweat, put on the cooler first and walk him for a while, then take off the cooler and rub him with a towel to dry him off and promote circulation to the skin. Remember, even in the cold your horse cools down his body by evaporating heat off his skin. Sudden exposure to cold will cause the blood vessels in the skin to contract and become smaller, decreasing the horse's ability to bring internal heat to the surface, evaporate it and cool off. If a horse is suddenly exposed to cold after becoming very hot during exercise, he may seem to initially cool down quickly, due to the contraction of the blood vessels. But if the cooling-out process is stopped while internal heat still exists and the horse is put away, he may break out in a sweat in the stall. This is a situation to be avoided because a sweating horse in cold weather, even with blankets on, will eventually become cold and may become ill.

If your horse does not cool down quickly during the cold months due to an excessive hair coat, it may be best to clip the hair on the horse's body. There is much controversy concerning body clipping, but it is in the horse's best interest to allow the cooling-out process to proceed as quickly as possible. This is difficult to do if his coat is acting as insulation. There are a variety of styles in which to body clip your horse, and you don't have to clip the entire body. I prefer to leave long hair on the legs, upper neck, and face for warmth. This is called a trace clip; it may not be acceptable for all types of showing, but it is used on many field hunters ridden in the winter.

Hot Weather

When you cool your horse down in hot weather, start the procedure under saddle. Ride with a loose rein, or allow your horse to have a relaxed, long, stretched neck. Keep him walking forward in a regular pace—do not allow him to become slow. This will help his blood circulation remove any residual waste products such as lactic acid, as well as his muscles relax gradually. The time will depend on how hot the horse is, the temperature, and his fitness level.

Once you remove his saddle you can make an assessment. If he is still extremely hot, hand walk him. If he doesn't start to cool down quickly, rinse him with cold or lukewarm water and remove the excess water with a sweat scraper. As the remaining water evaporates it dissipates the heat from the horse. Be sure to rinse the inside of the rear legs and on both sides of the lower part of the neck when you need to cool a severely over-heated animal.

WEATHER EXTREMES

Sometimes we don't give enough consideration to the effect of weather extremes on the horse's ability to perform. A horse needs to be conditioned to the type of weather in which he is expected to perform. In the southern US, we take as many precautions as possible in the heat and humidity of summer. Most three-day events and horse trials, as well as major horse shows, are not held during the hottest months of July and August. It would just be too hard on the horses and riders. Any competitive trail rides or horse shows that are held during the summer season are conducted with the utmost caution, with horses and riders monitored closely for heat-related problems.

Studies are ongoing to determine better ways to cool down a horse and help a horse maintain a high performance level during extreme heat conditions. These studies were initially begun in anticipation of the summer Olympics that were held in the very hot and humid climates of Barcelona and Atlanta.

Warm Weather Considerations

There are some general rules to follow when riding a horse in warm weather:

A warm-up period is necessary even when riding in warm weather. The horse needs a normal warm-up period to allow his muscles to function properly. The warm-up period will help you determine if your horse is tolerating the heat well. If your horse is breathing hard and covered with sweat at the end of a walk-trot warm-up period, he may not be in good enough condition to withstand much more exercise in hot weather. Some horses tolerate heat better than others, just as some people do. Never ride in competition in the heat unless you know that your horse will tolerate it. He could become dehydrated and seriously ill.

To assist your horse during exercise under hot conditions be sure to allow plenty of rest periods. If you are trail riding, even at a walk, stop and let your horse rest every 20 to 30 minutes—more often if you are going over difficult terrain. If your horse is in excellent condition, then your rest periods may not need to be as frequent. However, you need to monitor your horse's

WARNING SIGNS OF HEAT INTOLERANCE:

1. Excessive sweating, often turning to lather.

2. *NO* sweating. A horse ceases to sweat during exercise (after he has already been sweating).

3. A horse breathes very hard and is unable to slow down his breathing.

breathing to make sure he is not being overtaxed. A horse being schooled in the ring needs to stop every 10 minutes for a breather, allowing a loose rein so he may breathe as easily as possible.

If you notice any of these signs of heat intolerance while exercising your horse in hot conditions, you must take action immediately to cool him down. The easiest thing to do first is usually to wet the horse down with water, either with a sponge or with a hose. Continue to keep water on the horse during the cool-down process, so heat will evaporate from his body. Scrape the excess water off the horse and, if the horse is not too exhausted, walk him around a little bit.

Scraping the water off allows the heat to evaporate more quickly, so each time you soak the horse down scrape it off again.

If you have a thermometer, check the horse's temperature. In hot conditions, it should be 100 to 102 degrees Fahrenheit (37.8 to 38.9 Celsius). If his temperature is over 103 degrees Fahrenheit call your veterinarian. It may be necessary for the veterinarian to administer fluids intravenously to prevent your horse from dehydrating during the cool-down process. Replacing the lost fluid immediately will allow your horse's system to recover more quickly and help avoid other problems such as colic and laminitis (founder).

How do you prevent heat intolerance? The best plan is to be prepared and not work a horse that is out of condition in hot weather. Get your horse used to exercising in the heat gradually by monitoring his pulse and respiration while working him. Add electrolytes in his feed or water or, if your horse won't eat them, give him electrolytes in a dose syringe. (See *Electrolytes*, Chapter Five, p. 85.)

Cold Weather Considerations

Many people erroneously believe that horses can become dehydrated only in warm weather, but exposure to extreme cold can also cause problems with hydration. Often horses just don't want to drink during cold weather because the water is so cold. If your horse avoids drinking cold water, provide fresh warm water at least once a day in order to maintain his fluid balance. Or you can use a water warmer for buckets or tanks, which will keep your horse happy and avoid the problems associated with dehydration.

Other cold weather precautions include warming up, monitoring your horse's breathing, keeping your horse warm during exercise, and cooling down. The horse's muscles, tendons, and joints must be given adequate time to warm up

before regular work is performed. What is adequate time? That will vary from horse to horse. However, to give you an idea of the time required, consider how long it takes you to warm up when the temperature is 40 degrees Fahrenheit (5 degrees Celsius), or lower. When muscles and tendons are cold, their blood supply is decreased, so it's important to maximize this blood supply for optimum performance. Injuries can occur when cold stiff muscles are asked to do too much before they are thoroughly warmed up.

Joints are also more susceptible to injury in cold weather since a joint is filled with fluid that becomes slightly thicker in cold weather when the horse is not exercising. I recommend at least ten minutes of walk when starting out in cold weather below 40 degrees Fahrenheit (5 degrees Celsius). Start out slowly and gradually increase to a working walk.

Some horses become short of breath or seem to struggle for air when they breathe in cold air during exercise even though they are fit and easily able to perform the exercise under normal conditions. This can be due to a couple of reasons. First, if the horse does not like the feeling of the cold air when he inhales, he will not take deep breaths. The lack of air intake decreases oxygen exchange and a deficiency results. Second, the cold air may cause constriction of the blood vessels in the nasal passages and, some researchers feel, in the upper areas of oxygen exchange as well, decreasing the oxygen taken into the blood stream. As with hot weather, you should monitor your horse's respiration in cold weather too so you become familiar with his response to lower temperatures.

It can be a challenge to keep your horse warm while exercising in cold weather. If your horse seems very cold and shivers when you are starting out, he may need to wear a type of blanket known as a quarter sheet. To determine if your horse should wear a quarter sheet, try using one and monitor him carefully for excessive sweating. You may find that once he has warmed up he begins to sweat and no longer requires this extra protection. If so, use a quarter sheet that attaches to the saddle pad and can be removed once your warm-up is complete.

One of the newest methods to keep muscles warm is the use of a magnetic blanket. It can be used in cold weather before riding or put on between classes when showing.

TRACKING YOUR PROGRESS

A regular evaluation of your horse's progress will help you adjust your program to meet his needs.

Be sure to keep an accurate written record of the program, recording the overall plan, the type of exercise, times and distances covered, recovery rates, and changes.

Why keep a record? An accurate training record will help you to monitor your horse's progress in an objective way. Instead of saying "He worked much better today and seemed to cool out faster," you can know for sure by comparing your previous written record to today's workout. Don't play a guessing game because your horse might not be as fit as you think when competition time comes around, and an unfit horse could get injured.

TRAINING PROGRAM

Horse's Name: _____

Description of Fitness Plan: _____

_____

Goal/Competition Date: _____

Date	Type of Exercise	Time	Distance	Before Exercise		After Exercise		Changes from Previous Day
				Heart Rate	Respiratory Rate	Heart Rate	Respiratory Rate	

IO Nursing Your Horse

Horse owners now manage many of the medical needs of their horses. Many people live in areas where the nearest veterinarian is a long way away, or where there is a shortage of vets. It is a good idea to keep a supply of veterinary products on hand, as well as directions on how to use them properly. In addition, practice how to use these basic medical supplies so you don't panic when you have to apply them in an emergency.

You should also become observant, noticing small changes in your horse's demeanor. You should be able to tell the state of your horse's health and whether or not you need to intervene, or call the vet. If you suspect a gradual onset of a problem, start to keep a daily diary of the signs and symptoms so you have a written log to refer to when discussing the situation with your vet.

SYMPTOMS OF ILLNESS

If your horse starts to exhibit warning signs of any health problems or major behavioral changes, you should call the veterinarian to report them. Some symptoms, such as a decrease in appetite, are readily noticeable, but others are subtler. Here are some indicators that should be checked out with the veterinarian—at least with a phone call:

Abnormal Temperature. Normal range is 99.5 to 100 degrees Fahrenheit (37.5 to 37.8 Celsius).

Abnormal Pulse. Normal range is 35 to 45 beats per minute at rest (see p. 134).

Abnormal Respiration. Normal: 20 and below breaths per minute at rest (see p. 135).

Diarrhea, especially if watery. Prolonged diarrhea can lead to dehydration and may indicate the presence of a more serious illness.

Constipation

Not eating, or diminished appetite

Radical change in behavior, such as sudden aggressive tendencies

Excessive sleeping (change from normal)

Lethargy or lack of energy

Lameness or change in movement

Breathing problems or coughing

Difficulty urinating

Colic

An owner knows his or her horse better than anyone else does. Be alert to any indications that your horse is not feeling up to par and report them to your veterinarian immediately. You could be detecting a health problem early on, leading to a big difference in the severity of the prognosis.

DIAGNOSIS

Two methods being widely used by holistic veterinarians have proven quite useful in diagnosis and prescribing. In both methods, the body actually helps with the decision on which medication or other treatment to use. The methods—applied kinesiology muscle testing and pulse diagnosis—have one common denominator, which is that both tap into the body's innate intelligence for guidance. Although these methods are not a substitute for scientific expertise, I have found them invaluable in diagnosing and prescribing all types of treatments, from conventional to holistic. Pulse diagnosis, which I describe later, is fairly complex and best left to the veterinarian.

Within certain parameters, however, owners can use muscle testing in a number of ways, including determining the specific Bach Flower remedy (or combination of remedies) to use, ascertaining the best homeopathic remedy (and the specific potency) to use, or making sure a new supplement or food will not cause an allergic reaction. This method is not infallible and only responds to what the body needs at the time of testing. To test the accuracy check again in two hours using a different intermediary.

Applied Kinesiology Muscle Testing

Muscle testing utilizes a "muscle resistance" to determine whether a substance strengthens or weakens the body. When you are testing for an animal, a second person must stand in for the animal as an intermediate or surrogate.

My co-author, Norma Eckroate, has written a book entitled *Switched-On Living: Easy Ways to Use the Mind/Body Connection to Energize Your Life* with stress expert Dr. Jerry Teplitz, which gives the following step-by-step method for muscle testing. You will need a partner to do the procedure with you. Before you begin the actual muscle testing, you must test the normal level of resistance of your partner's arm muscles. If this method of testing is new to you, it will become clear as I proceed.

FINDING NORMAL RESISTANCE

Step 1: Face your partner.

Step 2: Your partner should raise one arm up from the side of the body so it is at a right angle to the body and level with the shoulder, with the thumb pointing toward the floor. Imagine a bird with a wing outstretched and you'll have the correct arm position. The other arm should remain at the side of the body.

Step 3: Now place one of your hands on your partner's extended arm, just above the wrist. Place your other hand on your partner's opposite shoulder.

Step 4: Instruct your partner to resist as you push down, firmly and steadily with a hard pressure, on the extended arm. Say out loud "Ready—resist," as you are about to push down on your partner's arm. You are not trying to force her arm down; her arm should stay fairly level during the pressure, however, you want to place a hard steady pressure on the arm in order to measure her normal level of resistance. You should press firmly for several seconds, and then release. [1]

When doing this testing method, do not look directly at your partner's face, because facial expressions can affect the outcome. (A smile is strengthening to your partner's resistance; a frown is weakening.) Also, remember that this will work only if you both understand that you are looking for a level of resistance in the arm muscles. This is not in any way like arm wrestling; you are not trying to overcome your partner, and, similarly, your partner should not try so hard to resist the pressure that she recruits other muscles to "fight back." When her arm muscle starts to fade, your partner should allow it to do so. (See figs. 10.1–10.2).

Muscle testing is being used more and more by veterinarians and horse owners. As I mentioned above, it is not infallible as a method of prescribing, but, when I must choose between two or more viable alternatives, I find muscle testing an invaluable tool. If two alternatives both check strong, I know that either will be effective. However, if one checks weak and the other checks strong, I know which one is best. I use muscle testing frequently and find it quite reliable.

Now you are ready to involve the horse in the muscle testing. Your partner becomes the intermediary who will touch your horse while he is being tested. (See figs. 10.3–10.4).

MUSCLE TEST USING INTERMEDIARY

Step 1: Face your partner.

Step 2: Ask the intermediary to place one hand on the horse and to hold the substance you are checking in that same hand. If the substance being checked is in a container, take the top off the container. Your partner should not know what substance she is holding. Ask her to stretch out her arm as she did in Step 2 above.

Step 3: Place your hand on your partner's outstretched arm, just above the wrist, and your other hand on her opposite shoulder.

Step 4: As in Step 4 above, ask your partner to resist as you push firmly and steadily down on her arm. Press firmly for several seconds, and then release.

If the resistance of the arm is made stronger while you are pushing down, the substance your partner is holding is a good choice. If the resistance is weaker, and the arm is easily pushed down, this substance is a poor choice, ineffective, or not agreeing with the horse's body. If more than one item gives a positive response, it is sometimes possible to discern that one feels even stronger than the others and is therefore the best choice.

In addition to using muscle testing to check medications, I have found a remarkable degree of accuracy when testing for food allergies. It almost always agrees with skin tests for allergies. Since skin tests are expensive, painful, and can take many efforts until the allergen is identified, I use muscle testing first. I have also used it to identify supplements that contained ingredients an animal is allergic to. Without the muscle testing, the animal would have been given the supplements, and we would not have known there was a problem with them until the animal's health was affected.

An excellent book on this subject is *Your Body Doesn't Lie* by Dr. John Diamond, who pioneered in the field.

Pulse Diagnosis

Pulse diagnosis is another method that is used by many veterinarians as an aid both in choosing a medication and in diagnosis. When a con-

---

1 Jerry V. Teplitz, J.D., Ph.D. and Norma Eckroate, Switched-On Living: Easy Ways to Use the Mind/Body Connection to Energize Your Life, *(Charlottesville: Hampton Roads Publishing, 1994), p.16-17.*

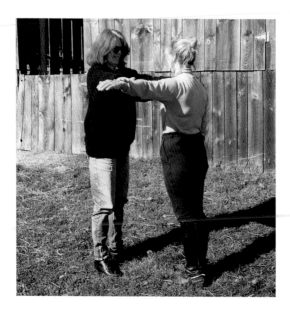

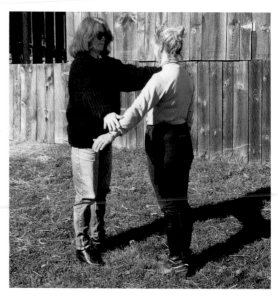

10.1 *First, test normal muscle resistance. Face your partner whose arm is outstretched. Place your hand just above the wrist of your partner's outstretched arm, and your other hand on your partner's opposite shoulder. Here, the partner is exhibiting good resistance under steady pressure; her arm is strong and is staying straight out.*

10.2 *The partner is now demonstrating poor arm resistance allowing it to be easily pressed down.*

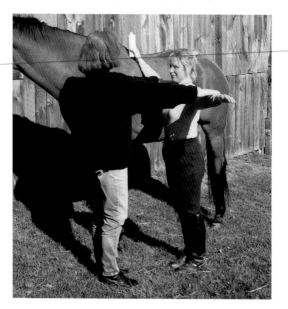

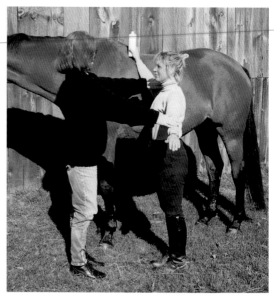

10.3 *Add the horse to the equation after you've tested normal resistance. Your partner—now your intermediary—stands holding the substance to be tested (remember to take the cap off) against the horse's side. Here the good resistance in the intermediary's arm indicates that this is a reliable substance for treating the horse.*

10.4 *If the result of the test is poor arm resistance, you will know that this is not an effective remedy for your horse.*

ventional medical doctor takes your pulse, he is only measuring one thing—the pulse rate of your heart. In traditional Chinese medicine, there are different pulses associated with each of the acupuncture meridians. The pulses are used to help pinpoint exactly which energy meridian is deficient. It requires considerable practice to distinguish the individual pulses and all of the variables possible for them. The technique must be taught by an expert as it can take years to develop the sensitivity to use it accurately as a diagnostic tool.

When doing pulse diagnosis, the vet checks all the pulses of an animal to find which one is weak. Then, while holding the proposed medication in one hand against the horse's body—it does not matter where—he checks to see if the weak pulse strengthens. If the medication is correct, a weakened pulse should return to near normal in the affected meridian; if the medication is not correct, the pulse will not react or it will worsen. This method has been found to be extremely accurate by the veterinarians who use it in their practice, and it is very helpful in selecting treatments.

ADMINISTERING MEDICATIONS AND TREATMENTS

The holistic veterinarian weighs a number of factors when choosing which specific treatments to prescribe for a sick or injured horse. For many medical conditions, there are treatment choices so the veterinarian will then consider which of the options is likely to be most effective while producing the fewest negative side effects. He must also consider any known allergies.

In addition to all of these factors, the veterinarian also must think about how the proposed treatments will be administered. After the veterinarian's initial visit, you, the owner, will most likely be giving any medication on an ongoing basis, so the veterinarian must make sure that you will be able to carry out his instructions accurately and without any danger to you or your horse. If the medication is in pill or liquid form, it often can be mixed into your horse's food, but some horses won't eat medicated food. In that instance, you can try an alternative method such as mixing the medicines with honey or molasses and giving them with a syringe, but you might need assistance if your horse objects to being dosed with a syringe.

Certain other medications can only be administered by injection. If your veterinarian proposes using one of these drugs, it's very important that he makes sure you are capable of giving injections and feel comfortable doing so. Otherwise, you will need to find someone else who can give the injections.

A final consideration is how often the medication must be given. If your horse lives at a boarding stable, this usually is not a problem because the stable manager or one of the staff members can give the medication as many times as necessary during the day. However, if you keep your horse at home, and you work at a job away from home, it could be difficult or even impossible for you to give medications three or four times a day.

When your horse requires medication as part of the treatment for an illness or injury, you should discuss all of the options thoroughly with your veterinarian. By working together, you will be able to develop a plan to insure that your horse gets the most benefit from the drug therapy.

MEDICATING YOUR HORSE

Giving Liquid Medications by Syringe

NOTE: If you are giving homeopathic remedies, please refer to specific guidelines in the *Homeopathics Appendix V* on p. 329.

To administer liquid medications it's best to use a syringe to prevent loss of medication and ensure accurate dosage. Syringes are available in a variety of sizes, from 1ml (the same as 1cc) to 60ml. If your syringe is marked in milliliters and you are following directions that call for a regular measurement, here are some conversions to help you:

1 drop	= 1/20ml
1 teaspoon	= 5ml (100 drops)
1 tablespoon	= 15ml
1 fluid ounce	= 30ml
1 cup	= 225ml

When liquid medications are prescribed, an allowance is usually made for a slight loss factor when administered. However, some medications require that the entire dosage be given very accurately. If you know that your horse is difficult and some medication may be lost be sure to check with your veterinarian to learn how accurate the dosage must be. With most liquid antibiotics it is okay to lose a tiny bit, but with some medications, it's essential that the dosage be precise.

When giving a liquid medication, hold your horse or place your horse in a position that will allow you to safely administer the medication and follow the steps listed below. Sometimes it's best to have someone help you, at least the first few times, until your horse realizes that there is nothing to fear when being given medication.

NOTE: If you have not medicated your horse before, be careful. Some horses have had bad experiences in the past and may overreact even though you are not threatening.

1. Talk to your horse about what you are going to do. Always use a soothing tone to explain the procedure. Have the medication ready.

2. Insert the syringe into the side of the horse's mouth and squirt the medication into the back of the mouth.

3. Once the syringe is emptied, close the mouth and keep the horse's head slightly elevated by holding your hand under his chin. Do not make fast moves—this may alarm your horse. Just talk softly and encourage him to relax and swallow.

Mixing Medication into Food or Water

NOTE: If you are giving homeopathic remedies, please refer to specific guidelines for giving homeopathics in the *Homeopathics Appendix V*, p.329.

If your horse is an enthusiastic eater, you may be able to mix some medications into his food. Many tablets are given—either whole or crushed—in the grain. However, picky eaters often detect the medication and refuse to eat. If you have a picky eater but still feel this is the best way to get the horse to take medication, try adding something to the grain to encourage the horse to eat it. I find that molasses, honey, and apple sauce have flavors horses like, and any of these foods will help to disguise the taste of the medication. Another alternative is to mix the medication with a dry fruit-flavored gelatin like Jello (jelly in the UK) and add the mixture to the grain. Orange is a favorite flavor with horses. Most of these gelatin products contain sugar, so avoid them if you know that your horse does not tolerate sugar. You may want to experiment to find out which of these alternatives your horse likes best.

Put the medication in only a part of the meal and serve that first. As soon as your horse has eaten the medicated portion of his meal, you can give the rest of it. That way if the horse isn't hungry you don't risk him missing out on part of the medication. Don't just put the food out and assume your horse will eat it when he gets hungry; this could be very dangerous if your horse is already ill. He could miss both a meal and the needed medication. If your horse will not take medication in grain, discuss other options of giving the medication with your veterinarian. Some medications that come as tablets can be pulverized and mixed with water or molasses then injected into the mouth with a syringe following the steps outlined above for giving liquid medications.

Very few medications are administered by mixing with your horse's drinking water. However, in case you encounter one that has to be given in the horse's drinking water, here are some suggestions. Be sure to introduce the medication gradually to the water. A sudden change in taste may cause the horse to stop drinking entirely. If the medication has an unpleasant taste, try adding another substance to disguise that taste. When using this method it's best to add the taste enhancer first, allow the horse to get used to that new taste, then add the medication.

I have had success using honey, molasses, Kool-Aid (a fruit-flavored drink made from powder), and apple cider. Although each horse has his own favorite flavor of Kool-Aid, orange and cherry seem to be favorites. Use a small amount—about 1/2 teaspoon per 1 cup (225ml) of water should be enough to flavor the water and cover up the taste of the medication. You don't want to use much because all of these choices are very sweet and Kool-Aid contains a lot of sugar. Add the flavoring in tiny amounts, gradually increasing it as the horse gets used to this new taste. Be aware that these mixtures will attract flies into the water bucket.

It's very important to monitor the water supply to ensure that the horse is drinking enough and not becoming dehydrated. Remember, your horse's instinct tells him not to drink odd-tasting water, so don't just assume that he will drink the medicated and flavored water. Try putting some in his mouth to taste. You can also try giving a taste to the horse next to him (providing that the horse will try it); often if a horse sees other horses eating or drinking something, he will try it too.

GIVING INJECTIONS

I recommend that horse owners become proficient at giving intramuscular injections so they will be able to do it if required for a treatment or in an emergency situation. (This is not as critical for owners in the UK where laws are different and veterinarians are usually in close proximity.) Many times I have received an emergency call from an owner living in an isolated area whose horse was in a life-threatening situation. Most of these owners are prepared with their own emergency kits, so they have been able to administer any necessary injections I prescribed to keep the horse comfortable until I was able to get there. It's also helpful for an owner to be able to administer injections while traveling. Occasionally a situation arises that requires tranquilization immediately, such as a traffic accident or a panicked horse stuck in its trailer. A friend of mine once had to contend with a panicked horse stuck in the escape door of the trailer. Unfortunately, she did not have a tranquilizer on hand, and the nearest vet was an hour away. The horse nearly died while struggling to free himself.

If you are inexperienced at giving injections and wish to learn how to properly administer them, ask your veterinarian to teach you. Most veterinarians are happy to demonstrate the procedure and give you a bit of coaching. However, before giving any injection, you should discuss the symptoms being treated with your veterinarian and get her approval.

The two types of injection procedures are *intramuscular* and *intravenous*. The intramuscular injection is administered in one of the large muscle groups on the horse's body. The most

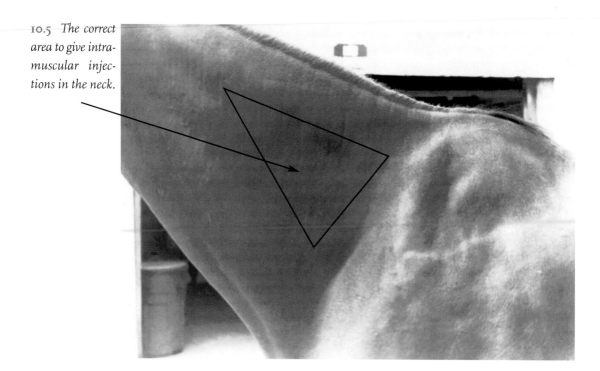

10.5 The correct area to give intramuscular injections in the neck.

common areas used are the neck and upper hind legs. Figure 10.5 demonstrates a triangular area where it is safe to give an injection in the neck. It's important that injections are given only in that area of the neck. The area below the triangle is where the neck vertebra or bones are located. If you inserted a needle into the vertebra, you might hit a bone and cause an irritation to the bone covering or periosteum. You also want to avoid the area above the triangle towards the mane because here the horse's neck is made up of dense connective tissue and a large ligament where there is less blood circulation. Medication given in this part of the neck would be absorbed too slowly into the bloodstream.

Injections are frequently given in the large muscle group on the back of the hind legs. Be careful when doing this because your horse may kick. The area marked on the photo is the best to use with most horses (fig. 10.6).

The hip area is not a good place for an injection because there is no drainage if an abscess

should develop due to an infection. When abscesses do occur in the gluteal region, the only possible direction of drainage is downward into the major muscle groups in that area. This can result in atrophy of the muscles and damage to the surrounding tissue.

Veterinarians sometimes advise using other injection sites if those commonly used become sore from repeated injections. The alternatives include the chest muscles in the front of the horse, the large muscle area above the front leg, and the large muscle area on the upper hind leg just above the stifle on the side of the leg. ***Caution:*** *Do not use these areas unless specifically directed to do so by your veterinarian and be sure to have the veterinarian point out the exact locations that are safe.*

Intravenous (IV) injections are given in the jugular vein on the neck. When giving an injection in this area there is a dangerous risk of accidentally puncturing an artery instead of the vein. This can cause a major problem because

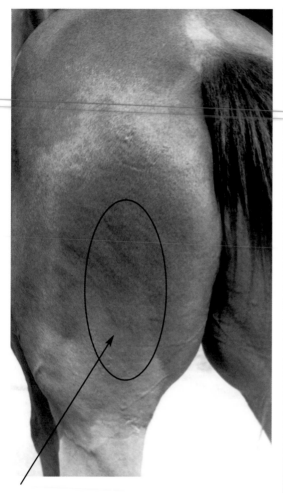

10.6 *The correct location to give intramuscular injections in the hindquarter.*

individual horse responds to injections. If you are inexperienced with horses, it's best to have a more seasoned person or your veterinarian assist you the first time you give an injection.

Normally, it is important that you give injections only under orders from your veterinarian, but in an emergency situation you should be able to administer a tranquilizer if necessary. Ask your veterinarian to calculate the correct tranquilizer dosage for your horse and keep this information among the papers in your emergency kit. Some owners routinely vaccinate their own horses. Keep in mind, however, that your veterinarian cannot give you a vaccination certificate, or sign an F.E.I. (Fédération Equestre Internationale) passport, for your horse unless she has administered the vaccine herself. Many boarding stables request a copy of a vaccination certificate prior to accepting new horses. In addition, vaccination certificates are often required for other reasons, such as when entering horse shows and for travel across state or country borders. If these factors are not relevant for you and you choose to administer vaccines yourself, you should discuss with your veterinarian which ones are best for your horse in order to avoid any adverse physiological reactions.

Reactions to Injections

Each horse must be monitored for at least ten minutes after any injection. Although it is rare, it is always possible for a horse to go into anaphylactic (allergic) shock. If he does, he must be treated immediately or he could die. Signs of anaphylactic shock include the following: the horse's mucus membranes (the area over the gums) become pale pink or white; the horse may wobble, start to sweat or lie down; or the horse may break out in hives. If your horse is known to be especially sensitive to injections in the past, has had allergic reactions to changes in feed or insect bites, or if you don't know, for safety's

some medications cause violent reactions if given in the artery. ***Caution:*** *Intravenous injection is a procedure that is best handled by veterinarians.*

Precautions When Giving Injections

Some horses barely seem to notice an injection while others object strongly, so you should always prepare by properly restraining the horse before giving the injection. Over time, you will develop a better sense of the way in which each sake it may be best to have the veterinarian administer all injections. Also, if your horse is insured, injections must be administered by a veterinarian only.

If a reaction to an injection occurs, call your veterinarian immediately. Tell him that while you are waiting you are going to start a homeopathic remedy by giving homeopathic apis 6C, or 12C, every fifteen minutes to help counteract the reaction. Keep giving it every fifteen minutes until the reaction subsides or your veterinarian arrives. (Be sure to follow the guidelines for administering homeopathics in the *Homeopathics Appendix V* on p. 329). In addition to the homeopathic, I also advise giving a few drops of Bach Flowers Rescue Remedy which is quite helpful in diminishing the effects of anaphylactic shock. It can also be given as often as every fifteen minutes.

The effects and lasting ability of any homeopathic or Rescue Remedy will vary depending on the type and severity of injury and other circumstances. So if you're using them in response to any allergic reaction or other emergency, remember to re-dose if immediate improvement is not evident, or if improvement has occurred but the reaction has started again, while you are waiting for the veterinarian to arrive.

BANDAGING FOR THE STABLE

There are various bandages and bandaging methods, including stable, exercise, polo, shipping, and other specialty wraps. All horse owners should have basic bandaging supplies on hand, and the knowledge to apply them.

Here, I'm going to discuss stable (sometimes referred to as "standing") bandages, since they are commonly used for many purposes: after strenuous work to prevent swelling ("stocking up"); to prevent a fractious horse from injuring himself in a stall; to protect an injury; and to hold a dressing in place.

(In Chapter Eight, page 129 I told you about *Bandaging for Exercise* and the process is similar). The materials you need are:

- 4 *pads* of cotton sheeting, or quilted fabric sized to fit the horse's legs.
- 4 non-elasticized *bandages* made of cotton or polyester with Velcro closures, or string ties. (If they do not have Velcro closures, you need masking tape, or safety pins, at the ready.)

To begin the bandaging process have all your supplies ready. The pads should already be neatly rolled, as should the bandages. Be sure the closures are rolled into the bandage correctly. There is nothing more frustrating than getting a horse's leg all wrapped and then discovering that the Velcro is the wrong way up!

Stand your horse in a clean place and be sure his leg is clean also. Wrap the pad around the leg so it is positioned smoothly between the knee (or hock) to just below the fetlock joint.

Start to bandage over the pad at mid-cannon on the outside of the leg tucking the end of the bandage under the edge of the pad. As you wrap, it's very important to remember to only apply tension to the bandage when passing over the *front* of the cannon, and not at the *back* of the leg, or over the *tendons*.

Make one wrap around the mid-cannon, and then begin wrapping downward over the fetlock joint until you've covered all but a half-inch of the pad that will be showing. At this point, wrap back up the leg to just below the knee (or hock), again leaving a half-inch of pad showing on top.

Now wrap a few turns back down the leg to use up the bandage. Always finish the bandage on the outside of the leg, mid-cannon. Fasten it securely with the closure you have at hand. If you are concerned that your horse might fiddle with the wraps, you can apply masking, or duct, tape over the closure for extra security (figs. 10.7–10.9).

When you use stable bandages to protect an injury, be sure to first clean the wound and apply any topical remedy. Then you can place gauze over the wound before bandaging in order to prevent the wrap from sticking to the wound.

For shipping, bandages are applied much the same as stable bandages. The main difference is that a shipping bandage should be wrapped low enough to cover the bulbs of the hoof and the coronary band. You do this to protect these sensitive areas in case the horse loses his balance in the trailer or van and steps on himself.

APPLYING POULTICES AND COMPRESSES

The purpose of a poultice is to reduce swelling by "drawing out" heat, inflammation, and infection from an injured area, and/or to increase the blood supply to aid in its healing—for example the tendons around the cannon bone. A compress is usually used for soothing an injury by applying a cold (sometimes ice cold to reduce inflammation) or warm medicinal substance to an inflamed eye for, instance. Poultices and compresses can be used anywhere on a horse's body and most horses enjoy their comforting qualities so they don't try to remove the bandages.

Poultices can be divided into two general types—hot poultices, also referred to as a "sweat," and cold poultices. A hot poultice is applied to increase blood supply to an area that helps a wound heal more quickly, and it is also commonly used to draw out an abscess, or small "foreign" body. Cold poultices are used to reduce fluid or swelling from an area.

Poultices are applied directly onto the hair and can be used anywhere that a bandage can be put on top of the poultice, or where the poultice matter will stay on by itself. You can put some gauze on underneath the poultice in order to keep the poultice ingredients in one place more easily before bandaging. A poultice should not be left on for more than 12 hours unless otherwise directed by your veterinarian. An exception would be a foot poultice that is often left on for a longer period to help draw out an abscess. However, you should still check with your veterinarian on the amount of time a poultice should remain.

When you remove a poultice make sure it is completely washed off. Sometimes you can brush a dried poultice off, but even then it is advisable to wash the area to be sure all of the poultice has gone so you avoid the skin becoming irritated.

Commercially made "hot" poultices are available. These are poultices containing an ingredient that "heats up" while bandaged on an injury. In the US a hot poultice is usually made of nitrofurazone applied directly from a jar and then covered with kitchen plastic wrap, a pad, and a bandage. In Europe many commercially available hot poultices contain ingredients such as bassoria and boric acid already impregnated into a thick padded bandage material with plastic backing. The bandage is cut to size, saturated with hot water, squeezed dry, and then placed on the affected area.

Cold poultices usually contain clay. They can be made from powdered clay that is mixed with water before applying, or purchased in a ready-to-apply form. Then, once the poultice is in place, some newspaper or a piece of a brown paper bag is placed over it to prevent whatever comes next—the cotton padding, quilt wrap, and main bandage—from absorbing the clay materials (figs. 10.10–10.13).

Types of home-made poultices which can be applied warm or cold include ingredients such as wheat bran, charcoal, linseed meal, or vegetables such as onions which draw out fluid. Herbal poultices can be made from fresh, dried, or powdered herbs. Hot poultices or compresses can be made by soaking the materials in an herbal tea (see the *Herb Appendix IV* on p. 321 for instructions on making teas. Look for chamomile, cliv-

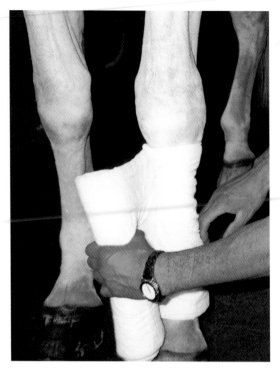

10.7

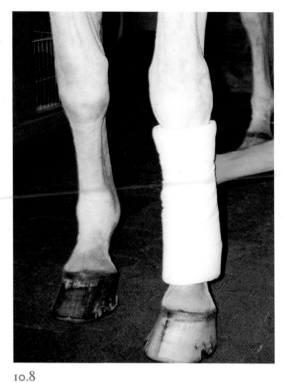

10.8

10.7–10.9 *You can learn to apply stable bandages with ease after a little practice (see p. 156). The secret is to go step-by-step, and position both your pads and wraps carefully so the result is a neat, secure bandage as shown here.*

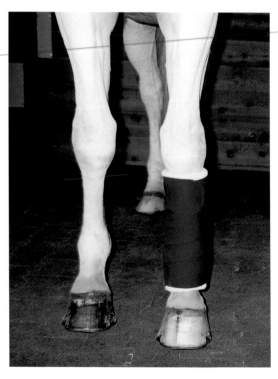

10.9

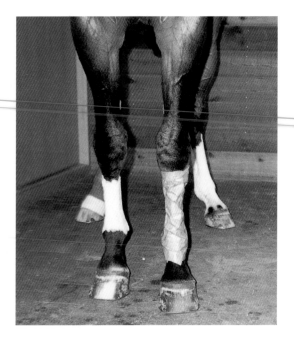

10.10 *Start the poulticing process by spreading an even layer of poultice over the cannon bone area as shown on this horse's right front leg. If you've used a cold poultice as shown on his left front leg, wrap a piece of newspaper or brown paper over the poultice.*

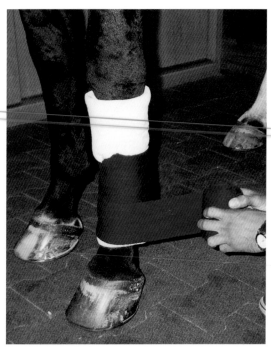

10.11 *Proceed just as you would to apply a stable bandage. Place cotton sheeting, or a quilted pad, over the paper, and begin wrapping downward over the fetlock joint.*

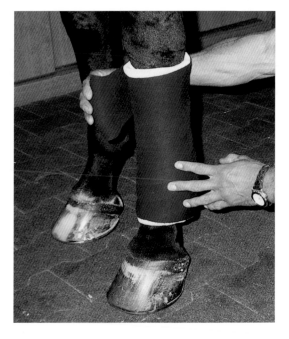

10.12 *Plan to come to the end of your bandage just below the knee. Secure the bandage on the outside of the leg. This is not only easier for the caretaker, but prevents interference from the opposite leg.*

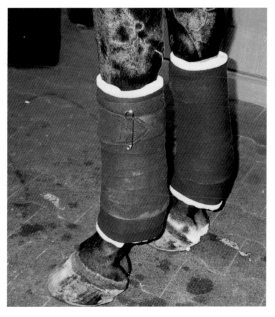

10.13 *Even if you are applying a poultice to one leg only, bandage both front legs, or all four. Most bandages purchased today have Velcro closures, but some people still prefer ties or safety pins.*

ers, comfrey, eyebright, kelp, marshmallow, and slippery elm).

Some fresh herbs—comfrey for instance, which works well on bone bruises—are best used whole, while others will need to be "bruised", chopped, or mashed. When you desire their specific healing properties, you can add certain herbs to commercially produced hot or cold poultices, or mix them with the clay varieties. NOTE: I have suggested a number of poulticing uses for different herbs and plants in the *Herb* and *Aromatherapy Appendices.*

The easiest way to make poultices or compresses from herbs is to place the herbs between two pieces of thin cotton cloth, cheese cloth, or gauze, then soak them in hot or cold water before bandaging or placing on. Some herbs may be difficult to work with because of their consistency. An alternative method of dealing with these herbs is to make a tea by adding the herbs to boiling water then leaving the tea to steep for 30 minutes. Dip your cloth into the tea and apply as a poultice or compress, hot or cold, as needed.

Kaolin and Epsom salts are frequently used as warm poultices for foot problems—a common example is for drawing out abscesses. *(Caution: Do not use these ingredients if an open wound is present.)* Kaolin comes in a can or tin that you place in hot water and warm up, then spread on gauze and apply to the foot before bandaging. I also suggest using Epsom salts mixed with other poultice ingredients such as wheat bran. Use one part Epsom salts to three parts wheat bran. Mix the ingredients altogether with hot water until the consistency is crumbly but not pasty, and then after it has cooled a bit apply to the foot before bandaging.

A HEALING ENVIRONMENT

When your horse has suffered an illness or been injured, the environment you provide will influ-

ence his rate of recovery. An extra dose of tender loving care will go a long way. Always be sure your horse is comfortable—notice that your sick horse may gravitate to a certain area in the stall or pasture because he is seeking warmth, coolness, or comfort, so be consistent in providing for his needs.

Here are a few considerations when caring for an ailing horse:

Check the area where your horse is recuperating. Is he resting quietly or pacing the stall? Some horses respond better to a restful stall or paddock away from the busiest part of the barn, while others prefer to be entertained by the hustle and bustle and attention of a more central area.

If your horse has to be in a stall all the time and/or is lying down often, check the bedding in the stall to be sure it provides enough support and absorption. Remember, horses can get pressure sores if they lie down on too hard a surface for a long period of time, so evaluate the bedding carefully. If your horse is having trouble rising after lying down, be sure the bedding is not slippery, as straw can sometimes be. For long recoveries, when a horse is going to be down more than usual, peat or shredded paper work well.

Check your horse's diet to make sure it is high quality and that the nutrients are digestible. Also, make sure that the amount of food is appropriate to your horse's needs. He may not need as much feed if he is not exercising.

Do not expect your horse to perform normal activities when ill. A sick animal cannot adhere to a regular training schedule.

Avoid taking your horse on extended trips when ill. Travel can be very stressful and sometimes makes the problem worse.

Pain

Treat your horse with just as much respect as you would want if you were ill or injured. Remember that just because horses can't talk and tell us about the pain they are experiencing doesn't mean they don't feel it. Most horses recover from illness or injury much more quickly than people and can return to exercise gradually. However, each case is unique. Watch your horse for signs of discomfort, including lack of appetite, stiff movement, or uncharacteristic behavior, such as not wanting to be touched or brushed.

If you suspect your horse is in pain, do not jump to the conclusion that medication must be administered immediately. There are times, with tendon or bone injuries for example, when it is best that your horse experience a little pain so he will limit his movement and allow healing to take place. If you medicate a horse that should not be moving around, he will be without pain and may exercise more than he should, possibly doing more damage. This can be a very fine line for some horses because any pain can lead to colic or laminitis. You need to consult your veterinarian whenever your horse is in noticeable pain.

Following a surgical procedure, horses are often very uncomfortable. The best medication to help relieve this distress is arnica, a homeopathic remedy that decreases inflammation and pain. It is very effective and is my treatment of choice both for horses and myself for many types of pain. A potency of 30x up to 30C is sometimes effective in alleviating pain and helping to diminish bruising and inflammation that occurs after minor surgery. Give these potencies five times the first day, then three times a day for the following seven days.

If the operation was major, such as surgery for colic, then a higher potency of arnica—200C, 1M, or 10M, may be called for. Give the higher potency of arnica three times a day for the first three days, then once a day for seven days. Higher potency homeopathics such as these are often only available through a homeopathic veterinarian or homeopathic pharmacist and they will also be able to advise you on the frequency of doses for your horse's specific needs.

Another alternative (or, in addition to the arnica) is to give phenylbutazone, sometimes referred to as "bute." Bute is available in tablet or paste form and does not interfere with arnica. Arnica will not upset the stomach as bute sometimes does and can be given long-term with no ill effects.

Caution: *Always consult your veterinarian before giving any medication for pain, especially following surgery.*

FASTING

Fasting is sometimes a normal response to illness; a horse instinctively stops eating while his body focuses his energy on recovery. During fasting, his body goes through a normal detoxification process as it expels wastes and cleanses organs, glands, and cells. But a total fast should be avoided. A horse's digestive tract depends on roughage to continue to function in a normal manner. If no food or water is taken, the food already in the system may move along too slowly. If the food stops moving altogether, it can become impacted in the digestive tract. That's why it is important to encourage a horse to at least eat small amounts of hay during most illnesses. Consult your veterinarian immediately if your horse is not eating or if you have any specific questions on feeding a sick horse.

Always supply plenty of fresh water to horses that are not eating well. Your veterinarian may recommend adding electrolytes to the water to support your horse's body during a stressful period. But don't just add electrolytes to the water and assume that your horse will drink it. Many horses are unaccustomed to the taste and may decrease their water consumption when the electrolytes are mixed in it. For this reason, it is important to monitor the water consumption carefully so the horse is guarded against dehydration. If your horse goes more than three hours without drinking, provide fresh water without electrolytes.

REHABILITATING AN ABUSED HORSE

When you take on a horse who has had a history of abuse, there are a number of things you can do to help heal the past emotional wounds and speed the rehabilitation process along. It's important to do whatever you can in terms of special considerations so the horse will not get upset. Take note of the horse's previous environment, and try to see his new one as he would perceive it. This includes the stable or pasture, the diet, any medications, and even what's in the water. For instance, a horse who is not accustomed to being kept in a stall may find the space too confining.

I recommend using Bach Flower remedies to help ease the horse through the transition. Learn as much as you can about the horse's behavior and then review my discussion of Bach Flower remedies in Chapter Three, and in the *Bach Flower Appendix III*, and/or research a book about Bach Flowers as to which remedies would be appropriate. If you have no information on the horse's history, and you can't predict how he will react to various situations, then try using Rescue Remedy. Another option is to put yourself in the horse's place and see how you would feel in the same circumstances. Write down your emotions and use the Bach Flower that best treats those emotions. If the horse will not allow you to put the medication in his mouth, put some drops in his water bucket or on a sugar cube. You only need a few drops.

Many abused horses need to gain weight and will require a new feeding program, but any changes to the diet should be made gradually. Do not get carried away and overfeed the horse. No matter how much weight the horse needs to gain, his body systems need time to adjust to the changeover from survival mode to weight-gain mode. Ask your veterinarian for assistance when considering what foods will work best. Diet can strongly influence the horse's behavior. If the diet is a little too rich at first, the digestive system may become upset and the horse will not feel well. Since it's difficult to tell when a horse is not feeling well, we may think that he is difficult to handle or has a bad disposition when in reality he has a mild stomachache. Worse, if the diet is changed too rapidly, the horse may get a case of colic and become severely ill.

A horse that has been abused in the past also may suffer from parasite problems, which could manifest as digestive upsets and failure to gain weight. Often it's a good idea to give abused horses the homeopathic remedy nux vomica in a low potency such as 6C or 12C, twice a day for a week. It seems to strengthen the liver and improve digestion, allowing digestive changes to occur more easily. Your veterinarian may want to follow the nux vomica with another homeopathic, such as ipecacuanha, calcarea carbonica, or carbo vegetabilis, that is more specific to the exact digestive problem that the horse is experiencing.

Linda Tellington-Jones' healing and training systems, TTEAM and TTouch, first mentioned in Chapter Three of this book, are also helpful in modifying the behavior of abused horses. I have seen many instances in which terrified horses settle down after some TTEAM work. Usually these techniques are done hands-on, or with a dressage whip that in TTEAM is called a "wand." But I have seen situations where horses have not allowed a person near them so that the TTouches had to be performed using a long bendable object like a lightweight plastic pipe. When the procedure was completed, the horses allowed people near them again and then the work could be done hands-on. Although these circumstances were extreme, the methods worked effectively resulting in difficult, upset horses being taught to enjoy human interaction and become confident and happy.

A HEALTH CARE KIT FOR HOME AND TRAVEL

You should always discuss any medication with your veterinarian before giving it to your horse, but every owner should keep certain medications and first-aid supplies on hand all the time. In the event of a sudden illness or injury, you should be prepared to administer basic first aid to your horse if necessary while you are waiting for the veterinarian to arrive.

In other non-emergency situations—for example, in the case of a lameness that has developed gradually—the veterinarian might tell you to give your horse a medication such as arnica to relieve discomfort if she is unable to schedule an appointment for your horse for several days. Remember again, however, if you are speaking to your vet, it's best not to give any medication without explicit instructions.

Listed below are the commonly needed medical items that I recommend my clients always keep on hand. The homeopathic remedies mentioned here are the ones most frequently used, and the potencies I have suggested are those that can be administered safely by the owner. For more information on homeopathic remedies, see Chapter Three; the *Homeopathics Appendix V* on p. 329; and in the lists of recommendations for *Horse Ailments* in Part Three.

Homeopathics

Apis 6C, 12C, or 30C. Use for allergic reactions, particularly hives. Also effective for reactions to insect bites.

Magnesium Phosphate 6C. Use for relieving muscle spasms and for mild cases of tying-up syndrome.

Arnica 30C. Use as an anti-inflammatory. Excellent for inflammation in joints as well as muscles, also bruising and hemotomas.

Nux Vomica 6C, 12C, or 30C. Use for digestive upsets.

Phosphorous 6C, 12C, or 30C. Use for respiratory problems. Also helps to stop excessive bleeding.

Bach Flower Remedies

Rescue Remedy. This product is a combination of five Bach Flower remedies (cherry plum, clematis, impatiens, rock rose, and star of Bethlehem). It is used to calm horses when they are under stress and is especially valuable in emergency situations. Although it does not replace the use of a tranquilizer in an emergency, it is very effective in restoring a horse to a calm, peaceful state of mind.

Aspen and Walnut. Both of these remedies help horses adjust to new situations. Use if traveling to a new location for a few days, particularly if your horse does not adapt quickly to new surroundings or becomes nervous.

To determine which other Bach Flower remedies you may want to have on hand, you can consult one of the numerous books available on the topic. Or read the insert from a package which gives short descriptions of all the Bach Flower remedies.

Herbs

Comfrey. Use in powder form to make poultices for horse's legs to assist in healing tendon problems and bone fractures.

Valerian Root. Use to calm horses.

Yunnan Paiyao (available in Chinese pharmacies). Use to control bleeding.

Supplements

Vitamin C , 500mg. or 1 gram tablets. Most horses like cherry chewable vitamin C tablets. Vitamin C provides excellent protection from viruses and also helps decrease symptoms of arthritis. Give 8 grams once a day for a 1,000-pound horse.

Vitamin E and Selenium. Use a brand specifically formulated for horses and follow label directions for dosage. These supplements are important if your horse regularly performs strenuous activities such as jumping or galloping. They can also be helpful if your horse becomes muscle sore or ties up.

Magnetic Therapy

Magnets are widely available in many forms and can be used for tendon, bone, or joint problems. If an injury has just occurred and is hot to the touch, do not use a magnet over the area immediately. Wait at least 24 hours until the inflammation is decreased in the injured area and then apply it. If you are competing your horse a great deal, take magnets with you when you travel. (See *Magnetic Therapy* in Chapter Three).

External Medications

Arnica Lotion. Use as a topical anti-inflammatory on tendons, bones, and hematomas.

BHI Traumeel. This ointment combines homeopathic arnica and other homeopathic remedies. It is used for the same problems as arnica lotion.

Calendula Gel. Use for skin irritations.

Antibiotic cream. Use for minor cuts. Keep only a small jar so it can be inexpensively replaced when outdated.

Hydrogen peroxide solution (regular 3% topical solution, not the 35% food-grade hydrogen peroxide described in Chapter Three). When treating a puncture wound use by pouring it into the wound after the initial cleanup is finished or as part of the cleanup. Always consult your veterinarian when your horse suffers a puncture wound.

Poultice and compress materials.

Injectable and Oral Medications

Flunixin Meglumine (Banamine). Consult your veterinarian about keeping this drug in your emergency kit. It can be given intramuscularly and is used to treat minor colic symptoms. If you have more than one horse, discuss each horse's appropriate dosage with your veterinarian and keep a record of this information in your kit along with the Banamine. If your horse colics, however, do not give Banamine without first consulting your veterinarian. The veterinarian can then make sure the correct dosage and medications are being selected and determine if an immediate veterinary call is required.

Phenylbutazone ("bute"). This is used as an anti-inflammatory. It is available in one gram tablets, and in paste form. It has a bitter taste so many horses will not eat the tablets even when ground up and mixed with feed. An alternative is to crush the tablets, mix with water or syrup, and administer by dose syringe. Do not use "bute" if your horse has, or has had, stomach ulcers since it can irritate the stomach lining.

Tranquilizers. Giving tranquilizers is not something I recommend for all horse owners, but if you regularly trailer your horse long distances, or if you do not have a veterinarian within fairly close proximity, it can be very helpful to have a tranquilizer on hand in case of emergency. Only those who are very familiar with the use of tranquilizers and have discussed the options thoroughly with their veterinarian should give them. There are many different kinds and the selection of which one you should have on hand will be up to your veterinarian. (See p. 63).

First Aid Supplies

- 1 sterile cotton roll
- 2 rolls of elastic self-adhesive wrap (known as Vet Wrap in the US)
- 1 roll of stretch gauze
- box of nonstick large-size gauze pads
- 1 roll of 1/2-inch wide adhesive tape
- 1 roll of 1 or 2-inch wide adhesive tape
- Bandage scissors
- Dose syringe, 60cc
- Brown paper bags (for poulticing)
- Plastic kitchen wrap

Documents

Records of vaccinations, and details of medications and dosages.

II Traveling with Your Horse

Shipping horses by van or trailer has become a commonplace activity, but along with the convenience of being able to travel with your horse come certain concerns. When traveling over long distances, horses may be exposed to a variety of potential health risks including dust inhaled while on the road, extreme changes in temperature or humidity levels, and confinement in trailers that are poorly ventilated. Long distance travel has been associated with problems such as dehydration, colic, diarrhea, constipation, founder (laminitis), and respiratory diseases. With careful planning, however, you can prevent most of these problems.

I have made two long distance moves with a horse and didn't hesitate to take him along either time. There are a few tips that can make your trip successful, whether it's a short trip or a long one. In this chapter I'll review feeding and watering during travel as well as other considerations of how to deal with travel stress.

TRAILERING YOUR HORSE

First, let's review the basics, starting with evaluating your horse. Does your horse trailer well? That's the most crucial question you need to answer before considering anything else. Most people learn the answer to this question when they first buy a horse and have to get him home. However, if your horse was purchased at the same stable where he still lives or arrived on a horse transport van, you might not. The best way to learn about your horse's behavior is to ask the people you buy him from. Be sure to enquire in detail, preferably before you buy him. If your future plans for the horse require significant amounts of travel—for instance, to horse shows or trail rides—his earlier experiences and attitude about trailering may be factors in your decision on whether he is the right horse for you.

If your horse is delivered to you by the previous owner, take a good look at the trailer or van he arrives in. Note whether it has a step up, or a ramp. Is it a slant-load, or side-by-side? What is your horse's attitude while in the trailer? Is he calm or kicking out? How does he respond to unloading? This information can give you clues to whether the horse is an easy experienced traveler or is uncomfortable in the trailer.

My own experience with trailering horses has been extensive, and the most important thing I've learned is that each horse must be treated as an individual. One of my old Thoroughbreds had raced extensively and traveled a great deal, so he was a very calm, adaptable traveler, who could be trailered long distances for several days without experiencing any problems—that is, once he got on the trailer!

Unfortunately, this horse had mostly been handled by men in the past and was far more difficult for a woman to load. I was able to improve his attitude but never to completely change it. It was exasperating and embarrassing for me when he would refuse to go on. Sometimes he would not only refuse but also sit down like a mule. If a man walked up, took hold of the rope, and told him to load, up he would jump right on the trailer instantly, as if he had suddenly changed into another horse.

This type of behavior serves to remind us of another characteristic of horses: remembering unpleasant experiences from the past. Since a horse's survival in the wild depended on memory, this trait is not easy to overcome with training, so the ideal plan is to train your horse correctly from the start. Avoiding unpleasant experiences with trailer training can be difficult because some horses seem to overreact to the situation. The goal is to get your horse accustomed to trailering with as few traumatic experiences as possible. However, many horses come with trailering problems, and you'll have to assess them as you go, deciding on the best method to deal with the specific problems as they arise.

When I got Charlie, I was told that he had only a few trailering experiences. It turned out that this meant he had been trailered a few times in a large open trailer used to haul cattle. When I went to pick him up in a standard two-horse trailer, the confined space of the stalls frightened him. He wasn't interested in leaving the only home he had ever known; his only concern was going back to the stable. Eventually I convinced him to load, but this experience didn't count as training. I wanted him to reliably load into the trailer, a goal I knew would take some serious time and a good training method. I used several techniques but it is the one taught by John Lyons and others that I recommend. This system teaches the horse to make the decision to load himself.

Attach a long, strong rope (or longe line) to your horse's halter. From where he stands behind the trailer run the rope through the inside of the trailer, out through the side door, and hold it back at the rear near the horse. You then tap the horse on his hind end with a whip (not whip him) and as soon as he moves forward a step, stop tapping and praise him lavishly. He quickly learns that stepping forward is the avenue of least resistance.

Before even attempting to train Charlie to load into the trailer, I worked with him to make sure he was paying attention to me. This may sound simple, but it's definitely not. Charlie and I also used TTEAM groundwork to make him more aware of his feet, including exercises such as leading him over poles and moving through objects (see Appendix VIII for TTEAM information). Charlie was a very large young horse, and he frequently tried to use his size and strength to his advantage. The groundwork helped him focus on what we were doing at the moment instead of thinking about returning to the barn or noticing what the other horses were doing. By doing this work first, Charlie was prepared for the actual trailer training process, which went smoothly and did not have to be repeated. He has remained a reliable loader.

The trailer training I used with Charlie is also very effective with horses that have had traumatic trailering experiences in the past. If you plan to retrain your horse, be sure you are prepared and experienced enough to handle the horse and also that you have adequate equipment. Unless you feel qualified to handle any situation that might arise, I suggest that you seek professional assistance. John Lyons and many others run training clinics that can teach you how to trailer train your horse by getting his attention and allowing him to make the loading decision on his own.

Once you have assessed your horse's trailering ability, you need to become familiar with his trailering habits. First learn how he travels. Some horses brace their legs in a particular manner, while others, like my horse Silver, "sit" on the butt bar. This information can help you understand the ideal way to make your horse comfortable when traveling. If your horse needs to brace his legs outward it's important that he have the space to do this. Many trailers do not have full center dividers (the type that go all the way to the floor) but just a center bar which allows horses room to spread their hind legs wider when traveling. This is a feature to look for in a trailer if your horse prefers bracing his legs that way.

Silver did not travel well in trailers that had butt chains instead of bars, since he could not sit comfortably on the chain. As a result, he shifted and moved throughout the entire ride. This was not restful for him and it was disconcerting for me as the driver of a trailer that constantly moved every time he shifted his weight.

Each horse reacts differently when he is uncomfortable in a trailer. Excessive movement,

kicking, and scrambling are some of the ways that horses indicate discomfort. Scrambling in a trailer can be difficult to describe if you have not experienced it. The horse seems to panic and begin running in place as he tries to find a way to brace himself. Sometimes I find that a horse will stop this behavior once he is switched to a trailer that better suits him. With others, this behavior becomes a habit. If your horse scrambles or exhibits behavior that resembles scrambling, such as climbing up the wall or into the manger, experiment with other trailers to see if his behavior improves.

One technique that often helps is to put a problem horse in a large trailer with no dividers and let him travel backwards. This usually results in a good trailering experience and assists with retraining.

Because horses can get into trouble if left untied in a trailer, the head should be tied. Trailer ties should be left in the trailer so they will always be there when you need them. You can buy special trailer ties that are equipped with breakaway snaps designed to come apart if enough pressure is put on them, allowing the horse to get free. However, despite the clever design of breakaway snaps, whether the breakaway snap is on the horse's halter or attached to the trailer, they do not always unsnap when a horse pulls back.

When you are tying the horse, be sure to leave enough slack in the tie so his head can be held in its normal position and some side-to-side movement is possible. If the tie line is high and too short forcing the horse to hold his head above the normal position, normal sinus drainage will not be possible. Since a lot of dust is kicked up in the trailer when traveling, this can make the horse more prone to respiratory problems.

When you make a stop during your journey, check the horse to see if he relaxes. Most horses stay in the same posture that they travel in, with their legs locked in a tense, rigid position. If he doesn't move his legs a little (more than kicking the trailer), his circulation could become impaired. So check your horse's posture before leaving and then again when you stop to see if he has changed his position. If he does not move much, it's wise to unload him every four to six hours and walk him around for some exercise. Be cautious when choosing an area to unload, particularly if your horse is not used to strange noises or sights. Many people use roadside rest areas for this purpose and they can work well, but keep an eye out for running children who might frighten your horse. You don't want to lose control of a horse so close to a road.

If your journey is going to last over four hours, it's best to know if your horse will urinate while traveling in the trailer. Many horses won't, so it might be necessary to stop and allow your horse an opportunity to urinate. (Even if your horse does urinate in the trailer, most horses will not urinate as often as they normally do, so it is wise to take him out for this purpose.) You will have to observe your horse to know his urinary frequency at home so you'll have an idea of what to expect. Most horses urinate every two to four hours during the day.

FEEDING WHILE TRAVELING

Most horses will eat in the trailer, although some will eat only hay and not grain. In any case, your horse should have an adequate supply of hay available to eat at will while on the road. Some trailers are equipped with a permanent hayrack in the front, but if you are using a hay net, it must be properly secured so that it does not swing around while the trailer is in motion. When traveling with two or more horses, it's best to place the hay nets between the horses' heads, but check regularly to make sure there is always sufficient hay in the nets.

It's very important to keep your horse's digestive system functioning normally while traveling, so do your best to keep him on his regular feeding schedule for grain. Also, carry hay and grain from your stable so there won't be a change in the feed when traveling. A different feed may cause digestive upsets, and you don't want to take a chance of an adverse reaction to the feed, especially when you're traveling.

Most horses rely on their food and water as sources for normal bacterial flora for the digestive tract. However, just as with people, additional stresses in their lives can cause the digestive process to be altered, resulting in an intestinal environment that is less hospitable to the normal bacterial flora. If this balance is upset and some of the normal bacterial flora dies, less desirable bacteria will grow in its place. These undesirable bacteria can survive in the digestive tract under these more stressful conditions, but may not be as efficient at digesting the horse's food.

Even when the horse is no longer in the stressful situation, the desirable bacteria may not be prevalent enough to regain its previous balance. This leaves the less-effective bacteria to digest the food, resulting in decreased utilization of the food by the body. In other words, you could be wasting food because your horse's body is not able to process all the nutrients available in the food, and your horse could be deprived of much needed nutrients, an important consideration for competition horses.

To avoid the loss of normal bacterial flora, you can feed your horse a product containing acidophilus and/or lactobacillus. These products, which come in powder or liquid form, are readily available in many feed stores or through horse supply catalogs and are reasonable in price. It is not necessary to feed this bacterial supplement on a constant basis once the stressful situation is over unless there is a specific need for it. Usually I recommend starting to use a bacterial supplement at least three days prior to the departure date. This will allow your horse time to adjust to a new additive in his diet (although most of these products are readily eaten) and to digest food at his optimum level before going through the stress of travel. Continue to feed the bacterial supplement throughout your travel and competition time, and for a few days after you return home. This is an easy, inexpensive way to maintain your horse's normal digestive process.

WATER

Another factor to consider when traveling is your horse's water consumption. Sometimes the trip is not long enough to worry about the water, but many trips require that water be offered. Some horses will not drink water away from home, either due to taste or a change in the container.

It's important to determine if your horse will refuse to drink strange water or water from a different container before you leave for a trip. If your horse is one of the finicky types, you have several choices. You can carry water with you or you can disguise the taste of the water so it always tastes the same. Carrying water is the best option if you have enough room and containers. Even if you don't have a picky drinker, it's best to carry water along during long trips or in hot weather in case of an emergency such as a breakdown. I suggest bringing water along any time you are taking your horse on a trip that's over two hours long. Be sure that the water container is clean each time it is used.

If you know your horse doesn't like the taste of different water, get him used to drinking flavored water before the trip. That way when new water is offered, the taste will always be the same. You will need to give flavored water in a bucket since it's difficult to keep an automatic water system constantly flavored.

If you suspect your horse is even slightly dehydrated while traveling, monitor him frequently by pulling up the skin on his neck. If the skin returns to its normal position, hydration is sufficient. However, if the skin stays elevated in a tented position, the horse is dehydrated. Find a veterinarian on your route immediately to check the horse and give intravenous fluids, or fluids via stomach tube to correct the hydration.

For more information on disguising the taste of water see p. 152, *Mixing Medications.*

REDUCING TRAVEL STRESS

Many horses become stressed when traveling and/or staying away from home despite their owners' efforts to make the trip a pleasant experience. Even though the feed and water are kept the same and the trailer is made as comfortable as possible, some horses just seem to worry more than others.

Among the signs that a horse is feeling stressed are poor appetite, pacing the stall, excessive sweating, and not lying down as much as he ordinarily does. Individual horses may show other signs of stress that are not as obvious, but an astute owner who knows her horse well should be alert to them. Unfortunately, poor performance may be one of these indicators.

If you know your horse tends to become upset when traveling, I suggest that you begin giving him electrolytes a few days before the start of your trip. Sometimes when the body is stressed, it uses excessive amounts of particular electrolytes, and feeding a steady supply of them will help ensure a constant replacement so no deficiencies occur. Although electrolytes are more commonly given only in the summer to counter the effects of excessive sweating, they can also be helpful during the winter months. Remember that when your horse is cold, he may decrease his water consumption. Since electrolytes are a form of salt, adding them to his diet will encourage him to drink more. As long as you follow the dosage instructions carefully, electrolytes are very safe.

Once you are on the road, however, unless you have already introduced electrolytes to your horse's diet, do not then add them to his water if he starts to show signs of stress. The sudden change in the taste of the water causes many horses to stop drinking altogether, compounding the problem.

Both Bach Flower remedies and homeopathics can also be helpful in relieving the symptoms of stress, whether at home or while traveling. See Chapter Three, Appendices III and V, and Part Three for more information on their use.

For additional discussion of electrolytes, see p. 85.

12 The Aging Horse

When is a horse old? There isn't really a definitive age when a horse is considered a senior because life expectancy differs for individuals. Ponies often live very long lives and can be useful into their late twenties, while most horses retire from use anywhere from their late teens to late twenties.

Statistics tell us that the average life span for most equines is about 25 years. However, today's advanced veterinary care allows many horses to enjoy more productive older years and longer life spans.

Each horse must be evaluated individually to determine if he is showing signs of aging. However, when a horse reaches the age of fifteen--no matter what his condition--I consider him a senior citizen and advise appropriate care, beginning with a thorough medical work-up. The parameters for testing vary somewhat with each horse, but at minimum you should request that your veterinarian perform routine blood work (CBC with differential and a complete chemistry profile), a physical that includes a heart checkup,

lameness testing, and X-rays of any known or suspected problems. From then on, horses that are still being competed regularly should have a veterinary exam at least once every six months to one year to ensure optimum health during their senior years.

X-rays are especially important if you plan to continue competing your horse. Having an X-ray of any pre-existing condition will help you and your veterinarian to monitor it better, and X-rays can provide important information that might help you in making a decision concerning your horse's future. For example, X-rays of a horse's hock taken at the age of fifteen can serve as a baseline against which future changes or degeneration are measured. Should the horse become lame a year or so later, the veterinarian can take a new set of X-rays and compare them to the originals to determine if, and at what rate, the hock is degenerating. He will also be able to see if there are any changes that could adversely affect the horse's performance. At the same time, if the horse's performance has declined but the X-rays indicate no change in the hock condition since the last exam, the veterinarian will know that he should check elsewhere for the source of the problem.

Some horses seem to age more quickly than others and may require checkups every six months before the age of fifteen. You and your veterinarian will have to be the judge of that. If you notice signs of arthritis, diminishing performance, or a change in attitude toward exercise, consult your veterinarian and discuss what might be done to enhance your horse's quality of life. Some simple changes that can be effective include a longer warm-up period, a nutritional supplement, or a homeopathic medication.

If you watch for changes in your horse's condition and address them right away, you are more likely to avert a major health problem down the road.

EXERCISE CONSIDERATIONS

A horse's exercise requirements change as he grows older. Understanding these changes and accommodating them will help the horse to continue performing up to his optimum athletic ability. The warm-up before the main exercise period is an important part of any horse's exercise program, and for older horses it plays an even more vital role. Older horses' bodies are less forgiving than those of young horses, and injury can result if the warm-up period is not adequate.

The muscles and bone structure of many older horses have developed over time to accommodate their main form of exercise. Therefore, it's important to understand which muscles are used the most by your horse and to design a warm-up period that targets these areas while, at the same time, warming up the lesser used muscles. The horse's joints must also be warmed up, and exercises should be chosen to gradually increase the movement in the joints. Some specific areas such as the stifles or the back may need extra attention, so you can incorporate into the warm-up a tightening and strengthening exercise like working your horse up a hill.

As your horse ages, it becomes even more important that you exercise him regularly in order to maintain him at a consistent level of fitness for the type of riding you do. Avoid letting him have extensive periods of time off because you may find that it becomes more difficult for him to regain his previous level of fitness after an extended break. Also, you probably will have to be more cautious in working to regain his optimum fitness level if he has developed any physical problems. In fact, if your horse has a minor soundness problem, for instance arthritic hocks, it's best never to completely rest him. When a horse loses muscle tone, such minor problems that were kept under control as long as the horse stayed fit will sometimes worsen.

If you are still competing your older horse, ride him enough to keep him fit but do not overschool at home. Save him for the competitions. Each horse is an individual, and it's difficult to gauge how hard the demands of a particular riding discipline are on any given horse. We do know, however, that the extra concussion of jumping or other active sports such as roping cattle, polo, or barrel racing can shorten a horse's useful life.

A variety of factors, including his conformation, his natural athletic ability, and his previous health history, will influence the rate at which each horse begins to show the effects of aging and use. Exercise your older horse regularly so that he stays fit, but use your best judgment as to how much exercise he can tolerate and be alert for indications that you are asking too much from him.

For more discussion of warm-up routines and other important considerations during exercise, see Chapter Nine.

COMMON HEALTH PROBLEMS OF THE OLDER HORSE

The most common debilitating health problem of the older horse is arthritis, which is discussed at length in the *Horse Ailments* section, Part Three of this book. Some common symptoms of arthritis are stiffness, not wanting to go forward, refusing to do what is asked, and a poor attitude.

The second most common health concern for older horses is a decrease in the efficiency of the digestive system, which may necessitate a change in diet. Among the symptoms to watch for are weight loss and/or a decrease in energy and occasional colic. Be sure to maintain a regular feeding schedule and provide plenty of fresh water. Have a dental examination done on your older horse every six months to check for sharp edges, broken teeth, or infected molars, all of which can have an impact on how well he digests his food.

Many older horses also suffer from a slowing down or malfunctioning of the glandular system. Older horses who maintain a heavy winter coat all year round instead of shedding their coats during the summer as normal may have a glandular problem. The most common ones are a benign pituitary tumor or a low thyroid condition. Signs of a low thyroid condition include an increase in the size of the crest area of the neck and fat pockets on the horse's sides and next to the top of his tail, as well as a long dull hair coat.

If you notice that your horse's coat is not shedding or has turned a different color, consult your veterinarian as soon as possible so your horse can be examined and treated. In the early stages of glandular problems I have found that horses treated with acupuncture and homeopathy begin to shed their hair or return to normal hair color, have increased energy, and perform better. Depending on the diagnosis, other medications are also available to treat many glandular disorders.

For more information on feeding and diet alternatives for the older horse, see Chapter Five.

PEPPING UP THE OLDER HORSE

When I examine an older horse, I'm commonly asked, "Is there anything I can do to make him feel better?" This is a challenging question because there are so many considerations, but let's take a look at some of the options.

Review The Feeding Program And Nutritional Supplements

My first response is to review the feeding program to make sure all the nutritional needs of an older horse are being met. Then I discuss supplements and review which ones have been tried in the past and which I feel might be helpful. Even if an older horse has no specific problems, a feed supplement can lead to an overall improved condition and more energy. I sometimes recommend feed additives such as yucca root, chondroitin sulfate, and special herbal formulations. There are many different commercial herbs marketed, and the decision on which ones to use will depend on the horse's specific needs.

For additional information on the use of herbal remedies and supplements, see Chapter Three and the *Herb Appendix IV.*

Review Parasite Control

Next, I review the worming schedule. If you do not know the recent history or care of your horse, there is always the possibility that parasites might not have been kept under control as often as they should have. This is particularly likely if the horse is suffering a digestive problem such as diarrhea, excessive gas, or mild colic.

If your horse usually experiences a digestive problem shortly before the scheduled worming treatment, it is possible that there is a build-up of parasites in his digestive tract that the horse is not tolerating. In some cases this happens due to scarring caused by excessive parasite migration in the past. Some horses can develop an allergic reaction to parasites. This is one of the reasons it is so important to monitor your older horse carefully, especially if he is having digestive upsets. A horse who suddenly develops a poor attitude or grouchiness may also be exhibiting symptoms of parasite build-up.

Massage For The Older Horse

I find that one of the best ways to pep up an older horse is a massage. Just as with people, years of work combined with age tighten muscles and cause general tenseness. Massage often gives older horses some relief from pain and allows them to become relaxed and supple again. Horses of all disciplines can benefit from regular massage and seem to enjoy the experience greatly. Look for a certified massage therapist in your area to do an overall massage, or learn how to do a gentle massage yourself.

See more on massage in Chapter Three.

Acupuncture For The Older Horse

I also generally recommend an acupuncture treatment for any older horse. My examination will reveal which, if any, specific areas need treatment. If there is nothing specific to treat, such as a sore stifle or arthritic hock, then I at least treat the horse metabolically to stimulate the immune system, liver, and kidneys. Owners often report a different horse after treatment, with maximum effects seen from one to three days later. Many owners have their horses treated with acupuncture just before shows because they find that the horses perform much better and have wonderful attitudes. Horses with cranky attitudes to start with often switch to a "can-do" attitude after just one acupuncture treatment.

I had a dressage horse that I showed until he was nineteen years old. He was always like a new horse the day after acupuncture. Any movement I asked for during exercise was willingly given and repeated without his usual difficult behavior.

It's a shame that acupuncture is usually only considered when a horse has a specific problem because it is also a wonderful health maintenance tool.

Detoxifying With Homeopathics

Older horses often require a bit of help in maintaining their liver's ability to detoxify the body. Homeopathics for this purpose can be very effective in making the older horse feel better and are particularly useful if the horse has been subjected to a lot of stress or given numerous conventional medications in the past.

There are a number of homeopathics used for this purpose but I prefer to choose one specific to each horse's unique situation. Consult a homeopathic veterinarian to find the correct remedy for your horse. If you purchase a homeopathic from a health food store, I suggest nux vomica in a low potency such as 6c or 12x or give ten times the dosage recommended on the label for people twice a day (as a general rule a horse weighs about ten times more than a human). If the homeopathic is in pellet form and the horse won't eat them, dilute them in a small amount of water and then give him the water.

DEALING WITH DEATH AND DYING

Whether due to old age, illness, or an injury, death is always hard to accept. In addition to dealing with death as a veterinarian, I personally have lost several old horses and a few young ones as well. No matter what the circumstances or age of the horse, it is always a heartbreaking experience.

Of course, anyone who owns an older horse knows at some point they will have to face the death of that horse. Even if you own a young and healthy horse, however, it is wise to be prepared for illness or injury, especially if you travel a lot. When you travel away from home, leave a complete itinerary including information on how to contact you in case of an emergency. You should also make sure that your veterinarian or the person left in charge of your horse has all of the pertinent information about the horse and knows how you would want an emergency situation such as colic surgery handled. Ideally, an owner should be contacted before any major procedure is performed, but in the case of a sudden severe injury or serious illness, your horse's caregivers may have to make decisions in your absence if you cannot be located quickly. Make sure that they are aware of your wishes about medical treatment, as well as about euthanasia and disposal of your horse's body in case of death.

The consequences of failing to plan ahead for an accident or sudden illness were evident in several cases I have handled in which owners were away on extensive trips and could not be contacted when their horses were severely injured. No one knew the horses' medical histories, whether the horses were insured, or how much money the owners were prepared to spend on medical treatment. Although it may seem uncaring to discuss finances when a horse's life is at stake, it is an unfortunate reality that many major clinics and university veterinary hospitals will not accept a horse for treatment without guarantee of payment.

Euthanasia

Making the decision to euthanize a horse is rarely easy. While euthanasia has long been accepted for animals and is commonly practiced in veterinary medicine, I prefer to consider it only in extreme circumstances. Since this is a very personal issue, I suggest that you explore your attitudes about it in advance so you will be prepared if the situation ever arises. Each veterinarian has his own preferred method to euthanize a horse, so discuss the procedures with your veterinarian beforehand so you will know what to expect. It is somewhat easier to deal with if you know the logistics involved and what to do with the body.

Most veterinarians use a euthanasia solution given by injection. The solutions that are now used to euthanize animals work in a matter of seconds—usually before the injection is completed. There is no pain or struggling. Consciousness goes first, so the horse is unaware of what is happening and slips into a sleep-like state, and then dies.

The injection method is the most common, but there are still some veterinarians who use a pistol or a rifle. Most people don't like the idea of using a gun, and I wouldn't choose this method except in the case of an emergency. However, if done correctly, death by gunshot is instantaneous.

There are services that will pick up and dispose of a dead horse. They are usually referred to as rendering services or animal disposal services. The other option is to bury the horse. A backhoe or other earth moving equipment is necessary to dig a hole large and deep enough and then to refill the dirt. If you are considering burial, check the local ordinances first to make sure it is legal to do so.

Grieving

When faced with the death of a horse, I assure my clients that it's okay to show their grief. After all, losing a beloved animal friend is one of the most difficult experiences a person can go through. It's normal to feel a strong sense of loss;

there is nothing to be ashamed of. However, when it's time for your horse to be euthanized, no matter how much you are grieving, you must say your good-byes and mentally let your horse go.

When the time comes, it's a good idea to have a family member or close friend present to help you through the ordeal. Also, to assist you through this experience emotionally, you can use Rescue Remedy, the combination Bach Flower remedy. Just a few drops in your mouth will help calm you.

In general, I encourage owners to handle this situation in whatever way makes them most comfortable. There is no "right" or "wrong" way to deal with death. Some of my clients have religious ceremonies performed during the procedure while others prefer not being present. Whether you are with him at the end or not, what is important is the help you have given your horse during his final weeks or days.

WHEN A CHILD LOSES A HORSE

As hard as it is for an adult to deal with the death of a horse or other animal, it can be even more difficult for a child. The concept of death is strange and terrifying for a child who has never before dealt with it. Rather than trying to shield the child from this experience, I find that involving the child is best.

If the horse is dying of a long illness, try to explain this to the child. Obviously the age of the child is a major factor here, but remember that even a very young child has some awareness of what's happening.

The child must wrestle with the same range of emotions that adults go through, from denial to guilt, anger, despair, and finally, acceptance. Ask the child what he is feeling and discuss these emotions with him. Above all, let him know that his feelings are normal. Over the next days and weeks, continue to ask the child from time to time what he is feeling about the loss of the animal. He may have gone from denial of the experience to guilt. Children often feel that they are the cause of bad things that happen in their lives. The child may remember a time when he did something wrong, such as hitting the horse, and feel that this is the reason the horse has died. This guilt must also be discussed so you can explain that his actions had nothing to do with the horse's death.

Asking the child to talk about these feelings is the only way to know how he is dealing with the death. It may be difficult for you to talk about the death because you are grieving too. However, your grief is a wonderful example to your child, showing him or her that it is okay to display your emotions and share them with others. If the child has lost a human friend or family member, it may be appropriate to mention that loss as a reference point. It can also help to perform a little ceremony after the horse's death, involving the child to whatever extent is appropriate for his or her age.

A number of books are available to help all of us deal with death and dying, including those by Elizabeth Kubler-Ross, a pioneer and leading expert on this subject. *The Fall of Freddie the Leaf* by Leo Buscaglia is an excellent book that helps to explain the concept to young children.

Part III

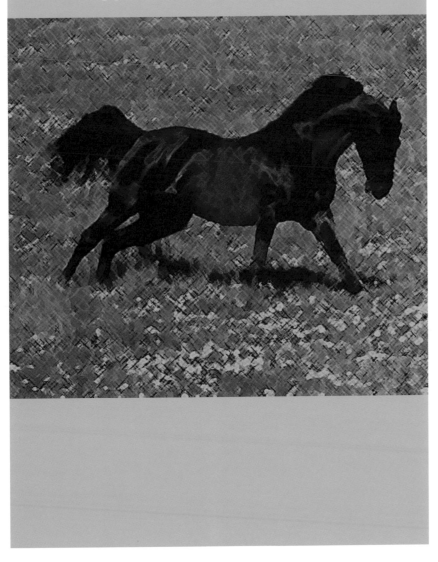

COMMON HORSE AILMENTS

This section of the book covers, in alphabetical order, many common (and not so common) ailments found in horses. Some are very serious, requiring immediate veterinary treatment, and for these I have suggested complementary remedies to use in conjunction (and after consultation) with the vet's first line of treatment. Other listings are for everyday ailments, many of which can be successfully treated by the horse owner with alternative therapies.

Not all therapies work for all horses, so I have listed a variety of options using many different remedies. I have pointed out where the order of suggested treatments is of consequence. I have also cautioned you where it is important to choose only a specific remedy and where there are contraindications present. It is difficult to decide which alternative treatment might work best for a horse. There is often no definitive answer, so the trial-and-error method may be the only way; however, except where I have mentioned, by trying different options you will be doing no harm to your horse.

Detailed information on how to use and apply various different therapies—acupressure, herbs, or homeopathy, for example—can be found in the appendices specific to these treatments, as well as in Parts One and Two of this book. Use the index for reference. Sources for medications, supplements, and other remedies can be accessed in the **Product Suppliers Appendix VI** *and are* listed in the index.

A-Z Common Horse Ailments

A

ABSCESSES

(See also *Hoof Problems; Lameness and Leg Problems: Hind Leg Hip Abscess*)

Abscesses are soft swellings that can be found anywhere on the horse's body. These areas are usually warm, painful to the touch, and filled with pus. Many abscesses result from invasive bacteria. The body fights these bacteria by surrounding them with white blood cells or pus. Many abscesses rupture by themselves, but if you suspect an abscess, rapid treatment can decrease healing time. Your vet may need to deaden the area in order to lance and clean out the abscess.

After drainage has been established, it must be maintained so that healing can occur inside the abscess. To achieve this, flush or rinse the abscess twice a day with a solution containing an antibacterial. A solution that works well for this purpose is made of three parts water to one part tamed iodine or regular 0.1 percent iodine (or Betadine). If your horse is allergic to iodine or an-

tibiotics, use a mixture of one part grapefruit extract and one part colloidal silver (both available in the health food store). Flushing the abscess daily for five to seven days usually helps the healing process. If you are treating the abscess yourself, be sure to wear gloves because the pus may contain bacteria that could infect any open cuts on your hands.

If your horse repeatedly develops abscesses in the same area, consult your vet. Recurrence can be an indication of a more widespread bacterial infection that must be tracked down to its source. Sometimes a specific source of infection can be found, such as a thorn that has worked its way deep into tissue. In other cases, the infection may have entered the bloodstream somehow and affected the entire body. Either way, it's important to eliminate the bacteria and the stress on the horse's immune system.

For information on treatment of hoof abscesses, see *Hoof Problems: Abscesses* on p. 217.

SYMPTOMS
- Soft swollen area that is filled with pus, warm and painful to the touch.

RECOMMENDATIONS

Vet Ask your vet to establish drainage in the abscess.

Clean Follow-up care should include daily flushing of the wound with Betadine solution as described above.

Laser Use of laser treatment around the area will promote healing.

Supplements Add antioxidants such as vitamin C (8 grams a day) to help deal with the increase in free radicals due to the abscess.

Aromatherapy
- Lavender. Stimulates healing.
- Juniper. Decreases toxin accumulations.
- Lemon. Stimulates immune system.
- Tea tree. Stimulates immune system to fight bacterial infection.

ALLERGIES

(See also *Skin Problems; Eye Problems*)

There are many symptoms that can be associated with an allergic reaction, including hair loss, mane and tail loss, itching, a change in coat color (usually to a lighter shade), hives, loss of appetite, loss of weight, dehydration, colic, and laminitis. Allergies have been a problem for a long time, but they have increased dramatically in recent years. Dealing with allergies can be one of the most challenging aspects of the veterinary profession. While the causes of some allergies are understood by medical science, others are still mysteries.

One of the most difficult aspects of treating an allergy is figuring out what agent is causing the reaction. Is it, for example, a reaction to an insect bite, a specific food, or a plant or fiber? Allergy testing can help determine the cause of a reaction, but it does not answer another important question: What factors contributed to the allergy occurring in the first place? Was the horse

inbred and therefore predisposed to having a poor immune system? (Inbreeding is a common occurrence these days within many breeds.) Are there harmful chemicals in the horse's environment that are a factor? Is the horse's body reacting to stressful surroundings or a stressful training schedule? Have so many vaccinations been given that the horse's immune system is affected? Is a diet of poor quality affecting the overall health of the horse? Is the horse allergic to a specific ingredient in the grain? These are just some of the questions that vets must ask to determine the best treatment in a specific case.

Skin testing is the method most frequently used to identify specific allergies. It is both reliable and specific, but it requires individual testing of each potential allergen. Because there are literally hundreds of possible allergens, this method can be prohibitively costly for many people. For these reasons I often use kinesiology muscle testing as an alternative (see Chapter Ten). However, although muscle testing works well, it is sometimes difficult to test all the substances or an interaction of several substances that might be causing the allergy. Your vet may also recommend blood tests for allergies that can be helpful in certain instances.

Research as well as observation has provided some answers and guidance in identifying the sources of allergies. It still can be difficult, however, to relieve the horse of symptoms, especially if he has multiple allergies or if his allergy is due to an interaction of several substances. Therefore, it is crucial that we understand the interaction of the various allergy-producing substances.

FACTORS TO CONSIDER

Stress

What is excessive stress to a horse? Illness, sudden changes in environment or diet, and weather changes are among the things that can cause stress. Each horse interprets the stresses in everyday life differently, and as a result, each one may respond differently; therefore, they also react differently to the same circumstances. When his stress level is increased, a sensitive horse will often have an allergic reaction.

Some horses demonstrate their stress through kicking, biting, pacing the fence outside, or walking around and around their stalls. Others, harder to diagnose, internalize their stress and you may not notice until some external symptom—such as hives—appears. Either way, you have to guess what it is that is causing the animal's stress. Make a list of possibilities—recent changes in diet, stabling, bedding, turnout, tack, or blankets. If you cannot pinpoint and/or alleviate the reason for the stress, try Bach Flowers as a remedy to help your horse cope (see Chapter Three, p.34, and the *Bach Flowers Appendix III*). If the decision about which Bach Flower remedy to choose is overwhelming, you can use Bach Flowers Rescue Remedy which will decrease a certain level of stress in horses.

Diet

When a horse is suffering from any type of allergic reaction, particularly a sudden reaction such as hives, I recommend first checking the feed with applied kinesiology muscle testing. If the muscle checking indicates that the feed is the source of the problem, you can make immediate changes to stop the reaction and then follow up and recheck with skin testing later. Corn (maize) is one of the most common grains that horses react to adversely. There are several reasons for this. When corn is freshly harvested, it can be beneficial in feed, but when it is stored for long periods and subjected to heat and humidity, it can develop fungal growth. Also, after the corn is cracked, it can rapidly lose nutrients and become rancid. Corn can contain mycotoxins, as well. When I suggest that corn may be the cause of an allergic reaction, owners often re-spond that the corn they have been feeding looks fine. However, since toxins and fungal growth are usually visible only through a microscope, the corn may have a normal appearance but still contain contaminants.

Once a horse develops sensitivity to a specific allergen—whether it is a feed, fungus or toxin—the reaction can recur anytime he is exposed to it. One of my own horses, while living at a boarding stable, was fed a large amount of moldy hay. Unfortunately, he would eat anything put in front of him even if the taste was a little strange. After eating the moldy hay, he lost his appetite, became dehydrated, and colicked. The mold was the same color as the hay, so at first it was difficult to identify the culprit but a close inspection and microscopic exam verified the diagnosis. Though he lost weight, he recovered after acupuncture and homeopathic treatment. Fortunately, he did not develop laminitis, which commonly happens after a horse ingests moldy hay or feed.

My horse remained normal for about one year. Then I begin to notice a recurrence of the same symptoms as those he experienced when he ate the moldy hay. The first thing I checked was the hay, but visibly there did not seem to be any mold. I checked it using muscle testing and found that the hay did seem to be the problem. Then I had it tested in a laboratory and a tiny amount of fungus was found at a microscopic level. Although a tiny amount of mold is usually tolerated by horses, and none of the other horses in the barn were ill, because of his history with this particular fungus, he was reacting to it. I treated him with a homeopathic that fit the signs he was showing for a few weeks and then he was fine. However, each year when this particular fungus began to grow the same symptoms would reappear due to the sensitivity he had developed.

So, if your horse is exhibiting allergy symptoms, especially hives, muscle test everything you are feeding him to help find the cause. If necessary, also have the feed tested in a laboratory for toxins or molds. If you are feeding a commercially mixed sweet feed, you will have to test individually each of the grains that are contained in the mix. Also check the hay since some horses are sensitive to the pesticide sprays that are used or, like my horse, a mold that is difficult to identify. If the feed is causing an allergy problem, or if you suspect it is, discontinue that feed and find a different source. Supplements can also contain grains, so if your horse has shown sensitivity to a specific grain, make sure that none of the supplements you are using contains that grain. If the allergic reaction continues after your horse has been on a new feed for a few days, have him checked by your vet.

Environment

There are some influences that we cannot see and therefore often fail to take into consideration when evaluating allergies. Take a close look at your horse's immediate environment to search for unseen or unnoticed allergens. Things to look for include insecticides sprayed into the air, pollen, smog, detergents used on saddle blankets and bandages, and disinfectants. I had never considered smog an allergen until living in Los Angeles and experiencing a smog-related allergy with one of my own horses. Smog-related allergies are often identified only after the horse is moved from the smog-filled environment to a smog-free area and an improvement is noticed. However, sometimes even a move is not totally effective. Horses that are sensitive to environmental pollution are sometimes also sensitive to other allergens in the air, and even a smog-free environment may contain other airborne allergens.

If your horse is allergy prone, do not use harsh detergents when laundering saddle blankets, bandages, horse blankets, or anything else that will touch his skin. Do your horse's laundry with a soap that is additive-free. Whether the horse spends most of his time inside or out, decrease the use of chemicals in his environment. Using an automatic fly spray system can stress a horse's system and should be avoided with the sensitive, allergy-prone horse. If this is not possible, remove the horse from the area being treated for at least twenty-four hours to help you assess how much your horse is reacting to the spray system.

Many horses react to products that are made of synthetic materials, such as plastics and polyesters. They are often the last place we look when trying to figure out what might be causing an allergic reaction. Most water and feed buckets are made of plastic materials, saddle blankets often contain synthetic material, and even some saddles are made of synthetics. If you suspect that a synthetic material may be at fault, replace it with a natural material. For instance, a plastic bucket can be replaced with one made of rubber or metal. A synthetic saddle blanket can be replaced with a wool or cotton blanket or a sheepskin pad.

Immune System Deficiencies

There is great concern over the question of immune system deficiencies. Research has shown that some breeds seem to have more problems than others with an increased frequency of disease occurrence and allergic reactions, which indicates that the immune system is not functioning properly. One of the comments I hear from older horsemen is "We never used to have all these health problems with our horses." They question why it is happening now. There are many possible answers such as influences from pesticides, vaccinations, and inbreeding, as well as other reasons that have not yet been identified. However, we must realize that the immune system has limits that need to be recognized and understood to keep our horses as healthy as possible.

Appaloosas are an example of a breed with a predisposition to allergies, as well as other health problems. The allergy problems are usually seasonal, starting in the spring and often lasting throughout the summer. Horses that are affected can have a variety of symptoms including eyes that constantly drain, itchy skin and loss of hair. Some of the imported warmbloods, particularly those from Russia and the Baltic countries, have also demonstrated a tendency towards immune system reactions. These horses generally overreact to insect bites, developing large swellings and, sometimes, hard areas around the bite. They can also react adversely to vaccinations.

SYMPTOMS
- Scratching and biting the skin.
- Drainage from the eyes.
- Hair loss from the coat or from the mane and tail.
- Change of coat color to a lighter shade.
- Difficulty gaining muscle; inability to get totally fit.
- Overreaction to insect bites and/or vaccinations.
- Hives (See also *Skin Problems*, p. 271).
- Recurring illness, particularly respiratory infections.

RECOMMENDATIONS

Acupuncture Stimulates the immune system.

NAET

Homeopathy A homeopathic remedy that is specifically prescribed for the horse by your vet or choose one of the following:
- Arsenicum album 6C or 12C, three times daily. Use when the itching is associated with dry swollen areas, or areas that involve open ulcerations of the skin.
- Sulfur 6C, two times daily. Use when the itching recurs on a seasonal basis.
- Apis mellifica 6C, three times daily. Use when allergies are related to insect bites.

Test Check the feed with muscle testing and, if necessary, laboratory testing.

Review
- Determine the cause of the allergy and eliminate it if possible.
- Investigate possible stress in the horse's environment and life, and how to reduce it.

Medication Investigate ways to keep your horse's immune system stimulated, such as a medication to help stimulate immune system response for a particular problem. For instance, a product called Equistim, from Immuno Vet, is an injectable medication used specifically to stimulate the immune system against respiratory illness.

Herbs Add to the diet herbs that stimulate the immune system and promote lymphatic drainage. You can refer to the list of immune-stimulating herbs in the section below on cancer, or try one of the following:
- Calendula. Give 20 grams (about 3/4 oz) daily in the food. Helps to alleviate stress.
- Nettle. Give 20 grams (about 3/4 oz) of the dried herb daily. Helps to stimulate circulation, has a high vitamin C content, and acts as a blood cleanser.
- Kelp. Give 15 to 30 grams (about 1/2 to 1 oz) daily. Helps to stimulate the thyroid gland, which affects the health of the skin and the hair coat.
- Meadowsweet. Give 20 to 30 grams (about 3/4 to 1 oz) daily in the food. Has an anti-inflammatory and soothing effect on digestion.
- Clivers. Give 15 to 20 grams (about 1/2 to 3/4 oz) daily. Helps drainage of the lymphatic system.

Herbal rinse A soothing rinse for the skin can be made by combining an equal amount of the herbs comfrey, chamomile, and witch hazel. Steep these herbs together in boiling water as if you are making a tea. After the mixture has cooled, strain the herbs from the liquid and retain the liquid. Place the cooled herbs in cheesecloth and apply as a cold compress over irritated areas for twenty minutes. After removing the compress, apply the rinse by wetting a cloth in it and patting the cloth over the affected area.

Supplement   Protease, a digestive enzyme (available in health food stores) has been found to be extremely effective in treating allergies. It is in powdered form that you can add to the horse's feed. Give twice a day. For a 1000- to 1200-pound horse (approx. 450 kgs) give ten times the amount recommended for an adult human.

Aromatherapy   Use the essential oil of lemon to stimulate the immune system.

Review the discussion of diet in Chapter Five and read the *Skin Problems* entry on p. 268.

SUGGESTED ORDER OF TREATMENT OPTIONS:

Acute cases:

Acupuncture

Homeopathy

NAET

Chronic "seasonal" cases:

Acupuncture Begin treatment just before the seasonal reactions start. A series of 3 to 5 acupuncture sessions will help prevent the allergic reactions from beginning.

NAET A series of treatments will be necessary.

Dietary changes

Environmental changes Dirt paddock instead of grass, for example.

ANHIDROSIS

The term anhidrosis refers to a condition in which the horse is unable to sweat. Sweating is an essential function because it is the way the horse's body dissipates excess heat. A horse with anhidrosis may stop sweating entirely or just in certain areas on his body, such as the neck. While seen most often in horses that are worked, anhidrosis is also found in horses that live outside and are not worked. Some horses are born with anhidrosis, others develop the condition gradually, and some stop sweating suddenly. There is no definite pattern for the development of the condition. Horses should always sweat when exercised. If your horse does not sweat when he is exercised hard enough to increase his respiratory and heart rate, check with your vet for information about anhidrosis.

The cause of anhidrosis is not known. When examining horses affected with anhidrosis, I always check the acupuncture points to determine which areas are out of balance. Usually the lung meridian is affected and sometimes other meridians as well. When treating anhidrosis, it's necessary to rebalance the body so all the systems are functioning properly. Acupuncture and/or homeopathy work well to obtain this goal and usually prevent a recurrence. Most horses with anhidrosis respond within two to three acupuncture treatments and begin to sweat. If your horse responds to holistic treatment, be sure to have him rechecked in two months to make sure the meridians are still in balance, particularly if the horse is involved in hard work.

One folk remedy that occasionally helps with anhidrosis is beer. Most horses like beer and enjoy it as a treat. One bottle of beer a day mixed in the feed may alleviate anhidrosis in minor cases. European beers seem to produce the best result because of their natural fermentation process; however any beer without artificial additives will work.

SYMPTOMS
• No sweating, or minimal sweating, often only in certain areas.

RECOMMENDATIONS

Exercise During the cool time of day or at night in hot weather. Sponge down with water frequently during the workout.

Stable Area In a cool environment if possible, and use a fan during hot weather.

Acupuncture

Homeopathy Treatment prescribed by your vet; works best if used in conjunction with acupuncture.

Chronic cases:

Start *acupuncture* and *homeopathic* treatments at least one month before onset of warm weather. Some cases will require continued treatments during the hot weather months.

ARTHRITIS

(See also *Lameness and Leg Problems—Front Legs: Arthritis of the Knee*)

Arthritis is a disease that is more common in older horses but may affect a horse at any age, particularly those horses that worked hard or suffered a trauma. Arthritis is frequently associated with the build-up of excessive bone-like material in areas where it should not be. This excessive build-up of bone can occur on a bone surface or a joint surface and is often the result of excessive wear and tear. Bone changes like this commonly form when an area is unstable or unsupported and the body attempts to strengthen the weak spot by adding more bone to it. In addition, arthritis can involve inflammation of a joint due to infection or trauma. Either the bone changes or inflammation can affect any area in the body.

Repetitive motion and concussion, particularly in large, heavy horses, can contribute to the development of arthritis. Constant jumping and galloping eventually take a toll on the horse's bones. Jumpers, hunters, event horses, and polo horses, for example, are used in a repetitive concussive fashion, making them prone to arthritis. Diet, as I discuss shortly, can also be a factor in the development of arthritis.

If your horse has always willingly performed for you, and then starts to display a bad attitude on a constant basis, it's probably because he's in pain. Arthritis can be very uncomfortable, even when it's only in a few small areas. Some horses just do not tolerate any type of pain, and these horses indicate the existence of a problem sooner. The area that is affected by arthritis usually varies depending on the horse's most frequent activity. For instance, horses used to rope cattle are commonly affected in the lumbar spine because of the many quick and sometimes unbalanced sliding stops that they must perform. Horses that jump fences often have arthritis in their joints because of the excessive concussion that must be absorbed when landing. Based on what your horse's most frequent activity is, you can figure out which areas might be stressed the most. You then can monitor these areas more carefully for signs of discomfort or change.

Pain is the most obvious consequence of arthritis, followed by loss of movement. In Oriental medicine the decreased movement of Qi, or energy, around arthritic areas is considered one of the main reasons for the pain. Pain may also develop elsewhere if the horse compensates by trying to avoid using the arthritic joint and thereby overstresses another area.

If you suspect your horse suffers from arthritis, X-rays are the best way to confirm its presence. Sometimes you can even feel a gritty, sand-like substance when an arthritic joint is flexed, or feel extra bone formation where it is not supposed to be. Once the diagnosis is confirmed, it's time to decide what can be done to alleviate the horse's discomfort. The choice of treatment depends on where the arthritis is located and how much the horse's movement is affected. To help me determine the best course of treatment for an individual horse, I like to start with an overview of the horse's lifestyle, focusing particularly on diet, exercise, environment, and treatments that have been prescribed in the past.

Diet and Its Affect on Arthritis

First, let's look at the horse's diet. Is this an old or young horse? Is the protein level excessive or not enough? What is the mineral balance in the diet? These questions must be considered to properly evaluate the arthritic horse.

Although arthritis is found in young horses (five years or less) and middle-aged horses (six to twelve years), the causes are highly variable and may, or may not, be influenced by diet. Young horses are most likely to have arthritic changes due to injury. In middle-aged horses the cause is usually performance-related with bone surfaces suffering from repeated concussion or strain. Yet, with horses of any age, dietary requirements should be monitored to help decrease a horse's tendency toward developing arthritis and to keep further arthritis progression to a minimum.

Young horses should not be fed excessive amounts of protein. Usually a ration with 12% protein is adequate. Excess protein when combined with excess calories can lead to the development of bone problems such as osteochondritis dissecans (OCD, see p. 225). It's a good idea to check the protein balance of a young horse's diet to make sure he is not deficient in any of the essential amino acids (the building blocks that make up protein) that are needed for growth. Cereal grains alone do not provide all the essential amino acids that a young horse needs. If you are formulating your own rations from individual grains, and not feeding a premixed feed that's been professionally balanced, be aware that your youngster's diet will need the addition of a legume hay (alfalfa, or clover), or possibly soybean meal. If essential amino acids are not provided bone may not develop properly.

Fat is now being fed more, particularly to middle-aged horses requiring more calories for optimum performance, and to aged horses to maintain a healthy weight. It is a good source of slow release energy; however it is important to remember that fat is not a source of protein, calcium, and phosphorus as are cereal grains. A good rule of thumb to go by if you are supplementing your horse's diet with fat is to find other sources of protein, calcium, and phosphorus if fat replaces more than one-eighth of the grain ration. Consult your vet or an equine nutritionist to help you balance the ration correctly. If protein is insufficient, or the calcium and phosphorus ratio unbalanced, bone health could be compromised.

As a horse ages and digestion becomes less efficient, higher levels of protein, calcium, and phosphorus are needed to maintain the horse. If these levels are not provided then a horse becomes more prone to injuries and may not have the proper nutrients for tissue to repair itself. By providing properly balanced nutrition we can decrease the odds that arthritis may occur.

Minerals and Supplements

The mineral balance and source of minerals is important. The horse's system must be able to break down and absorb the minerals in the diet in order for them to be properly utilized by the body. Over-supplementing the diet with one or more minerals can imbalance the system and also predispose the horse to arthritis. The mineral that is most often the culprit is calcium. Calcium must be balanced correctly with other minerals, particularly phosphorus, when added to the diet. Some horses, particularly those in the southern United States, require extra calcium supplementation because not enough calcium is supplied naturally in their feed. However, in areas where alfalfa hay is fed, sometimes the opposite is true since alfalfa hay contains high levels of calcium. Many horses that have been imported from Europe were bred and raised to best develop and exist on a lower calcium-to-phosphorus ratio than those in the United States. When too much calcium is provided in their diet, it may predispose these horses to health problems, including the possibility of developing arthritis.

Horses with bone problems like arthritis can benefit from supplements that help to enhance performance. Supplements marketed specifically for this purpose include vitamin C, yucca, chondroitin products, and glucosamine. In addition to its role as an antioxidant, vitamin C can also promote the growth of cartilage. For this reason, all young horses can benefit from additional vitamin C in the diet. (For discussion of the antioxidant role of vitamin C, see Chapter Five.)

Chondroitin products and *glucosamine* are compounds that occur naturally in the cartilage that cushions the joints. Glucosamine stimulates production of the building blocks of cartilage, while chondroitin products block the action of enzymes that break down old cartilage. Supplemental forms of these compounds are given to support cartilage and improve the health of joints. Chondroitin products are available alone or combined with glucosamine. There are two sources of these supplements: some are obtained from cattle (bovines) and others from green-lipped mussels.

These supplements are available in powder and liquid form, and some contain many additives. The liquids seem to be easier to absorb from the gut tract—an important consideration for the older horse. Glucosamine is also available in an injectable form that is very effective with some horses. It usually takes from two weeks to a month to see any results.

Herbs

The herb yucca comes from the root of the yucca plant and contains a substance called saponin. Saponin is a plant form of glycoside that improves the performance of horses with bone problems, particularly arthritis. Yucca root powder varies in quality depending on the amount of saponin in the root and the manner in which the herb is processed. Liquid yucca usually contains a pure source of saponin that is well liked by most horses and seems to produce improvement more consistently than the powdered form does.

Exercise

Once the diet has been checked and corrections made, it's time to look at exercise. Is the horse getting adequate exercise on his own? If your horse depends on you to exercise him daily then you must be sure to provide this exercise. Even arthritic horses require exercise to maintain their flexibility.

When a horse with arthritis is allowed to stand around, he gets stiff and then experiences more problems when he is suddenly asked to exercise. A constant exercise program designed with the horse's limitations in mind can help in keeping him moving freely and will make him much happier in his work.

Acupuncture

Acupuncture often gives great relief from arthritis pain. Usually several treatments are necessary to get the problem under control, after which maintenance treatments often allow the horse to function normally. The common conventional treatment for arthritis in the hocks is injections of hyaluronic acid and steroids. These injections are sometimes unavoidable. Even if arthritic hocks are being injected as often as once a month, acupuncture will often give additional relief and sometimes reduce the number of hock injections needed.

A few years ago, I treated a 13-year-old Hanoverian gelding with extreme degenerative arthritis in both hocks. In the past, this talented horse had been maintained by injections in his hocks every four to six weeks, but the injections were no longer giving him relief. After a complete exam, I suggested acupuncture to make him more comfortable and improve his performance. Reluctantly, the owner agreed and I did one treatment. That weekend, the horse was taken to a large top-rated hunter show. He won all six of his classes, and everyone who saw him perform remarked that they had never seen him move so well. After a few more treatments, he required acupuncture only once every three months and his hock injections only once every four months to maintain top performance. Acupuncture certainly agreed with him.

Homeopathy

I have also found homeopathy to be extremely effective in treating arthritis. Each case differs greatly in terms of which remedy is effective, but once you find the remedy that works for your horse, it can help to maintain him in a pain-free state. It's usually best to consult a vet who practices homeopathy and can assist in selecting the appropriate remedy. However, if there is not one in your area, try one of the remedies listed under the *Recommendations* heading below.

Magnetic Therapy

Magnetic therapy can also be helpful in relieving the pain of arthritis. Magnetic therapy increases the circulation to an area, keeping it well-nourished and reducing stiffness and swelling. Used alone, magnets are not as effective as acupuncture, but they provide an excellent maintenance tool. For treating arthritis, I find a combination of acupuncture, homeopathy, and magnetic therapy to be a most effective treatment program.

When you apply a magnet, you will notice an increase in temperature under the area where the magnet is used. There may be sweating in the area as the circulation increases. Many owners who used to put their horses in standing wraps to decrease lower-leg swelling after a hard performance are now getting much better results by wrapping magnets around the legs under the standing wraps. A hunter with arthritic hocks was brought to me for treatment. It was this mare's last show season before retirement. She was past her routine hock injection time because her show schedule had been so hectic, and her performance was diminishing. The owners did not want to inject her hocks and possibly overstress them at the next show, so needed an alternative to keep her comfortable. I used a combination of acupuncture treatments and magnetic therapy to relieve her pain. The magnets were kept on her hocks between acupuncture treatments. The treatments were effective, and she performed very well at the final two shows.

Later, when presented to another vet for her hock injections, the mare was examined and her hocks were given a flexion test. She responded with no lameness at all on one hock and only a slight lameness on the other. The examining vet was sure that the injections were not needed, but the owner suggested X-rays to assist in the evaluation. The X-rays showed advanced arthritis throughout both hocks. This astounded the vet who repeated the flexion tests with the same results. The owner then explained about the acupuncture and magnetic therapy the horse had been receiving. On hearing this additional treatment history, the vet agreed to inject the hocks but recommended that the alternative therapies be continued as well.

Shoeing

If your horse is arthritic, it can also be helpful to talk to a farrier and discuss any alterations in the shoes that might decrease the concussion the horse is feeling. It may be as simple as adding a high concussion-absorption pad under the shoe or trying some of the shoes made of new materials on the market that absorb concussion so the horse's joints are not jarred as much when exercising. Shoes made of neoprene with an aluminum core are one example. Although they are a bit challenging to put on because the blacksmith's hammer tends to bounce off some of the neoprene shoes, they can make a big difference in a horse's performance. In addition to relieving the symptoms of arthritis, these shoes can give horses with ringbone and navicular disease a new lease on life. Horses with problem hocks also often benefit from this type of shoe.

SYMPTOMS

- Painful, stiff movements, or limping; pain and stiffness worse in cold weather.
- Movement improves with exercise.
- Not wanting to go forward.
- Refusing to cooperate with training.
- A bad attitude on a constant basis in a horse that previously had been cooperative.

RECOMMENDATIONS

Diet Feed a diet suited for your horse's use, breed, and age, as outlined above and in Chapter Five. Avoid excessive protein in the diet. Rebalance the protein, calcium, and phosphorus levels if fat makes up more than one-eighth of the grain ration.

Exercise Long, slow warm-up when exercising.

Turnout As much pasture turnout as possible.

Homeopathy You can choose one from among the following possibilities:

- Arnica montana 6C, 12C, 30C, 6X, 12X, or 30X. Give three times a day for pain and inflammation. Can be used with other homeopathics.
- Rhus tox 3C, 6C, 30C, 6X, 12X, or 30X. Give three times a day. Use when any of these conditions are present: hot, painful swelling in the joints; the condition worsens in damp weather; the condition improves during exercise; the condition involves tendons or tendon sheaths.
- Bryonia 12C, 30C, or 30X. Give three times a day. Use when any of these conditions are present: joints are hot, swollen, and stiff; condition worsens with movement; pressure on affected area is painful.
- Hekla Lava 6C, 12C, 30C, 12X, or 30X. Give twice a day. Use when there is inflammation in the navicular bursa or coffin joint. This remedy is very helpful when treating ringbone.
- BHI Arthritis. Use three times a day. (Available in health food stores.)
- BHI Zeel. Use three times a day. (Available in health food stores.)

Acupuncture Acupuncture and moxibustion treatments are very effective in relieving the pain associated with arthritis and increasing the movement of the affected area. While acupuncture must be done by a *veterinary* acupuncturist, you can learn to do indirect moxibustion treatments yourself. (See the section on *Acupuncture* in Chapter Three.) Indirect use of the moxibustion stick over the affected area can be very helpful in relieving pain.

Topical

- Arnica lotion. A strong tincture of arnica in an alcohol base that is rubbed on the affected area. Decreases inflammation.
- DMSO. Best results with DMSO are obtained for joint arthritis. Use only medical grade from the vet; others have impurities that can be carried into the body with the DMSO. The horse's skin must be very clean when DMSO is used. It can be used after arnica lotion. (Always wear rubber gloves when applying DMSO as it is absorbed through your skin also.)
- BHI Traumeel. An ointment (with arnica as the main ingredient) that is anti-inflammatory. Extremely effective for acute flare-ups. This ointment has a cream base and may be messy. (Available in health food stores.)

Caution: *Avoid counterirritants such as HEET, Mineral Ice, liniments, and sweats. Long-term use causes skin irritation and results are very transient.*

Magnetic Therapy The increased circulation from treating with magnetic therapy can help to keep inflammation to a minimum. Consistent use is helpful in some cases of arthritis.

Aromatherapy
- Chamomile. Eases discomfort and reduces inflammation. Also use topically as a compress or poultice.
- Juniper. Decreases the accumulation of toxins in the joints. Topically it may be combined with rosemary and used as a massage oil.
- Rosemary. Reduces arthritic pain. Use as a compress, or massage oil. **Caution:** *See contraindications for rosemary listed under* Aromatherapy in *Appendix II, p. 308).*

Supplements
- Vitamin C can provide relief for many of the movement symptoms of arthritis. Start with 4 grams and increase the dosage gradually. Most horses can tolerate a dosage of 8 grams per 1,000 lbs (approx. 450 kg). If manure appear loose it is an indication that you have exceeded the correct dosage, so decrease the amount if you notice loose piles of manure. Be sure to feed vitamin C with the regular meal to avoid excessive acid in the stomach (vitamin C is ascorbic acid). If your horse will not eat vitamin C powder, try adding herbs with high vitamin C content to his diet, such as 10 grams (3/4 oz) of rosehips and 10 grams of nettle a day.
- Chondroitin products can be very helpful when arthritis is affecting the joints. Works best when combined with glucosamine. Use according to directions on label.
- MSM (methylsulfonylmethane), a naturally occurring nutrient which provides bio-available sulfur to the tissues. Use alone or in conjunction with other supplements. Seems to work well particularly when arthritis involves the spine. Give according to label directions.
- Antioxidant supplements such as vitamins A, C, and E, and beta carotene are helpful in relieving some arthritis pain, especially when the arthritis is throughout the body. Give these supplements according to label directions.

Herbs Yucca works well in some cases of arthritis. The liquid form is most effective; or use one 100 percent pure yucca for best results. If the yucca root contains a high amount of saponins and has been properly processed, 1/4 to 1/2 teaspoon a day will be sufficient. If the powder clumps together, it has not been processed correctly and does not seem to be effective when fed to horses. This is probably because the active ingredient, saponin, has been affected in the processing. I have also found that yucca pellets do not seem to be effective, perhaps due to the heat used in the process of manufacturing the pellets. (NOTE: Yucca may test "false-positive" in a drug-screening test).

SUGGESTED ORDER OF TREATMENTS
The best combination of the treatments will vary depending on the severity and location of the arthritis. I outline a typical program below. (NOTE: Remember to change your choice of homeopathics, supplements, and herbs after using the same ones for 2 to 3 months, since their effects may diminish.)

Acute flare-ups:
Acupuncture
Homeopathy
Supplements and Herbs: MSM and Yucca
Topical Products

Chronic management:
Acupuncture and Moxibustion
Dietary Management
Exercise
Homeopathy and Herbs

B

BITES

Horse Bites

If your horse is bitten by a horse and swelling and bruising are the only signs (there's no break in the skin), a five-to-ten-minute cold-water hosing will help to slow the circulation and reduce the swelling. Allow the affected area to dry, then rub it with arnica tincture. If the bruising is severe and the horse is sore, it's best to give homeopathic arnica in a potency of 30C three to four times a day as well. This procedure can be repeated for several days if minor soreness persists. If the area becomes extremely hot or swollen, consult your vet.

Bites that actually break the skin need to be thoroughly cleaned using an iodine disinfectant. Hydrogen peroxide is often used, but it has a limited ability to kill bacteria, so iodine is preferable. If you are washing out a deep bite, dilute one part iodine with three parts water and wash the area a number of times until all debris is gone. Because of the high number of bacteria that are associated with bite wounds, it is almost impossible to get rid of all of the bacteria, even with extremely thorough washing.

In most cases, the vet will not suture a bite wound unless absolutely necessary to avoid trapping bacteria inside the wound. If the wound is severe and must be sutured, care must be taken to arrest infection. In these cases antibiotics are sometimes unavoidable and are rightfully used. Arnica tincture is helpful around the edges of an open bite wound, and homeopathic arnica in a potency of 30C can be given to help with pain and inflammation.

Bites From Other Animals

Bites from small animals, such as a dog or a wild animal that a horse might encounter in a pasture,

should be examined immediately. Anytime you suspect that a horse has been bitten by a wild animal, check his vaccination record and see if a rabies vaccine has been given within the last year. Rabies is widespread in some areas of the United States. As much as I dislike vaccinating horses for rabies, the alternative is worse. Most horses kept in pastures, particularly in areas with active rabies, should be vaccinated annually or according to your vet's recommendations. Refer to Chapter Four, p.71, and my discussion of rabies there.

Rabies is a very contagious, dangerous disease that can be spread to humans. Although usually spread through infected saliva, there are other less common avenues of infection such as through the air, so do not take any chances when dealing with an animal bite. (See **Caution** below). If the skin has been broken, use rubber gloves when cleaning the area. Over the years I have observed a few horses with rabies. Do not ignore any bites that you suspect may have been from a stray dog or cat that may not have been vaccinated against rabies, or wild animals.

While I was in veterinary school, a horse was brought into the clinic that was thought to have some form of encephalitis, a disease affecting the spinal cord and brain. After inflicting considerable damage to the examining area of the clinic, the overly excited horse was confined to a quarantine stall. Since encephalitis is not often seen, many students examined the horse. When the horse later died, a diagnosis of rabies was confirmed. All 25 students who had been directly exposed to the rabid horse had already moved away from the area and had to be tracked down so they could be treated. This unfortunate episode could have been avoided if greater care had been taken in handling the case.

SYMPTOMS
• If a bite has not broken the skin, the only signs may be swelling, bruising, and soreness. In se-

vere cases the area may become extremely hot and swollen.

- Puncture wounds appear like small holes sometimes surrounded by bruising.
- Bites can look like lacerations.

RECOMMENDATIONS

Caution: *If you suspect a bite was from a wild animal and you live in an area where rabies is a problem, consult your vet immediately BEFORE cleaning out the wound. Also, be sure to wear protective gloves whenever you touch or clean the wound so that you do not come in contact with the infection.*

Clean When cleaning the wound, first use a detergent-based soap and follow with a solution of one part iodine to three parts water. Repeat the cleansing until all debris is gone.

Bach Flowers Give Rescue Remedy if the horse is upset.

Topical

- Arnica tincture should be applied around the edges of an open bite wound but not on the wound itself.
- Apply an ointment containing the herb calendula.

Homeopathy Arnica 30C can be given three to four times daily if swelling and pain persist.

Aromatherapy

- Tea tree. Stimulates immune system to work against bacterial infections.
- Thyme. Make an infusion to clean the wound. (See *Aromatherapy Appendix II* for instructions.)

Antibiotics May be warranted if the wound is severe and must be sutured.

Insect Bites

Insect bites are probably one of the greatest nuisances that horse owners face. While most horses tolerate mosquito and fly bites quite well, some horses are allergic to certain types of insect bites

and must be treated right away to stop them from reacting. The signs you will notice are swelling and heat around the bite area, with sweating, trembling, a decrease in pulse, and pale gums. The less common insect bites, such as spider bites, are more likely to cause these reactions. If your horse starts to have an allergic response to an insect bite, call the vet immediately.

The quicker you treat the problem area, the more successful you are likely to be. If left untreated, some insect bites, such as those from brown recluse spiders, can cause a terrible mess and possibly result in scarring. Consult your vet for the best treatment for whatever type of insect bite that you suspect occurred. If you do not know, then administer homeopathic apis in a potency of 6C every hour, as well as arnica 30C three to four times a day.

(Also see *Allergies* on p. 185 for more on allergic reactions to insect bites; *Fly Bites* on p.206; *Reactions to Insect Bites* under Skin Problems on p. 274; and in Chapter Six for insect control methods.)

SYMPTOMS

- An area of skin may swell and be hot to the touch.
- Symptoms of shock: sweating, trembling, a decrease in pulse, pale gums.

RECOMMENDATIONS

For severe allergic reactions or anaphylactic shock:

Vet Call your vet immediately.

Bach Flowers Give Rescue Remedy.

Homeopathy Give apis 30C every 15 minutes for up to 2 hours.

For regular treatment of an insect bite:

Homeopathy Give apis 6C and arnica 30C every hour. Arsenicum alba 6C can also be given three times daily if the horse's skin is hot surrounding the bite area, and the horse is restless.

Cold Treatment If the area is hot, stimulate circulation with a cold water hosing for 5 to 10 minutes.

Vet If swelling persists or symptoms worsen, call your vet.

Poultice A clay poultice can help reduce swelling and cool the area. Apply poultice to areas surrounding the injured area. Do not apply to the wound directly.

Snakebites

Since many riding trails are in areas inhabited by poisonous snakes (such as pit vipers), snakebites are a concern to most horse owners. Depending where you live, snakes may also be a problem in the barn area since rodents live in many barns and snakes eat rodents.

When I moved to San Antonio, Texas, the first thing I was told when I moved my horse into the barn was never to reach behind anything into an area I couldn't see, particularly my tack trunk, as snakes were extremely common. I soon learned just how common they were while trail riding with a friend. We were trotting along on a well-marked trail through a brushy area when we heard a noise and stopped our horses. When we turned around we saw a large rattlesnake writhing and thrashing all over the ground. Apparently we had mistaken the snake for a branch, had trotted over it, and one of the horses had actually stepped on it. Neither of us had even recognized the large snake directly in our path.

Horses are occasionally bitten by a poisonous snake so you should check your horse carefully if you have been riding in an area known to be populated by snakes. Snakes have very sharp fangs and bite very quickly. The horse sometimes doesn't even feel the quick impact of the fang, so many horses don't react when bitten. Other horses just seem to spook and then settle down. Finding a snakebite may also be difficult, unless you actually saw the snake bite the horse.

The fang marks can be quite small, and it's possible that only one fang actually hit the horse.

Often the first indication an owner has that the horse has been bitten by a snake is finding a large swollen area. If you search carefully, you can usually find the fang marks which will look like tiny holes in the skin. The distance between the fang marks will usually indicate how large the snake was—the wider the distance between the fangs, the larger the snake. This can be helpful information, since it might give the vet an idea of how much venom could have been injected into the horse.

Because a horse can go into shock from a snakebite, call your vet immediately. Even though a horse's large body can sometimes handle the toxins and tolerate a snakebite, the effects vary depending on the amount of venom injected by the snake. If the horse is bitten on a leg the situation is less life threatening than if he is bitten on the nose. When bitten on the nose, swelling can occur that might block the horse's ability to breathe, making the situation more serious with immediate treatment necessary. If bitten on a leg, the local area may swell and become hot. *Do not* cut open the area over the fang marks as seen in old Western movies. Let your vet administer any invasive treatment later if necessary.

If you have suction cups (which come with many snakebite kits), follow the directions on the kit to help draw the venom out. ***Caution:*** *Never try to suck out venom with your mouth. The venom is injected deeply, and very little is actually at the surface to suck out. Also, if you should have any open lesions in your mouth, any venom that you suck can be absorbed into your system, thus poisoning you. If you are poisoned too, you're not going to be much help to your horse.*

While waiting for help, keep the horse as calm as possible. Do not continue riding or walking the horse, as the toxin is spread throughout the body by circulation. Keep the area cool to help diminish swelling and slow circulation of the blood and toxin. Expect possible infection and tissue damage around the area of the bite.

Older remedies used for snakebite include the use of garlic both internally and as an external poultice, but I have never seen a case where garlic was effective as the only treatment of snakebite.

SYMPTOMS

NOTE: Symptoms of snakebites are variable depending on how much time has elapsed since the bite and the amount of venom injected.

- In some cases, snakebites lead to a large swollen, hot area that, upon close examination, will reveal tiny holes in the skin.
- Possible symptoms include shock, weakness, total collapse, or the horse may seek seclusion standing in a corner of his stall, separating himself from other horses in the field, or not coming in at feeding time.

RECOMMENDATIONS

- If you suspect a snakebite, call your vet immediately.
- If you have a snakebite kit, use the suction cups and follow directions on the kit to help draw the venom out.
- While waiting for the vet, attempt to reduce the potential for shock by keeping the horse as calm as possible.
- Keep the area of the bite cool with ice packs (or hosing if ice packs not available) to help diminish swelling and slow circulation.

Homeopathy Give the following homeopathics together every 30 minutes for two to three hours; then continue with the frequency as listed below:
- Arnica montana 30C hourly.
- Apis 6C for swelling, given three times daily.
- If the horse has been bitten on the nose, give lachesis 1M hourly.

First Aid Apply a tourniquet above a leg bite to decrease the spread of the toxin but do not tie it so tightly that the arterial circulation is stopped. Release the tourniquet every 15 minutes for 1 to 2 minutes to allow normal circulation. After treatment remove the tourniquet.

Antibiotics Usually warranted to prevent infection that often accompanies snakebites.

FOLLOW-UP CARE

Clean Daily cleaning of the bite area is usually necessary, depending on the severity of the bite.

Moxibustion Do around the area of the bite to help to speed healing. Start only after the initial inflammation has subsided (at least 3 days after the bite) and do not perform this treatment if infection is present.

C

CANCER

Cancer is a complex disease. It is not just an isolated tumor or affected type of cells (such as leukemia cells), but a condition of the entire body system that has allowed these cells to develop in the first place. Sometimes, people find it difficult to comprehend that the entire body is involved when the cancer is manifested in the form of an apparently isolated tumor. That one tumor, however, is the body's way of saying that something is very wrong and it isn't able to prevent the mutated cancer cells from multiplying. The challenge is to treat the cancer and keep it in remission while you are also supporting the body system.

Practitioners of conventional veterinary medicine have generally treated cancer in horses in much the same as cancer in humans is conventionally treated, primarily with surgery and chemotherapy. However, there are many approaches to cancer treatment and certainly many differing opinions. I will give you some options and the reasons behind them to help you make your decisions. I advise that you learn as much as you can about all the possibilities and then make your treatment choices in conjunction with your vet's recommendations.

Melanoma

A melanoma is a tumor seen most often in gray horses, usually around the tail or head area, but it can occur elsewhere (see fig. III–1, p. 198). Melanomas appear as raised areas under the skin—as discolored lumps on the underside of the tail and around the anus, or raised, knobby lumps on the underside of the throat. The old medical texts refer to melanoma as a disease of old horses, but it is now being seen in younger horses as well. It is not known why melanoma has begun to occur in younger horses, but it is possible that since this tumor has a genetically linked predisposition, there may be a connection to stress on the immune system.

Years ago most horses did not travel as much as they do now, nor did very many of them have show careers, live in crowded stables with no turnout, or eat hay treated with herbicides and pesticides. Nor were they given vaccinations. It is difficult to say if one of these stresses is the reason we are seeing more melanoma in younger horses; it is more likely that melanoma is caused by a combination of stresses.

Melanoma can metastasize widely throughout the body, so if treatment is recommended it should be started as soon as possible. Holistic medicine bases its approach on supporting and healing the failing body, which allows the body to respond and fight the cancer. With any type of cancer, I prefer a treatment plan that considers the current state of the body and strengthening it to prevent cancer cells from continuing to form.

A new treatment with autogenous vaccines helps control development of more melanomas and stop the progression of existing ones (melanomas first seen under the tail area often spread to the digestive tract). A biopsy is performed on a melanoma, or on all melanomas if there are several, and a vaccine developed specifically for that horse. More than one vaccine may be required. This treatment has proven to be effective in some cases.

Cimetidine, a generic pharmaceutical drug used to treat stomach disorders such as ulcers in people, has been effective in the treatment of some melanomas. Cimetidine must be used for quite a long period—possibly up to six months or more—so this treatment is a long-term commitment. Check with your vet if you are considering using cimetidine to treat your horse's melanoma.

Acupuncture will stimulate the immune system and balance the body's energy so it can function more efficiently. Homeopathy can be used to stimulate the immune system specifically against cancer and is also a good supportive measure. There are also a wide variety of herbs that have been used to help combat cancer. In my experience herbs have been very helpful, but each case must be carefully evaluated.

The late Dr. Lawrence Burton developed a cancer therapy in the 1960s called the Immune Augmentative Therapy that is basically homeopathic in nature. It is based on comprehensive lab work in which four proteins which block the growth of cancer cells are isolated from the blood and then given as a series of injections. This program has a remarkable record and I have had good results using it. The therapy includes three to four injections given daily by the owner, plus re-checks and follow-up lab work which can go on for a number of months. Its main drawbacks are the owner-intensive requirement and the fact that the horse may develop intolerance to the injections. This therapy works well with other holistic treatments. Nutritional supplement

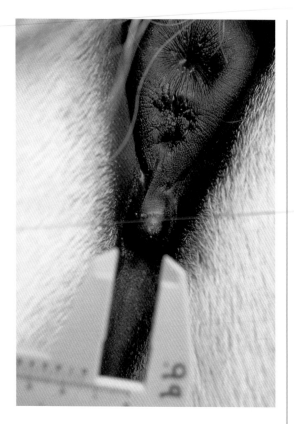

III–1 *A perineal melanoma.*

recommendations and nutritional advice are included in this program. Dr. Burton's work is being carried on at the Immunology Research Center in Freeport, Grand Bahama Island, for human patients and in New York for animals by Dr. Martin Goldstein, a vet (see Appendix VIII).

Many other alternative cancer treatments are still being perfected. Before instituting any alternative type of treatment, check into it carefully. Consult a vet who knows alternative medicine for advice. The wrong type of treatment could cause a worsening of the condition.

SYMPTOMS

- There are no specific symptoms for cancer, which makes it difficult to diagnose. Affected horses may lose weight and/or appetite, or just become lethargic, but even standard blood tests, so sensitive to many body changes, fre-

quently remain normal until cancer is in an advanced stage. You need to watch for changes in your horse's normal behavior and check his body regularly for unusual lumps. The detection of cancer starts with an owner's observation skills, and keeping a record of your horse's health in a journal will help you notice changes. When you have any doubts that all is not normal discuss the matter with your vet.

RECOMMENDATIONS

For Melanoma:

Surgical Removal

Drug Treatment Discuss giving cimetidine with your vet. It should be started when melanoma is first detected and continued as necessary for 6 months to a year.

For all types of cancer:

Diet High quality.

Supplements

- Shark cartilage is a recently discovered cancer treatment that shows some promise. Response depends on the purity (refinement) of the product and the type of cancer being treated, so check with your holistic vet to order it. Follow label directions.
- Include a vitamin and mineral supplement in your horse's diet.
- Increase vitamin C in the diet. While dosage varies, as a general guideline give 8 grams daily to a 1,000-pound (approx. 450 kgs) horse.

Homeopathy Choose one of the following:

- Thuja occidentalis 30C, three times daily. Use when tumors are being treated, particularly those that involve soft tissue.
- Nux vomica 6C. Give three times a day. Use when liver enzymes are elevated or when using conventional chemotherapy treatment.

Herbs Immune stimulating herbs:

- Echinacea acts to stimulate the immune system. Give 10 to 20 grams a day.

- Boneset to stimulate the immune system. Give about 1/4 cup (4 tbsp) daily. Use of this herb may result in a slightly loose stool. Another property of this herb is vasodilation, so consult your vet if your horse is taking other medications to make sure there is no interference.
- Garlic stimulates the immune system and can be effective in reducing some tumors. Garlic can be added to the feed as well as made into a paste and applied directly on external tumors. Give 8 cloves of crushed or chopped garlic a day (fresh garlic is best) or 20 grams of garlic powder.
- Fenugreek is often used in conjunction with garlic as a treatment for cancer and tumors. This herb works well to stimulate appetite and help improve the horse's general condition. Horses that are allergic to alfalfa may react to fenugreek. **Caution:** *Do not feed to pregnant mares or use when the cancer involves the reproductive system since this herb produces compounds in the body that are similar to the reproductive hormones.*
- Cat's claw is a herb from the rainforest that stimulates the immune system; however, it can be expensive. Make a tea by adding 2 tbsp of cat's claw to 1 liter of boiling water. Let it steep for 10 minutes and then remove the herb and feed 1/2 cup (100ml) of the tea on the grain twice a day.
- A commercial herbal mixture for immune stimulation is available from Hilton Herbs under the brand name Ditton.

Electrical Therapy This treatment was developed in Sweden for human cancer patients. In animals most applications have been to external tumors. Although effective, electrical therapy is not widely utilized since it breaks down tumors very quickly and, as a result, overburdens the body with toxic products.

Aromatherapy
- Jasmine (*sambac var.* only). Helps skin tumors.

- Lemon. Stimulates immune system.
- Litsea Cubeba. Stimulates immune system.

Bach Flowers
- Gorse. Relieves depression.
- Olive. Helps relieve the feeling of exhaustion—mental, physical, and of the spirit which often occurs during a long physical illness.

CHOKE

A case of *choke* is an emergency, and a vet should be called in immediately. It occurs when an object or clump of feed becomes lodged in a horse's esophagus. Dry feeds, such as beet pulp and wheat bran, which expand when exposed to moisture, are associated with causing choke, as are whole apples, pears, and carrots. Horses who eat very quickly or "bolt" their food are also predisposed to this condition.

SYMPTOMS

The signs of choke will vary depending on the location of the blockage and may include any of the following:
- Head and neck held out in an extended position.
- Saliva may drip out of the mouth, or you may see saliva on the walls of a stall and on fence boards when a horse with choke flings his head around as he attempts to relieve the blockage.
- The horse cannot swallow.
- The horse coughs repeatedly.

RECOMMENDATIONS

Vet Call your vet immediately.

Bach Flowers Give Rescue Remedy to help calm the horse.

Diet Take food and water away from the horse.

Homeopathy
- Magnesium phosphorica 12C. Give four times, 15 minutes apart, to help relax muscle spasms.
- Arnica montana 30C. Give three times a day for 3 days to reduce the inflammation.

Acupuncture Use to relieve choke when regular veterinary treatment has not been successful, and when the location of the blockage is particularly difficult. The acupuncture will help to relax the area around the choke, which should help the material to pass.

COLIC

Colic is one of the most common health problems we have with horses. Because a severe case can be fatal, it's extremely important that all owners are familiar with the signs and possible causes of colic. Don't wait until your horse experiences colic to learn about it.

Colic in horses is similar to a stomachache in humans. The two most common types of colic are spasmodic and gas colic. Other forms of colic such as impaction, or a displaced internal structure (large intestine, small intestine, or spleen), though seen less often, are far more serious and may require surgery. Signs of colic include: looking and biting at the sides, pawing, stretching out the hind legs when standing, restless walking or circling, lying down and getting up, and rolling. Additional symptoms of gas colic include a tense abdomen, noises from the abdomen, and the passing of gas. If your horse appears to be in distress, check immediately for the signs mentioned above. In more severe cases, you may also see signs of sweating, increased respirations, and increased pulse (over 100 beats or more, per minute). See Chapter Nine.

If you suspect colic, contact your vet immediately and follow the recommendations he gives you, and if he agrees, give one of the homeopathic or herbal remedies outlined below. If possible, do not allow your horse to lie down or roll. Slow walking is often helpful unless your horse is very stressed and in great pain. If so, keep him as quiet as you can until the vet arrives. Homeopathics are often helpful to treat colic before and after the vet arrives. Always check with a vet

when colic symptoms appear and do not rely only on homeopathic treatment. There are many different types of colic and some colic can have different stages. You may not be dealing with a simple spasmodic colic, so it's better to be safe than sorry. Remember, colic can be fatal.

If your horse experiences any of the symptoms of colic, it's important that you be prepared to deal with them until your vet can get to your horse. If you live in a remote region, ask your vet about standard treatments for colic that you can keep on hand. If you show and travel a lot, it's also a good idea to have an emergency kit that includes colic treatments in case of an emergency without a vet available.

There are a number of causes of colic such as stress, dehydration, food changes, hormonal shifts, parasites, and many others. Some causes are specific to different regions of the country, such as parasites that infest a certain area or soil that is mostly sand which the horse ingests. Once you become familiar with the common causes of colic, you should take steps to avoid them. If you are unfamiliar with colic, ask your vet to explain it to you further.

SYMPTOMS
- Restless walking or circling.
- Looking or biting at sides.
- Tense abdomen.
- Pawing.
- Lying down or rolling.
- Severe signs: sweating, increased respiration, and increased pulse.

RECOMMENDATIONS
Caution: Call your vet immediately.

Acupuncture After your vet has determined the type of colic from his examination, he can use acupuncture to stimulate the bowel. Acupuncture is particularly useful with impaction colic.

Acupressure and/or Moxibustion Do over acupuncture points associated with the large intestine as it can be soothing for spasmodic colic. The easiest point to use is BL_{25} (see *Acupuncture/Acupressure Appendix* I, and Chapter Three for *Moxibustion*).

Homeopathy Choose one of the following:

- Nux vomica 6C, 12C, 30C, 12X, or 30X given every 2 hours for up to 4 doses. Use when a spasmodic colic or gas colic is present. These types of colic are indicated by signs such as the horse turning around frequently and looking at his stomach, or repeatedly trying to pass manure. (In an emergency situation, you can use the potency up to 1M that is available from a holistic vet.)
- Carbo vegetabilis 30C given every 2 hours for up to 6 doses. Use when colic occurs after eating or exercise, excessive gas is being discharged, and the manure smells rancid.
- Ipecacuanha 30C given every 2 hours for up to 4 doses. Use when colic is associated with a feed change or when the colic may be due to the use of very coarse hay. The horse will have no appetite or thirst and will stretch out the hind legs behind him.
- Calcarea carbonica 6C or 12C given three times daily. Use when horse has eaten something he is allergic or reactive to such as moldy hay. Assists horses that have become lethargic and are not eating all their feed.
- Belladonna 6C or 12C given every 2 hours for up to 4 doses. Use in severe cases of colic when the horse is excitable and sweating. The skin may be hot to the touch. The horse will have no interest in food.
- Aconitum napellus 6C, 12C, 30C, 12X, or 30X. Give every hour until signs of colic are gone. Use when colic is first noticed. The horse may want to drink water and will be restless. NOTE: This remedy can be used together with any of the other remedies listed here.

Herbs

- Comfrey to reduce inflammation of the stomach lining. Give 25 grams a day.
- Marshmallow works to coat and soothe the digestive tract. Give 20 grams a day.
- Slippery elm works to coat the digestive tract. Give 2 to 4 tablespoons, three times daily for 5 days. I suggest mixing the slippery elm with 3/4 cup (175ml) of yogurt and/or 2 tablespoons of honey.

NOTE: Instead of mixing the above herbs in the feed, you can make a tea from one or more of them with 1 liter of boiling water. Allow to cool, mix the tea with the grain twice a day.

- A commercially available herbal mix for digestive disorders such as those available from Hilton Herbs.

Aromatherapy

- Combine lavender and hops. Relieves cramping in the digestive tract, especially when the colic is due to nervous tension.
- Lemon. Calms, particularly when the horse has a fever.
- Litsea cubeba. Decreases gas.
- Melissa. Relaxes.
- Sandalwood. Decreases diarrhea that sometimes occurs with colic.

Bach Flowers Impatiens. Prevents re-occurring mild colic.

Parasite Control Colic can be prevented by control of the parasites that cause damage to the digestive tract. (See *Worms and Worming*, p. 101.)

Feeding If you live in an area where the soil is primarily sand, do not feed your horse on the ground. Use products marketed to help minimize the amount of sand in the large intestine. They are usually made of psyllium seed husks and help to push the sand out of the digestive tract so it does not build up.

Exercise Always cool your horse completely following exercise before giving food or water.

CUTS AND PUNCTURE WOUNDS

Horses seem to be prone to getting cuts on a regular basis, and most horse owners keep a few common salves and ointments around to treat them. Small abrasions usually heal easily and are not much of a problem, but large or deep cuts are of concern. Cuts over prominences, such as shoulders and knees, can be difficult to heal because of the constant pull of the skin on the area. Cuts become of particular concern if a horse is prone to developing excessive granulation tissue (known as proud flesh), over the cut area in an effort to heal it (see fig. III–2, p. 203).

Puncture wounds are extremely dangerous because they may be undetected for some time, and without treatment can fester into an infection. Deep puncture wounds can also harbor non-aerobic bacteria (bacteria that do not require air), and these bacteria may be deadly. Tetanus is one example—the reason why regular vaccinations for tetanus are recommended for horses, which I discussed in Chapter Four, p. 68. (See also *Puncture Wounds* under *Hoof Problems*, p. 220).

RECOMMENDATIONS

If the wound is still bleeding:

First Aid
- Apply pressure to the area. For gaping wounds, use bandage material and press inward with your hand using continuous pressure. A pressure bandage can be applied to leg cuts with extensive bleeding. Pressure bandages can be made using a clean gauze pad and a bandage such as vet wrap. Place the gauze pad over the area that is bleeding and wrap with the vet wrap. Do not wrap so tightly that circulation to the leg is stopped.
- Pack gauze into a large bleeding cut, using sterile gauze if possible. Then apply pressure over the top of the gauze with your hand. In an emergency situation, when bleeding is very severe and the cut is large, any padding that can be used to pack into the cut area will work.

Vet Call a vet as soon as possible to handle large cuts since some of the blood vessels may have to be treated surgically.

For treatment of severe swelling, see Swelling *on p. 284.*

Homeopathy
- Phosphorus 30C every 15 minutes for up to 2 hours or until bleeding is under control.
- Hypericum 30C. Give 4 times over a 24-hour period. A higher 1M potency may be used if available. Use when a wound is severe, nerves have been injured, and when the horse is in great pain.
- Ledum 12x, 3C, or 6C. Use for deep puncture wounds.

NOTE: Hypericum and ledum can be used together if the injured horse has not had a tetanus vaccination, or the vaccination is not recent.

Aromatherapy
- Eucalyptus and Lavender. Use together for healing purposes.
- Tea tree. Stimulates immune system to fight bacterial infection. May also be used topically as a healing agent.
- Thyme. Make a thyme-based infusion to clean wound. (See *Aromatherapy Appendix II*.)
- Chamomile. Soothes the irritated skin around the cut.

Herbs Give the Chinese herb Yunnan Paiyao orally to help control excessive bleeding. However, limit its use because it can cause severe side effects if used repeatedly. (If it is used on a regular basis for a horse with a repetitive bleeding problem such as bleeding in the lung when galloping, do not use it more than twice a month.)

Topical/Ointments:
- Calendula ointment. Stimulates healing. Apply twice a day over affected area. (Available in health food stores.)

- Hypericum ointment. Treats puncture wounds, extremely painful wounds, and those involving nerves. Use twice a day. (Available in health food stores).

To cleanse the wound from a cut:

First Aid Evaluate the area first. If the cut is over a day old, appears to have sealed over, or is crusty, and it shows no signs of infection, then it's usually best to leave it alone and let nature take its course. If a cut is fresh or appears hot, or has pus in it, clean the area.

Clean Clean the wound with water first, followed by a disinfectant. Do not overuse water because it can cause cell damage and slow the healing process. You need to clean the area thoroughly but not over-flush it. Iodine is one choice to flush the wound. When using iodine (usually available in 7 or 10 percent solutions), dilute it with water in a ratio of one part iodine to three parts water. If the cut is a puncture wound, rinse it out with hydrogen peroxide first, then follow with iodine. Some of the bacteria deep inside the wound will be killed by the oxygen that is emitted by the hydrogen peroxide. If your horse is sensitive to disinfectants and iodine, wash out the wound with warm water mixed with a little hypericum tincture (available in health food stores). Then, instead of using hydrogen peroxide, rinse the wound with a tea made of the herb, slippery elm. You can also pack the wound with a paste of slippery elm. Simply grind the herb and then mix it with just enough water to make a paste.

Medication

- Once the cut is cleaned, allow the area to dry, and examine the cut for any other problems, such as discoloration that might indicate bruising or foreign bodies, such as splinters. An ointment (preferably one containing the herb calendula or hypericum) or antibiotic cream (available in most horse supply stores) should

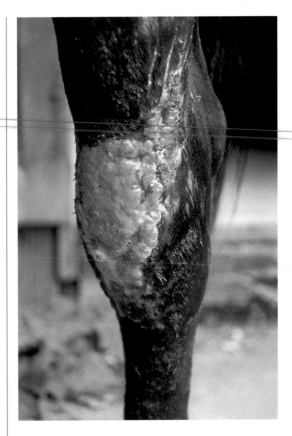

III–2 *A hock laceration two weeks after occurrence showing granulated tissue commonly known as "proud flesh."*

then be applied to the cut to protect it and keep it clean. Do not assume that all the medications sold for cuts will promote healing—some won't. If you are unsure which product will work best for your horse's cut, consult your vet for advice.

- The decision on which medication to use depends on several factors. If the cut is infected, a topical medication may not be able to take care of the infection in the surrounding tissue. Instead, an injectable or oral type of antibiotic prescribed by your vet may be necessary. If your horse is unable to take antibiotics, use colloidal silver (available at a health food store). The dosage is 2 to 3 teaspoons a day. A laser can also be used around the cut to stimulate healing and especially helpful if the horse cannot tolerate antibiotics. Consult your vet about its use and a treatment schedule.

Cuts on the Leg:

Bandage

- The healing process for a cut on the leg may be slow due to poor circulation in the area and constant movement. If you're not sure about whether or not to bandage, consult your vet. If the cut area needs to be kept clean, a bandage may be a good idea. But be careful in hot humid climates—bandages can cause problems by creating a warm moist environment that allows bacteria to flourish.
- The decision about bandaging will depend on several factors including the size and location of the cut and the attitude of your horse. Some horses will not tolerate bandages and seem to delight in tearing them off, ignoring all of the hard work—not to mention the expense—of putting on the bandage.
- If the horse does not tolerate bandages but must wear one, a neck cradle can be used to prevent him from tearing off the bandages. Neck cradles are made of long pieces of wood tied together and fitted around the horse's neck so that he cannot reach down to the bandage. Cradles are available from many tack shops and horse supply catalogs. If you're familiar with the "Elizabethan" collars used in similar situations for dogs, it's the same idea but using wood instead of plastic.

D

DIARRHEA

Diarrhea can occur suddenly or be a chronic problem. When diarrhea comes on *suddenly,* check the horse's overall condition: Is his temperature high? Is he eating? Is he in any distress or pain—biting at his sides or walking around constantly? There are several serious syndromes that can cause sudden diarrhea and the threat of one of these should be eliminated first. Salmonella poisoning and Potomac Horse Fever are examples of diseases that cause sudden diarrhea and can be life threatening, so evaluate your horse immediately. If he shows signs of illness in addition to the diarrhea and, in particular, if he shows signs of shock (pale gums, sweating, decreased pulse and respiration), call a vet immediately. If the diarrhea is severe, a horse can dehydrate and fluids may need to be given. We always want to think that a serious disease couldn't happen to our own horse, however horses have a knack of doing just what we think they won't, so don't overlook any possibilities.

If the diarrhea comes on suddenly but there are no other signs of illness, monitor your horse closely. The most common causes are too much grass or a reaction to food. If a horse is not used to eating grass and is suddenly allowed to eat a large amount, diarrhea is often the result, along with the possibility of more serious complications such as colic and laminitis. This condition is usually temporary and improves when the grass has moved through the digestive tract. When you return the horse to grass, be sure to do it more gradually.

Feed reactions can occur when feed is changed too rapidly, when a new feed provides more nutrients than a horse has been used to, or when a horse is allergic to a feed.

If your horse has *chronic diarrhea,* there are a variety of possible causes such as malabsorption syndromes, liver disease, stress, and an antibiotic treatment that upset the bacterial flora. Review your horse's history to help determine what changes, stresses or illnesses have occurred in your horse's past that might have brought on a state of chronic diarrhea.

Some horses can be very sensitive to change. You might be unaware of a small change in the environment that your horse has interpreted as stressful, even if it's happened during a regular occurrence, such as a weekly trail ride or horse show.

Parasites are still a frequent cause of diarrhea, and are often overlooked when reviewing the horse's health. A routine worming program will eliminate the parasites but not the damage that excessive parasite infestation can do to the digestive tract. Even when the parasites are gone the diarrhea may persist due to the damage that has been caused.

Do not take anything for granted when evaluating the possible causes, because isolating the cause of the diarrhea may be helpful in choosing in the treatment or in preventing future problems. If you are unable to find a cause, it's best to consult your vet for suggestions. He may recommend blood work and a checkup.

SYMPTOMS

- Soft or runny stools of an acute or chronic nature.

RECOMMENDATIONS

Caution: *Consult a vet immediately if your horse shows other signs of illness along with the diarrhea.*

Parasite Control Review your parasite control program and have a fecal check done if you are unsure if the program is effective.

Diet Check feed for any changes that might have caused a reaction.

Turnout If just starting a turnout program, decrease the time allowed on grass.

Supplements Feed a bacterial supplement product containing lactobacillus and/or acidolphilus to replace the natural flora in the diet (see p. 86).

Acupuncture Helps rebalance the digestive tract and often successfully treats the problem.

Homeopathy Choose one of the following:

- Nux vomica 30C given three times a day. Use when the diarrhea is associated with an excessive amount of gas, when the diarrhea is worse in the morning, or when the liver enzymes on the blood work are elevated. Also when the horse is jaundiced in conjunction with the diarrhea.
- Podophyllum 6C or 12C given three times a day. Use in chronic cases of diarrhea. Works best in cases where diarrhea is watery and contains mucus. Also can relieve diarrhea due to ovulation pain in mares.
- Ipecacuanha 3C given three times a day. Use if the horse is straining with the diarrhea or if the diarrhea has a frothy or slimy consistency.

Herbs The same herbs that treat colic are helpful for diarrhea (see p. 201).

Review

- Any recent sources of stress such as antibiotic therapy or illness to help determine the possible cause and do what you can to eliminate it.
- Your feed program to help determine if it's supporting your horse when chronic diarrhea is present and that it is not a cause of the diarrhea.

Vet Consult your vet if the horse has not responded to any treatment that was given and the case becomes chronic.

E

EAR PROBLEMS

The most common ear problems that affect horses are ear infections and fly bites.

Ear Infections

When infected, the ear is usually red and uncomfortable. Constant scratching of the affected ear is the most common symptom. Sometimes there is a discharge that can be white, yellow, or brown, depending on the organism causing it. There are two basic types of ear infections—bacterial and fungal. Bacteria and fungus make up the normal flora in a horse's ear canal. Ideally, a balance is maintained between them, but if something happens to alter the conditions in the ear, either the bacteria or fungus might have more favorable conditions and multiply at a greater rate. As a result, one of the organisms predominates and grows out of control. Then the ear is "infected" and causes the horse discomfort.

Horses with long, heavily haired ears should be checked regularly for ear infections since the hair can trap moisture and allow for an overgrowth of bacteria or fungus. However, be careful when checking your horse's ears—especially if you suspect an infection is present—since an infected ear is sensitive to touch.

Do not try to diagnose and treat an ear infection by yourself. Several different types of bacteria and fungus can grow in the horse's ear, and it's very difficult to tell a bacterial infection from a fungal infection. It is very important to select the correct medication to control the conditions. Treating the incorrect organisms will result in a worsened condition and longer recovery time. Sometimes it may even lead to a chronic condition.

Ear infections rarely go away by themselves, so get treatment as soon as possible.

SYMPTOMS
• Scratching and rubbing in or under the ear.
• Red or white patchy area inside the ear.
• The horse will not let the ear be touched; may not want the halter or bridle put over the ear.

RECOMMENDATIONS

Vet Consult a vet if you notice a problem with the ear. Do not treat the condition yourself. Incorrect treatment may make the problem worse.

Acupressure On points around the ear may be helpful. Use points BL_{10}, TH_{17}, GB_{20}, and TH_{21} (see Appendix I). However, be careful because most horses with ear problems become sensitive to touch around the ear.

Prevention of Ear Infections:
• Do not get water in the ears when bathing.
• If your horse is prone to infections keep a fly mask with ear covers on him to prevent debris from entering the ear.
• Do not clip the hair in the ears.

Caution: *Do not apply ear medication unless the ear is infected and a vet has prescribed it.*

Fly Bites

When flies congregate on the tips of a horse's ears and repeatedly bite the area, the result is often a bloody, hairless area on the outer edges of the ear. The eye area can also be attacked by flies. This can cause an inflammation at the corner of the eyes. Both conditions are painful and irritating, causing the horse to scratch his head. Sometimes this scratching then creates even worse problems.

SYMPTOMS
• Hairless areas on the tips of the ears; some may be bloody and raw.

RECOMMENDATIONS

Topical
• Use a fly repellent on the ears and around the eyes and a fly mask to keep flies from landing on them. (Do not apply repellent over the top of the eyes because it might run into the eyes when exposed to heat.)
• If necessary, commercial products are available that have an insect repellent in a sticky petroleum jelly-type base to keep the flies away, so further damage can be avoided.
• A sunscreen can be used to protect the area around the damaged ear from sunburn.

Turnout For pasture horses in severe conditions, cattle ear tags with fly repellent can be attached to the halter. (If using a halter in the pasture, make sure it's the type that will break if the horse catches it on anything.)

Acupressure Do on points around the ear to stimulate healing. Use points BL_{10}, TH_{17}, GB_{20}, and TH_{21} (see Appendix I). If the eye is affected by fly bites as well, also do acupressure on point BL_1 and BL_2.

Review Read the section on *Insect Control* in Chapter Six.

ENCEPHALOMYELITIS

(See Chapter Four, p. 69)

EQUINE INFLUENZA

(See Chapter Four, p. 70)

EQUINE PROTOZOAL MYELOENCEPHALITIS (EPM)

Equine Protozoal Myeloencephalitis (EPM) is a disease that has been recognized for many years but its impact has been underestimated. In the past, neurological symptoms such as toe dragging, back soreness, intermittent lameness, asymmetrical lameness, bucking, head tossing, and incoordination were thought to be the main symptoms of EPM. Now, vets are aware that a variety of other symptoms can be indicators of this protozoal infection. In fact, sometimes the first change noticed by owners is a behavioral change, particularly irritability or spookiness. Other signs mentioned by many owners include a change in the hair coat, a dull coat, or hair that does not lay down flat. Often, the coat appears normal one day, and then the next day these symptoms suddenly appear. In its worst form, EPM can cause severe neurological signs such as staggering, paralysis, or muscle atrophy, often affecting only one side of the body. From this varied list of possibilities, it is obvious that EPM is difficult to diagnose based on symptoms alone.

EPM is caused by tiny microscopic parasites called protozoa. The type that causes EPM in horses is called *sarcocystis*, although there is another genus of protozoa, *neospora*, which has also been found to cause neurological symptoms in horses. It is not known how common *neospora* infection is in horses.

Sarcocystis is thought to be carried by opossums and birds, and it is disseminated in their feces. Once in the horse's system through eating hay, grass, or some other food that has been contaminated by *sarcocystis*, it is thought that the immune system usually kills the parasite. If the horse's immune system doesn't kill the parasite, it makes its way to the nervous system, where it can affect the brain, spinal cord, or both and cause lesions at several locations. Because several different locations and areas of the nervous system can be affected at one time, the signs of EPM vary from horse to horse and also vary in intensity.

There are currently two blood tests and a spinal test that are used to diagnose EPM. Although they are helpful when diagnosing a suspected EPM case, the tests are still imperfect for a final diagnosis. One blood test, the Western blot, checks for antibodies produced by the horse. A positive result tells us only that the horse has been exposed, and not if EPM is actually causing the current problem. A negative result may mean that EPM is not the problem or it may also mean that the horse's immune system has not yet mounted a response to the parasite. The other blood test, called the PCR, tests for a segment of DNA in *sarcocystis falcatula* (formerly *S. neurona*). This test seems to be the most reliable early in the infection or after the immune response has decreased. The spinal test requires that a spinal tap be performed and spinal fluid withdrawn from around the spinal cord. This spinal fluid is then tested for antibodies. If positive, it confirms that *sarcocystis* is present in the spinal cord area and is most likely the cause of any neurological problems. If the spinal fluid is contaminated with blood during the procedure, the test will not be accurate. Bear in mind that the spinal tap is not 100 percent reliable even when the procedure is done correctly. Often all three tests are performed so the results can be compared later to evaluate the effectiveness of the treatment after it is complete. If the antibody numbers are still high, then treatment will have to be continued.

Although testing is preferred, many owners decide against these procedures because of the expense as well as the risk involved in transporting their horses to a clinic or veterinary school. Check to see if a vet will perform the tests at your stable since more are doing this safely in the field. There are many factors to consider when making the decision to test for EPM so it's best to consider each case individually. I explain the pros and cons of the testing procedures to an owner and let him make the decision to go forward with them or not. The cost of the tests varies depending on your location, but the cost of all three generally is about the same as 20 to 30 days of the medication that is currently used to treat EPM. If a horse is showing severe neurological signs, immediate treatment is initiated at the same time the test is performed since it takes about a week to get the results once the tests have been performed. This is too long to wait when neurological symptoms are rapidly worsening.

Even though the tests are not totally accurate, the results can be helpful. For instance, if the spinal fluid does contain the antibodies that indicate the presence of EPM, the horse can be retested after being given a course of the medications. If the second test is no longer positive, the treatment is then discontinued.

The treatment involves daily doses of pyrimethamine and a sulfa drug for at least 90 days, or 45 days past the disappearance of symptoms. Many horses are now treated for six months to decrease the chance of a relapse. The current treatment does not kill the parasites but rather prevents them from reproducing while the horse's immune system itself responds and kills them. Unfortunately, the immune system does not always completely kill all of the parasites and some horses' immune systems do not respond well. These horses do not recover. Other horses suffer spinal cord lesions during their bout with EPM which cause permanent neurological problems. New treatments are under study and hopefully in the near future a better alternative will be found.

One important piece of information that has come out of the research on EPM is that stress has a marked effect on the horse's ability to deal with the parasite. The more stress on the horse, the more likely that he will be unable to fight off the protozoa. So the best way to assist in the prevention and treatment of EPM is to support the horse's immune system, especially in stressful circumstances. Each horse has a different interpretation of what constitutes stress. Therefore, it is important for an owner to consider his horse individually and do the best to practice preventive stress relief in circumstances that might be upsetting to the horse, such as moving to a new location, going to a horse show, or dealing with illness or injury.

If your horse has EPM or has been treated for EPM in the past, it is important to stay informed about current developments in research through your vet or the internet, which has a number of web sites devoted to EPM.

SYMPTOMS
- Lameness, bucking, head tossing, stumbling, toe dragging, and back soreness are all possible signs.
- Neurological signs such as incoordination and ataxia.

RECOMMENDATIONS

Tests

- Diagnostic testing for EPM, if desired, should be carried out before or as soon as possible after treatment is started.
- There is a high correlation between EPM and stomach ulcers so check your horse for their presence and treat if found.

Drug Treatments Treat the horse with pyrimethamine and sulfa drugs. It is important to give these drugs consistently and not on a stop-and-go basis which could result in a poor response to the treatment. Use the prescribed dosage and give the medication on an empty stomach. Pyrimethamine affects the level of folic acid in the horse's body, so also give 40 mg of folic acid as a daily supplement at least 12 hours apart from the medication.

Bach Flowers Keep stress to a minimum. If you think a situation is potentially stressful, give Rescue Remedy to help the horse cope with the situation.

Herbs Support or stimulate the immune system. There are a variety of herbal formulas available commercially for this purpose. When using herbs in this manner, do not feed them constantly; instead, give them for a month, then stop for two weeks. Then, if you feel it is necessary, repeat the cycle. One example of a commercially available herbal mixture is Ditton, from Hilton Herbs.

Acupuncture Treatments are helpful to stimulate the immune system. I recommend acupuncture in combination with the standard medical treatment for EPM.

Homeopathy Use homeopathics to help relieve symptoms while the horse is undergoing treatment with the standard medications for EPM. It is important to note, however, that homeopathic remedies are not a cure for EPM. Choose one of the following:

- Rhus toxicodendron 3C to 30C three times a day for 7 days. Use when neurological symptoms are present but not extreme, when back soreness is present. In severe EPM cases, particularly those not responding to medication, consult a homeopathic vet for a higher potency such as 200C and for dosage recommendations.
- Kali bichromicum 3C to 30C three times a day for 5 days. Use when EPM is causing lameness, toe dragging, or staggering.

Aromatherapy Lemon: Stimulates the immune system.

Supplements

- Vitamin E. Give 8,000 to 9,000 IU of vitamin E daily for its anti-inflammatory effects and to promote healing of damaged nerve tissue.
- Tahitian Noni (available in health food stores), also known as Hawaiian Noni, is very effective. It seems to boost the immune system and combat the symptoms of EPM. Most horses eat it readily (it tastes like strong, unsweetened, grape juice), so you add it to their feed. The dosage is 5 tablespoons (75ml) for each 1000 lbs the horse weighs. Give twice a day for at least 4 days.
- Colloidal silver (available in health food stores). I recommend giving colloidal silver if the horse is not responding quickly to the traditional medical treatment or if neurological symptoms recur. Do not overuse since colloidal silver can affect the liver and cause the very stress you are trying to avoid. Give 1 to 3 teaspoons a day, depending on the size of the horse.

Exercise Do not ride a horse with EPM if he is showing dangerous neurological signs such as staggering or falling down. Any horse affected with EPM must be ridden with a great deal of caution since many horses cannot control their movements, or their movements are unpredictable. Once on treatment, exercise is recommended and helps to improve the horse's symptoms at a quicker pace. Do not overstress or overexercise an affected horse.

Chiropractic Adjustments should not be done until after treatment is started because they can increase symptoms such as a sore back or lameness.

Massage Should not be done because it can increase symptoms such as a sore back.

Diet If you live in an area where EPM is prevalent, consider using heat-processed feed, as high temperatures will kill any sarcocystis in the feed. Check your grain and hay for signs of fecal contamination.

Stable Area Keep your barn clean. Check the feeding areas frequently for signs of fecal contamination from wild animals and, if found, clean it up immediately. Try to keep birds out of the barn.

In cases where horses do not tolerate the regular medication, alternatives such as a combination of acupuncture, homeopathy, and supplements can be used as a primary method to treat EPM. However, I do not recommend this plan unless working closely with a vet experienced in treating EPM using these techniques.

EQUINE ROTAVIRUS

(See Chapter Four, p. 72)

EQUINE VIRAL ARTERITIS

(See Chapter Four, p. 71)

EYE PROBLEMS

Eyes are an interesting combination of resilience and delicacy—some structures in the eye are incredibly tough, whereas other areas are rather fragile. The outer covering of the eye, the cornea, consists of layers that are relatively strong and dense. The internal areas are more susceptible to injury and more difficult to treat and repair due to their location. The body maintains a certain pressure inside the eye to enable it to work properly. A complex physiology controls that pressure. If it is decreased or increased, damage can result.

Time can be a critical factor when treating eye injuries, so when your horse has an eye problem, get it checked as soon as possible. An eye that has received a direct blow will often swell, resulting in increased pressure. Medication can help to relieve this pressure and prevent damage. If your horse receives a severe blow to the head, even if there is no noticeable external damage, internal eye injuries may have occurred. The back part of the eye has a large blood supply that can hemorrhage when severe concussion occurs, altering the pressure and causing injury to other areas.

Let's look at the common problems that affect the eye: allergy-related eye problems, eye infections, corneal abrasions and ulcers, cataracts, and blindness.

Allergy-Related Eye Problems

Problems such as red, watery eyes can be the result of allergies—much like those experienced by humans. This problem is noticed most often in the spring and fall when certain plants are blooming and breezes blow the pollen around. Medication can reduce the symptoms, and cold laser also seems to afford some help. Cold laser is a laser that functions in a lower frequency range and does not cause tissue damage to the skin when it is used directly on it.

SYMPTOMS
• Red, watery, itchy eyes

RECOMMENDATIONS

Herbs The herb eyebright *(euphrasia)* is used to treat eye inflammations and other problems. Use an herbal eye wash product (see *Product Suppliers* in Appendix VI) or dilute 5 drops of eyebright tincture in 2 tbsp (28ml) of optical saline solution. If you are not able to find a tincture or herbal eye wash product, the loose herb can be used. Make a tea by putting 1 teaspoon of eyebright in a small pot with 1 cup (225ml) of distilled or spring water and let it boil for 5 minutes. Strain the mixture through cheesecloth and throw the loose herb away. When the tea cools, wet a cotton ball in it and then squeeze a few drops into the affected eye. Or, you can put the solution into a clean eyedropper and then use it to administer a few drops. You can repeat this treatment several times a day if necessary.

Laser Your vet may treat with cold laser.

Acupuncture Give treatment to increase circulation around the eye and stimulate the immune system.

Aromatherapy Lemon. Stimulates the immune system.

Chiropractic Treatments can also help to activate the immune system.

Eye Infections

One of the most common eye problems, an infection, can go unnoticed and cause damage to the eye. The eye may appear red and watery and may be painful, itchy, and sensitive to light. An infection can be caused by bacteria, a fungus, or a virus that can be spread by touch or by air. Bacterial infections are generally more responsive to treatment than those caused by a fungus or a virus. Luckily, fungi and viruses are not as common in horses. Your vet can use cold laser to stimulate the energy and circulation to the eye, hastening the healing process. A variety of antibiotic ointments and drops are available to treat infected eyes and can be prescribed by a vet. Most horses respond well to these treatments.

Be extremely careful when treating your horse's infected eye. If it is a bacterial infection, the bacteria could be contagious to your eyes. Although this is very rare, it's best to use common

sense and wash your hands thoroughly when finished.

SYMPTOMS
• Red, watery eyes; may be painful, itchy, and sensitive to light.

RECOMMENDATIONS

Herbs See entry for the herb eyebright *(euphrasia)* above under *Allergy-Related Eye Problems.*

Homeopathy Euphrasia eye drops are available in health food stores. They can be used two to three times a day.

Topical Your vet may prescribe antibiotic ointment or drops.

Laser Treatment with cold laser can be helpful in combating an eye infection.

Acupressure Can be used to stimulate the circulation around the eye. Use points BL_1, BL_2, TH_{23}, GB_1, and ST_1 (see Appendix I).

Stable and Turnout Keep a fly mask on the horse's face to prevent flies from irritating the eye and to keep the horse from rubbing the eye.

Corneal Abrasions and Ulcers

A scratch to the outer surface of the eye is called a corneal abrasion. It usually results in extreme sensitivity, redness, and sometimes a cloudy area. This condition is painful, making the eye sensitive to light, and your horse may guard the eye or try to protect it. You will notice this because he will be reluctant to have you examine his eye, and may also keep it closed most of the time—particularly in direct sunlight. Some abrasions are not visible to the human eye and can be seen only when the vet stains the eye with a fluorescent dye that collects in the scratched area. Once diagnosed, the eye can be treated with an antibiotic. Cold laser treatment can also be used to stimulate circulation and increase the rate of healing.

A corneal ulcer is sometimes caused by an untreated abrasion or a foreign body in the eye, such as a thorn (see fig. III–3, p. 214). The ulcer is an unhealed area, usually circular in shape, which affects several layers of the cornea. Generally there is a cloudy area surrounding the ulcer, which can spread across the cornea, giving the eye a bluish-white appearance. Although the ulcer can be difficult to heal, there are many new medications that can assist healing even ulcers of long standing. Often an antibiotic is used, and cold laser is very helpful in stimulating healing. One of the successful medications now being used for corneal ulcers is cyclosporin, which is dropped in the eye several times a day.

Eye medications containing steroids should not be used for corneal abrasions or ulcers.

SYMPTOMS
- Red, watery, painful eyes. Horses may try to rub eyes.
- Sometimes a cloudy, bluish-white appearance around the abrasion.

RECOMMENDATIONS
- Follow recommendations for Eye Infections above.

Cataracts

Cataracts affect your horse's ability to see clearly. This condition may occur with age or it may be congenital. It involves a cloudy or bluish coloration to the lens of the eye (see fig. III–4, p. 214). Cataracts that develop with age may continue to worsen. Congenital cataracts do not usually progress, but stay the same over the course of the horse's life. All horses with cataracts should be evaluated by an ophthalmologist to help determine how safe they are to ride. Surgery to remove cataracts and new techniques in treating them are fairly successful in people and small animals. Veterinary ophthalmologists are beginning to use these techniques for horses.

Another condition that is not understood is a type of cataract characterized by the *sudden* development of a bluish, cloudy appearance to the cornea that sometimes disappears when the diet is changed. Not much information is available concerning this condition in horses, but it is thought to possibly involve an interaction of protein metabolism. Total remission as a result of the changes in diet is possible in some cases. Because of the lack of current research and information concerning this problem, the best recourse is to consult your vet or a veterinary ophthalmologist. Cataracts influenced by protein in the diet are most commonly seen in older horses.

There are few medications that help with cataracts. However, vitamin C and zinc eye drops seem to give some aid in slowing or even stopping the progression of cataracts that develop with age. In some cases, vitamin C eye drops actually help to diminish these cataracts.

SYMPTOMS
- Cloudy, bluish, or hazy appearance in the eye.

RECOMMENDATIONS

Vet Confer with a veterinary ophthalmologist about recommended treatments. There are new techniques being developed all the time.

If the cataracts are influenced by protein in the diet:

Nutritional Supplement Add a special dietary supplement called Professional Nutrition. This supplement is fed with high-quality oats and hay and helps dietary cataracts in some cases.

Blindness and Impaired Sight

Uveitis (also known as moon blindness, and periodic ophthalmia) is the most common inner-eye disorder and a leading cause of blindness (see fig. III–5, p. 214). Many horses who are missing the sight in one eye still can be used for riding. The degree to which these horses adjust depends on the individual horse's temperament and when the eyesight was lost. If a horse was not very trustworthy before the loss of the eye, a sight deficit may cause a worsening of behavior. Some horses with blindness or impaired sight can be spooky and should be handled with care. Do not walk up on the sightless side and surprise a horse. Always speak to a horse first and let him know where you are.

Complete blindness is challenging for horses and requires a controlled environment and special handling to help them cope. Some horses do very well and are completely trusting. I have even known some that compete in shows successfully. If you are considering showing a blind horse check with the association running the shows you compete in since some have rules against showing blind horses.

SYMPTOMS

- Spooky, runs into things, performs better in one direction than the other.
- Likes to be approached on one side only.

RECOMMENDATIONS

- Have a veterinary ophthalmologist evaluate the eyes.
- Keep the horse in the same surroundings he is used to.

FRACTURES

(See also *Lameness and Leg Problems* Front Legs: Knees, *Chip Fractures*; Hind Legs: Upper Leg Area, *Pelvic Fractures*)

Fractures of smaller bones may be so minor that they are not even noticed or they can be more serious and result in lameness. Fractures of large bones are much more dramatic and frightening. Historically horses with fractured legs were considered finished but today many fractures can be repaired. Nowadays the problem often is not how to fix the fractured leg but how to deal with the horse while you're treating the fracture. Anyone who has experienced a major

fracture knows the pain involved. Horses often panic in response to this pain and cause further damage to the fractured area. Of course, a horse doesn't understand that standing still is best for him. His nature as a flight animal is to run away from anything threatening or causing pain and this instinct often takes over, making the horse very difficult to control.

When a horse has a fracture to a major bone in a leg, keep him as still as possible until the vet arrives. If you have a tranquilizer on hand, consult with your vet over the phone about tranquilizing the horse while you are waiting for his emergency visit. Using a tranquilizer may not be advisable since some horses may be in shock due to the pain.

Give Bach Flower Rescue Remedy while you are waiting for the vet. It can be used every fifteen minutes until the emergency has subsided. It is safe to use when a horse is in shock, and safe in combination with a tranquilizer.

In addition to the horse's reaction to pain, several other factors influence the likelihood of success in fracture repair, such as the weight of the horse and his attitude during recovery. The weight is a factor if the horse cannot put any weight on the affected leg. Nature did not design horses to stand on three legs so the unaffected opposite leg will be overburdened during the healing process. Therefore, it's important to support that leg as well as the fractured one.

The horse's attitude must be considered since some are better patients than others. Horses with volatile temperaments who do not tolerate long periods of stall rest may not be good candidates for fracture repair.

RECOMMENDATIONS

Vet Call your vet immediately. Give a tranquilizer if recommended by your vet after he has details of the injury.

Keep your horse as still as possible. Since most horses are frightened and in pain, he will try to

III–3 *A corneal ulcer that has been stained with fluorescein stain for diagnosis.*

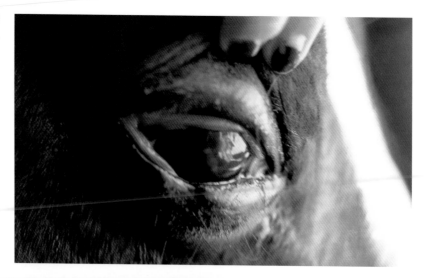

III–4 *A cataract.*

III–5 *Uveitis, also referred to as "periodic ophthalmia" or "moon blindness" is one of the most common inner eye disorders and the leading cause of blindness.*

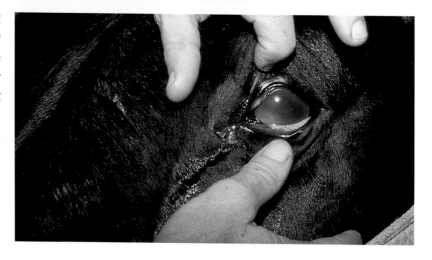

move around, so holding him, rather than tying him, is preferable.

Bach Flowers Give Rescue Remedy.

Homeopathy Use *both:*

- Phosphorus 30C. Give immediately to help control internal bleeding. Repeat dosage in 15 minutes.
- Arnica montana 30C. Give three to four times daily for 5 days.

LONG TERM RECOMMENDATIONS

Acupuncture Helps to stimulate circulation in the affected area.

Magnetic Therapy By applying magnets around the affected area you can stimulate circulation. Do not use magnets if any metal pin or other device has been inserted to stabilize the fracture.

Massage Helps the affected area. It is most useful when performed on the opposite leg where the horse has to transfer all the weight from the fractured leg.

Bandage Support opposite leg with a standing bandage.

Chiropractic Once fracture is healed, check to see if horse needs an adjustment.

H

HEART PROBLEMS

We think of horses as strong animals and do not associate them with heart problems. Unfortunately, heart disorders do exist in horses, and they often go unnoticed. Horses can have heart murmurs, arrhythmias, and a variety of other complaints.

Horses that are regularly galloped and raced or are competed in endurance or three-day eventing are monitored more often than horses that are primarily ridden on trails. Heart problems are most often noticed and diagnosed in perform-

ance horses during a routine check, although sometimes a specific health problem alerts the vet to check the heart. Symptoms are variable and may include shortness of breath, occasional coughing, poor condition, and a slow return to a normal heart rate following exertion.

Since horses have such deep chests and large lung fields, evaluating the heart with a regular stethoscope is often not very effective because it's hard to hear the heart distinctly. If you suspect your horse has a heart problem, have him evaluated at a clinic that is properly equipped for it. Large clinics and universities usually have the facilities required to perform and to interpret the results of the necessary tests.

The consequences of ignoring a heart disorder can be severe. Many horses are very loyal and will not stop even when their heart is causing them problems. Remember that horses interpret this situation differently than we do. They don't know they should slow down when their chest hurts or if they don't feel good. Some horses will just go until they drop, even when you're on them.

SYMPTOMS

- The symptoms of heart problems are variable, and in some cases there may no signs of a problem. Signs sometimes seen include: shortness of breath, coughing, increased respirations, and slow return to a normal heart rate following exertion.
- Sometimes condition is poor. Horse may be underweight and have a poor hair coat.

RECOMMENDATIONS

Exercise If a heart problem is suspected, limit the horse's exercise (with a rider) until a complete evaluation is performed.

Test Have a complete heart evaluation done by a veterinary specialist at a large clinic or university.

Acupuncture Sometimes helpful, depending on the type of heart problems. Consult a veterinary acupuncturist after a final diagnosis is made to determine if acupuncture will help your horse.

Homeopathy Very effective. Assists other treatment. However, the homeopathics are very specific for heart problems and need to be suggested by a vet on a case-by-case basis.

Aromatherapy
• Ylang Ylang. Decreases heart rate.
• Litsea Cubeba. Regulates heart rate.

HEAVES

(See *COPD* under *Respiratory Problems*)

HEMATOMAS

A hematoma develops when an injury causes a blood vessel to break, allowing blood to escape into the surrounding tissue. Eventually, the blood forms clots that will, over time gradually be broken down by the body. Small hematomas are commonly called bruises. When first formed, hematomas near the surface, such as on a leg or just under the skin, appear as a soft mass. Depending on the type of injury that caused the hematoma, there may also be some heat and inflammation in the surrounding area (see fig. III–6, p. 219).

Hematomas are usually the result of a sharp blow, such as a kick, from another horse. Once formed, the clot can take anywhere from a few weeks to a month or more to break down completely. Often the area is painful since the clot has invaded a tissue area that wasn't designed to accommodate it. When the blood clot displaces the surrounding tissue, the tissue may be damaged or adhere to its new location, leaving an empty space when the hematoma gets broken down and is reabsorbed by the body. The empty space that remains is a soft area which can fill with surrounding body fluid or adhere to nearby tissue causing a dimpled look on the skin surface. Immediate treatment of hematomas not only helps to ease the horse's pain but can also help to prevent the appearance of these dimpled areas.

When treating a hematoma make sure all bleeding in the affected area has stopped.

SYMPTOMS
• Soft mass that is felt under the skin. Heat or inflammation may be present.

RECOMMENDATIONS

Bandage Make sure bleeding has stopped; apply pressure bandage if necessary.

Herbs Give Chinese herb Yunnan Paiyao to help control excessive bleeding. However limit its use because it can cause severe side effects if used repeatedly. I recommend using it twice a month as a maximum.

Homeopathy Use *both together:*
• Phosphorus 30C. Give immediately to help control bleeding. Can be repeated every 15 minutes if necessary.
• Arnica montana 30C. Give three to four times daily for 3 to 5 days.

Bach Flowers Give Rescue Remedy as a topical preparation on the affected tissue, and orally as a calming treatment if needed.

Aromatherapy Geranium: Heals bruises.

Moxibustion Once inflammation is gone (about 2 to 3 days), apply moxibustion indirectly over the area to help dissipate the hematoma.

Topical
• Apply arnica tincture liberally over hematoma and surrounding area 2 to 3 times daily.
• Administer a cold compress made from the herb comfrey to help break down the red blood cells. Use fresh leaves, slightly crushed, placed directly on the bruise and cover with cotton and a wrap to hold in place. An alternative is to make a tea by placing the comfrey in a liter of boiling water. After the tea cools, remove the herbs from the liquid and place on the bruise with a bandage to hold them in place.

HOOF PROBLEMS

(See also *Navicular Disease*)

Horses can suffer from a variety of hoof problems, many of which cause lameness. To understand why this is so, let's review briefly the design and physiology of the hoof.

The horse's hoof is often compared to a human fingernail and toenail, but it is actually a much more complex structure. The blood circulation to the hoof is very limited, and the blood flows through the laminae which are layers of tissue that line the inside of the hoof wall. If the tissue under one of your nails is injured, the skin around the nail provides an alternative pathway for blood to circulate through the injured area. However, the soft tissue inside the hoof has no room in which to expand, so when the hoof is injured, there is no alternative pathway in which the blood can circulate. The decrease in circulation reduces the system's efficiency in flushing out infections and inflammation and also allows congestion to build up inside the hoof. The combination of these effects can be very painful and can cause serious, often permanent, damage to the internal structures of the hoof.

Now, let's discuss some of the more common hoof problems that horses experience.

Abscesses

An *abscess* is formed when an infection causes pus to be produced inside the hoof, usually in a confined area or "pocket" surrounded by inflamed soft tissue. In some cases, the abscess will migrate up the hoof wall and break out at the top near the coronary band (a condition sometimes known as *gravel*) (see fig. III–7, p. 219). As the abscess develops, intense pressure builds up inside the hoof, and because the external structures of the hoof are rigid and unable to expand to relieve the pressure, the condition quickly becomes very painful, often resulting in sudden severe lameness.

When the abscess is close to the surface, either on the sole of the foot or at the coronary band, it may be noticeable as a soft, warm area. Since the area around the abscess is usually very tender, you should be careful when examining it. If the abscess is deep inside the hoof, you may not be able to find any outward signs of it at the time that your horse first becomes lame.

If you suspect an abscess—even if you cannot find a soft area on the sole or at the coronary band—soak the hoof several times a day for 15 to 20 minutes in warm water and Epsom salts to try to draw out the abscess. When the abscess begins to drain, follow the recommendations for care given below in order to prevent the hoof from becoming re-infected. If the abscess does not break through within a few days, your vet may be able to establish drainage by cutting open the affected area so healing can begin (see fig. III–8, p. 219).

The most common cause of an abscess is a tiny piece of gravel or sand that has worked its way up into the hoof.

SYMPTOMS

- Acute or severe and sudden lameness
- Hoof may be warm and soft in the area of the abscess.

RECOMMENDATIONS

Topical/Soaking Soak the hoof in warm water and Epsom salts to draw out the abscess.

NOTE: If the abscess does not break through within a few days, call your vet.

Clean and Poultice Once draining has been established, clean and medicate it daily by flushing it with 0.1 percent iodine, poulticing it with hot linseed meal for one hour, then packing the area with cotton or gauze. Continue until abscess no longer drains and the hole starts to "fill in" from the inside.

Homeopathy After the abscess has begun draining, give hepar sulfuricum 30c twice daily in addition to steps above.

Aromatherapy Tea tree: Stimulates immune system against bacterial and fungal infections.

Acupuncture Helps increase circulation to the leg and correct any system imbalances.

Bruised Soles

Horses, particularly those with wide, flat feet or soft soles, most often get a *bruised sole* from stepping on a rock or some other hard object. The other common culprits are incorrectly fitted shoes, or ones that have become bent.

SYMPTOMS

- Lameness. It may be sudden (when caused by a rock), or gradual (from a shoeing problem). This lameness may worsen when the horse is going on hard ground, and improve with soft footing.
- You may see a bruise on the sole of the foot.
- You may find the sensitive area with a hoof tester. Be aware that if the horse is fairly to very lame this could be an abscess forming. See the section above.

RECOMMENDATIONS

Poultice Poultice the affected foot with comfrey (see Chapter Ten and *Herb Appendix IV*).

Topical/Soaking Soak the foot in Arnica lotion twice a day. Use 1/4 cup (50ml) of the lotion mixed into 2 pints (1 liter) of lukewarm water.

Homeopathy Arnica 30C. Use twice a day for 5 days to decrease the inflammation until signs of the bruise are gone.

Aromatherapy Geranium. Use as an inhalant once a day, every other day, for a total of 3 treatments.

Topical Venice turpentine, or iodine. Use to re-harden the sole before returning the horse to work. Do not treat the frog area.

Coffin Joint Inflammation

The coffin joint is the lowest joint of the leg, located inside the hoof. This joint can become inflamed from trauma such as concussion on a hard surface. Once irritated, the joint can be difficult to heal since the blood supply to the area

is limited. A chiropractic adjustment can alleviate minor coffin joint pain when needed.

SYMPTOMS

- Lameness

RECOMMENDATIONS

Test/Vet Diagnostic work-up to confirm the diagnosis.

Acupuncture

Homeopathy Choose *one* of the following:

- Arnica montana 30C given three times daily to decrease inflammation.
- Aconitum napellus 6C, 12C, 30C, 12X, or 31X given three times daily. Use when the movement throughout the lower leg seems stiff and the area around the front of the coronary band is warm.

Aromatherapy Juniper: Decreases any toxins that may have accumulated in the joint.

Magnetic Therapy Small core magnets can be imbedded into the hoof wall to maintain circulation, or a slightly larger magnet can be placed under the hoof and held in place with tape.

Chiropractic Adjustment of the coffin joint.

Supplements Give chondroitin sulfates and glucosamine according to label directions to decrease inflammation.

Medication In severe cases, the joint can be injected with hyaluronic acid by your vet.

Corns

A corn is bruise on the sole near the heels (the "angle of the bar" point—see diagram on p. 220) usually resulting either from improper shoeing (too small a shoe, or heels left too low), or from shoes being left on too long, when the hoof grows out over the shoe putting pressure on the sole near the heels.

SYMPTOMS

- Sore feet.
- Bruising at the "angle of the bar" (see diagram p. 220).

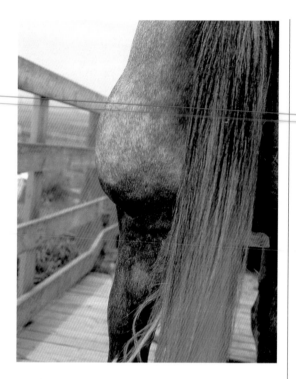

III–6 *A severe hematoma.*

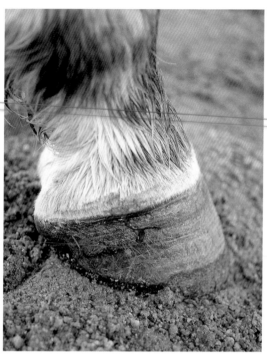

III–7 *An abscess breaking open at the coronary band.*

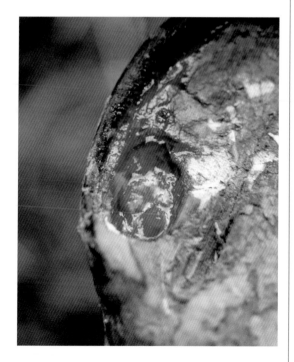

III–8 *A sole abscess. This one has been pared out to relieve pressure and allow it to drain.*

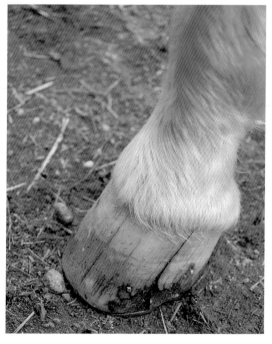

III–9 *A dry, shelly rear hoof with sand cracks.*

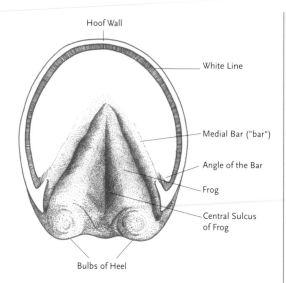

III–10 *Parts of the hoof.*

RECOMMENDATIONS

Review Correct the shoeing problem and use pads if necessary. Make sure feet are shod regularly.

Topical/Soaking Soak affected foot with 1/4 cup (50ml) arnica lotion in 2 pints (1 liter) of warm water for 20 minutes twice a day.

Dry Hooves

A dry hoof can crack or become brittle and split easily (see fig. III–9, p. 219). If your horse's hooves are dry, review your basic hoof care. (See the section on *Hoof Care* in Chapter Seven). If the dry hoof problem is severe, consult your vet because the dryness may be due to a nutritional deficiency or other disease. Lack of trace minerals is one of the most common nutritional deficiencies that contribute to dry hooves.

A disease condition that is frequently mistaken for dry brittle hooves is a fungal infection. Fungal infections can affect different areas of the hoof, commonly working their way into the hoof lamina structure between the outer and inner walls of the hoof. So if your horse has a dry or brittle hoof condition, especially with hoof wall separation, and hoof conditioners are not helping, check with your vet and farrier concerning other possible causes.

SYMPTOMS

• Dry, brittle, or split hooves.

RECOMMENDATIONS

Topical Apply a hoof ointment, formulated to soften dry hooves. There are a number of different types, from lanolin-based creamy products to petroleum-based, gel-like products and oils.

Supplements

• Try feeding a hoof supplement containing biotin and methionine.
• Trace minerals (available at the feed store) should be added to the diet.
• Salt should be available at all times.
• If the problem persists, ask your vet to examine the hooves to determine if there are other causes.

Puncture Wounds

Puncture wounds in the hoof are all too common and can result in severe consequences. The actual puncture site will be obvious if the "foreign" object, such as a nail, is still lodged in the sole, but when it has fallen out, the hole may have closed over and be difficult to find. In this case, wash the sole and frog area before you inspect the bottom of the hoof. The penetrated area may appear as a tiny, dark line, a bruised area, or a spot with many tiny red lines. You may find no visible sign at all—particularly if the penetration occurred in the frog, which is soft and spongy and tends to close over the hole quickly.

Many crucial foot structures can be injured—the deep digital flexor tendon, navicular bursa, navicular bone, coffin joint, and the coffin bone are all at risk, so never ignore a puncture wound.

SYMPTOMS

The signs vary according to the depth and location of the wound.

- Early signs: slight, or no lameness.
- Progressive signs: heat, lameness, digital pulse, sweating and colic symptoms from pain, swelling of the deep digital flexor tendon, and discharge from the wound site.

RECOMMENDATIONS

Clean Remove the object from the wound and flush the hole with hydrogen peroxide to deter anaerobic bacterial growth.

Review Consult your records for the date of your horse's most recent tetanus vaccination. (Horses are very susceptible to tetanus, and a puncture wound can put a horse at risk for this potentially fatal infection). If the horse's vaccination is not up to date, and the puncture wound is deep and/or caused by a rusty item he will need a tetanus antitoxin vaccination. When he has this ask your vet for a homeopathic tetanus nosode to help him overcome any side effects from the shot. (See also a discussion of *Tetanus* in Chapter 4, p. 68).

Vet If you suspect a puncture wound but cannot find the hole, call your vet at once. He may have to find the closed-over infection site using hoof testers. Once he finds it he will establish drainage by reopening the hole and flushing out pus and any foreign matter.

Antibiotics (or alternatives) An antibiotic flush may be recommended. For a horse sensitive to antibiotics, iodine can be used instead. And if the horse does not tolerate iodine, colloidal silver, or an aromatherapy infusion of the essential oils of lavender and thyme mixed equally, can be used.

Bandage Pack the puncture wound with cotton or gauze following treatment and keep the area bandaged. This will allow the hole to heal from the inside and close up gradually. You do not want the hole to close over on the outside before the interior has healed because infection could reoccur.

Acupressure Use to stimulate the immune system and the blood flow to the affected hoof. Start acupressure 5 days after the initial treatments:

Front feet. Points to use:

TH_1, TH_5, LI_1, SI_1, HT_9, LU_{11}, PC_9, GV_{14}

Hind feet. Points to use:

ST_{45}, GB_{44}, LIV_1, SP_1, BL_{67}, KI_1, GB_{34}, GV_4

Homeopathy Use arnica, hypericum, and ledum the first day, accompanied by aconite if needed; then arnica with either hypericum or aconite whichever fits your case as outlined below:

- Arnica 30C. Use when inflammation and pain are present three times a day for 3 days, then twice a day until pain is relieved.
- Hypericum 6C. Helps with pain and promotes healing—three times a day for 3 days.
- Aconite 30C. Three times a day when the injury is acute, when the horse has a fever, and if the coffin joint is inflamed.
- Ledum 6C. Use on the first day. Give every 4 hours (total of 4 doses in the day).

Aromatherapy

- Mix an equal combination of diluted essential oil of lavender and thyme as an inhalant to stimulate the immune system. (**Caution:** See Aromatherapy Appendix II *for contraindications to thyme).*
- Lavender. Works well on its own, stimulating the immune system and healing abscesses.
- Lemon. Use when infection is severe and accompanied by a fever, colic, or digestive upset.

Seedy Toe

Seedy toe occurs in the white line area—where the inner sensitive laminae meet the outer insensitive hoof wall laminae—when the laminae separate and a space is created between them (see diagram p. 220). This cavity allows the entry of bacteria or a fungus, and provides a warm, moist environment for infection to grow. Evidence of the condition is often a white line area filled with soft, gray, crumbling hoof horn (see fig. III–11). If the condition goes untreated, the infection can progress from ground level up the hoof.

SYMPTOMS

- Affected hooves sometimes have uneven hoof growth.
- If the cavity extends up the hoof, the hoof may sound hollow when you tap it.
- Lameness can result if a large area of the hoof is affected.
- There may be no outside, or obvious, symptoms at all.

RECOMMENDATIONS

Clean   Clean out the hollow cavity between the laminae with an antibacterial cleaner, or 7 or 10 percent iodine. This may require some of the hoof wall being cut away, so work with your vet and farrier and decide on a treatment regimen according to the condition of the hoof.

NOTE: Do not put the horse's shoes back on until the infection is cleared up.

Magnetic Therapy   Use hoof magnets on the outside of the hoof wall to increase the rate of hoof growth and increase the circulation to help deal with the infection.

Aromatherapy   Lavender and thyme: Mix an infusion of the two herbs together. Use as in inhalant once a day for 5 days, then every 3 days until the condition clears up. Or you can use it as a cleanser in the hoof cavity if the horse is sensitive to antibacterial cleaners or iodine.

Acupressure/Laser   Treatment stimulates the immune system, and blood flow to the hoof:

- Front feet. Points to use:
  TH_I; TH_5; LI_I; SI_I; HT_9; LU_{II}; PC_9; GV_{14}.
- Hind feet. Points to use:
  ST_{45}; GB_{44}; LIV_I; SP_I; BL_{67}; KI_I; GB_{34}; GV_4.

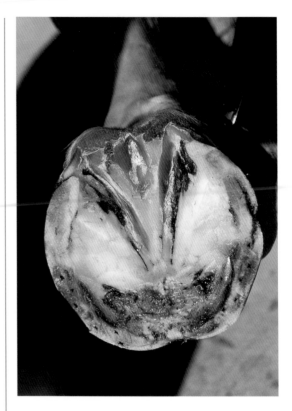

III–11   *A severe case of seedy toe.*

Supplements   Supply your horse with free choice trace minerals. These are also available at most feed stores in a loose salt form, and may be left out in small buckets, or separate feeders.

NOTE: Biotin, methionine, and MSM are frequently advertised as dietary additives to heal this condition but I have seen very few horses improve with just these products alone.

Caution: *You should not poultice, or soak, a foot with seedy toe. Many cases of white line disease involve a fungus, which only worsens when exposed to a warm, moist environment.*

Sore Feet

Many different conditions can cause or contribute to "sore feet"—a lameness that originates in the hoof but cannot be specifically diagnosed. If your horse is lame, and the discomfort appears to be in his foot, first check carefully for any obvious signs of a problem such as deeply penetrating thrush around the edges of the frog. Have your farrier or vet check for possible hoof abscesses or a shoe nail that may be causing the soreness. You should also have your vet examine the foot thoroughly for possible navicular disease or coffin joint soreness or inflammation. These are just a few of the problems that can cause foot soreness.

Often, the vet will isolate the foot by using a nerve block as a way of confirming that the foot really is the source of the lameness. If the problem is in the foot, the horse will appear sound while the nerve block is working but will then become lame again when the effects of the nerve block wear off. Unfortunately, however, these cases can be frustrating because sometimes a definitive cause for the lameness cannot be found despite the use of extensive X-rays and other diagnostic procedures. In these instances, your observations and watchfulness can sometimes help your vet in making a diagnosis.

RECOMMENDATIONS

Supplements Mineral salt: Give either as free choice or added to the feed in a powdered form. *Do not* rely on salt blocks that are licked since a horse does not receive enough salt to replace what he loses during exercise from licking a salt block. There are many free-choice mineral systems on the market that you can try.

Acupressure Treatment will stimulate circulation and relieve inflammation in the hooves.

Homeopathy In many cases a homeopathic remedy will aid circulation and decrease inflammation. Choose one of the following possible remedies:

- Arnica montana 12C or 30C twice daily. Use when inflammation such as navicular bursitis is suspected.
- Hekla lava 6C, 12C, or 30C three times daily. Use when foot soreness involves the bones in

the hoof, such as pedal osteitis (inflammation of the coffin bone).

- Calcarea Fluorica 30C once a week for 4 to 6 weeks. Use when extra bone formation is present and is suspected as the cause of the lameness. An example would be pyramidal disease, extra bone growth in the area of the extensor process on the third phalanx (coffin bone).
- Bryonia 30C three times daily. Use when there is heat present in the hooves, coronary band, or pastern. Swelling may be present from the coronary band to the fetlock.

Topical/Soaking Soak the sore hoof in Arnica lotion or an Epsom salts solution daily.

Magnetic Therapy Magnets can be applied to the bottom of the hoof, or small core magnets can be applied on the hoof wall. Magnets will increase circulation to the hoof.

Thrush

Thrush is a foot infection around the frog, or middle, triangle-shaped area on the underside of the hoof. Thrush is usually associated with dirty hooves, but it can be picked up in damp stabling conditions and during the week or so before a horse is due to be shod. The frog area has grown so air is not circulating around it as earlier in the six-week shoeing cycle. Bacteria are the most common cause of thrush although it can be caused by yeast or fungal infections as well.

It is important to treat thrush as soon as possible. If caught early, thrush, like most bacterial infections, responds readily to treatment. When thrush goes unrecognized or untreated for a prolonged period of time, the infection can work its way down into the sole. Once the infection gets into the lower layers of the frog, it can be difficult to completely clear up because of the small pockets formed in the deep areas where most topical treatments won't reach.

Many treatments for thrush have been tried over the years, but unfortunately this common infection of the hoof can still be challenging to treat successfully. There are no commercial holistic thrush treatment products. Most home remedies, such as bleach and strong iodine tinctures, dry out the hooves too much and usually don't get rid of the infection completely. However, a holistic remedy I have had success with is a mixture of colloidal silver and calendula ointment.

Some horses that wear shoes constantly develop contracted heels, a condition which results in the decrease of the space on either side of the frog. These horses are more prone to thrush because the frog area does not receive as much air and bacteria has more of a chance to grow. If your horse is having a problem with contracted heels and chronic thrush, you can either find a farrier who is able to correct the heel problem while keeping the shoes on the horse (this requires a skilled farrier), or have your farrier remove the shoes. Removing shoes and turning a horse out on pasture to bring his feet back to the way nature intended them is the ideal way to correct contracted heels. However, it's not always possible to do this. In cases where shoe removal isn't possible (sometimes because the feet chip easily), work closely with your farrier to correct the problem. Even horses turned out on pasture without shoes will require treatment for thrush if it's present.

Remember, all the thrush treatment in the world cannot replace good, regular hoof care by you and your farrier. Many cases of thrush can be prevented if this advice is followed.

SYMPTOMS
- Foul odor given off by the hoof, particularly around the frog area after it is cleaned out.
- Hoof is soft and may have black areas on either side of the frog.
- Horse may be lame.

RECOMMENDATIONS

Clean The first step in treating thrush is basic hygiene. Pick out the hooves daily, and keep the horse in a clean, dry environment to thwart the growth of bacteria infecting the foot, which grow well in a warm, moist environment.

Shoeing The next step is to have the farrier trim the frog and perform any hoof care that is necessary to help ensure a successful treatment.

Topical There are many treatments for thrush, some of them old remedies. Remember, horses have been domesticated a long time and many remedies have been tried. It's impossible to discuss every treatment available, but let's look at a few:
- A mixture of one part colloidal silver and three parts calendula ointment is a natural alternative to commercial products. (Both of these products are available in health food stores.) Use this mixture twice a day on the affected hoof for 7 to 10 days.
- Prepare a dilution of either tea tree oil or lavender oil by adding 5 drops of the oil to approximately 1/3 cup (30ml) of a suitable carrier oil such as grape seed oil, sunflower oil, or walnut oil. Paint the whole area with this mixture two or three times a day. Scrub the feet with a salt solution before each application. (This recommendation comes from *A Modern Horse Herbal*.)
- Kopertox, the trade name of one of the best known topical treatments in the US for minor thrush, is commonly available in most equine supply stores, or feed stores. Kopertox should be used about 5 days in a row to make sure the infection is totally gone. Be careful with Kopertox since it stains easily.
- Thrush Buster is another popular commercial product in the US. Many of my clients swear by this remedy and have had great success using it.

- Bleach is a common household product that is sometimes used for thrush. However, I don't recommend it because it dries out the hoof and frog area and usually doesn't work anyway. Also, if there are any pockets of thrush that connect with the more sensitive internal structures of the hoof, bleach can cause significant damage to them.

- 7 percent iodine is used by some people. If the infection is relatively mild and has not penetrated into the deep layers of the frog, iodine can sometimes be effective in getting rid of the thrush. 7 percent iodine is a strong solution, however, and it can dry out the hoof if used repeatedly.

- Cattle mastitis medication is another treatment that has come into use more recently. These medications come in tubes with a plunger and resemble a large syringe. The type of mastitis medication that has been used most successfully to treat equine thrush is one from the cephalexin-based antibiotics. These are extremely strong antibiotics and are recommended only in the most advanced, chronic cases of thrush. If the infection is that severe, I strongly advise you to have your vet examine your horse to make sure there are no other problems present before treatment is begun.

The most common and effective way to apply mastitis medication is to clean out the hoof area thoroughly, apply it as close as possible to the affected area, and then apply several gauze layers over the top of the area to pack the medication in the hoof. Apply duct tape over the bottom of the hoof and leave the medication packed in the hoof for 2 days. Then repeat the process once or twice to ensure that all areas of infection are gone. For severe, chronic thrush, this treatment has been found to be very effective.

Aromatherapy

- Lemon. Stimulates the immune system.
- Lavender. Heals fungal and bacterial infections.

L

LAMENESS AND LEG PROBLEMS

(See also *Arthritis; Fractures; Hoof Problems; Laminitis; Navicular Disease*)

When horses become lame, their owners are often concerned that the lameness is a sign of a serious condition that will be permanently disabling. Keep in mind, however, that the structure and function of horses' legs is very complex, and consequently, lameness can be caused by a wide variety of problems. Although some lameness problems are severe enough to result in permanent disability, most can be successfully diagnosed and treated.

Some conditions that cause lameness can occur in both the front and the hind legs. Others are specific to either the front or the hind legs but not both. In this section, I will discuss first conditions that can cause lameness in all four legs. Then I will discuss the types of lameness seen only in the front legs, and last, types of lameness found only in the hind legs. I discuss the various conditions under specific leg-part headings. For general reference see the diagrams on pp. 228, 229, 233.

LAMENESS AND LEG PROBLEMS IN BOTH FRONT LEGS

Joints

Osteochondritis Dissecans (OCD)

Osteochondritis dissecans, referred to as OCD, is a condition that affects the joints in the horse's body. Through a series of reactions, an area on the surface of the cartilage becomes roughened and may no longer cover the underlying joint surface, creating a lesion on the cartilage. Because of this roughness on the surface, the joint is painful when movement occurs over that area. Plaques or pieces of cartilage may also break off in the joint. OCD can even end a horse's career, depending on the exact location of the lesion or fragment.

Some horses have a genetic predisposition to OCD, but it is almost impossible to predict which horses will be affected. Although generally associated with Thoroughbreds, OCD occurs in warmbloods also. With the increasing use of warmbloods, OCD has become a problem that many owners have to deal with.

Each case of OCD is different and must be evaluated by your vet so a prognosis and treatment plan can be established, but dietary changes can often be very helpful in the treatment program. If you are aware that OCD is prevalent in your horse's breeding line, you may be able to reduce the odds that it will occur by controlling his diet. Have your feeds tested and evaluate the protein, carbohydrate, and fat content as well as the calcium and phosphorus levels. The calcium and phosphorus levels are especially important since these nutrients affect the cartilage in the joints. Horses that require the closest monitoring are those who are accustomed to a different calcium phosphorus ration in their diets from that which is being fed. For example, European horses have been bred and raised with a calcium-to-phosphorus ratio of 1:1 or 1:2. In the US this ratio is usually 1:3 or even 1:4. When European horses are imported to the US, these dietary differences are sometimes overlooked, and problems such as OCD can result.

Other dietary supplements used to treat OCD include glucosamine HCL, chondroitin sulfate, manganese, and vitamin C, all of which help the cartilage maintain and repair itself. A brief description of the make-up of cartilage will help you to understand why these supplements are helpful. The cells in the cartilage are constantly synthesizing two substances—collagen and proteoglycans—which help the body to con-

tinually replenish the cartilage when mechanical force or stress is placed on the joint. Proteoglycans are made up of hyaluronic acid and glycosaminoglycans, and they provide the framework for the collagen to follow. Hyaluronic acid is also the main component responsible for the high viscosity of synovial fluid. When treating cases of OCD it is helpful to supply glycosamine and hyaluronic acid so that these components are available if the body needs them to aid in the healing process. Hyaluronic acid is available as an intramuscular injection through the product polysulfated glycosaminoglycan (sold as Adequan in the US). Glucosamine, chondroitin sulfate, manganese, and vitamin C mixed together are readily available in commercial mixes. If your horse has OCD, I suggest that you provide a supplement containing these, as well as discuss Adequan injections with your vet.

Treatment of OCD will vary with the severity and location of the cartilage lesion. Some severe cases require surgery, which can be very successful if performed in the early stages before extensive damage is done to the joint. In other cases, the implementation of dietary changes and the use of supplements can heal the condition over time. Many Europeans favor at least six months of stall rest, a simple yet often highly effective method of dealing with OCD. The horse stays in his stall for six months with no exercise on a greatly reduced ration of feed. This method of treatment is becoming more popular in the US as records are showing that many cases respond poorly to surgery. (The famous show hunter Rox Dene, a Thoroughbred/warmblood cross, had OCD when she was young. She was given this stall-rest treatment, and went on to become one of the most successful competitive hunters in the country).

SYMPTOMS

- Lameness may be intermittent. Usually there is no heat or swelling involved. Lameness does not improve as horse is warmed up.

RECOMMENDATIONS

Test Have an evaluation to diagnosis OCD

Diet Check to make sure protein, carbohydrates, fat, and calcium and phosphorus levels are correct for the individual horse. If necessary, consult an equine nutritionist to help design a diet for your horse.

Acupuncture Helps in some cases.

Supplements
- Add 8 to 10 grams of vitamin C to the diet daily.
- Feed a supplement containing chondroitin sulfates, glucosamines, and manganese. Give according to label directions, since dosage will vary depending on the concentration of the nutrients in the product.

Herbs Give the herb yucca. Dosage will vary according to purity of the product. 100 percent pure yucca can be given in a dosage of 1/2 to 1 teaspoon per 1,000 lbs (approx. 450 kgs). (NOTE: Although yucca itself is not a prohibited substance it will sometimes give a false-positive for other—illegal—substances, so it's best not to give at least 72 hours before horse shows.)

Medication Discuss with your vet the possibility of giving intramuscular injections of hyaluronic acid.

Inflammation of the Joints

The joints that make up the horse's legs, shoulders, knees, fetlocks, pasterns, coffin, hips, stifles, and hocks can become irritated and inflamed. Sometimes joint inflammation is associated with overwork or exercising on hard ground but it can also occur for no known reason since horses are active and can easily injure themselves. Although inflamed joints can be difficult to treat and often require a period of rest, there are some new ways to deal with this problem, which are listed in the recommendations below.

First confirm the diagnosis of joint inflammation with your vet to rule out any possibility of OCD, arthritis, or a bone fracture involving the joint. Then, review your horse's exercise program to determine if you are doing anything that might contribute to the problem such as exercising on a hard surface or performing movements such as sudden stops and starts or pirouettes that could be irritating to the joints. The best course of action is to eliminate the type of exercise that is contributing to the problem until the inflammation in the affected joint subsides. Sometimes preventive measures can help so you will avoid the problem of joint inflammation altogether.

Preventive measures include: avoiding hard surfaces; regular injections with polysulfated glycosaminoglycan (Adequan) given intramuscularly to help lubricate the joint; concussion absorption pads under the horse's shoes; stretching exercises or riding exercises to strengthen the horse in specific areas; laser or magnetic therapy as prescribed by your vet or physical therapist.

If the inflammation becomes chronic and returns as soon as your horse starts work again, check the diagnosis with your vet. It is possible, for instance, that the horse's back is sore which is influencing his stifle. If there is no question about the inflammation of a specific joint you will need to review your treatment. Is it correct and have you done it for a long enough period? Why did the therapy not last? Further therapy and treatment may be required.

SYMPTOMS
- Lameness
- Heat and swelling may be present around the affected joint.

RECOMMENDATIONS

Exercise
- Evaluate the horse's exercise program and try

to determine any movements that might be aggravating the problem. Eliminate or reduce these movements.

- Work your horse on a concussion-absorbing surface. Do not work your horse on a surface that is too deep or too hard since either can pull on the joints and cause irritation as well.

Shoeing Use concussion absorbing shoes and/or pads to decrease the referred concussion coming up from the hooves.

Acupuncture Helpful in decreasing, controlling, or altogether eliminating, joint inflammation.

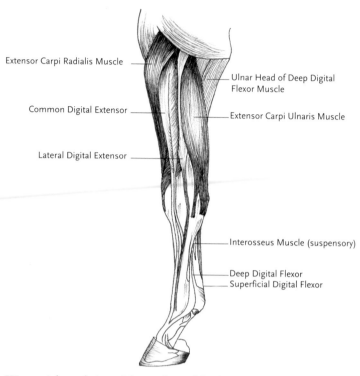

III–12 *A lateral view of the tendons of the foreleg.*

Extensor Carpi Radialis Muscle

Common Digital Extensor

Lateral Digital Extensor

Ulnar Head of Deep Digital Flexor Muscle

Extensor Carpi Ulnaris Muscle

Interosseus Muscle (suspensory)

Deep Digital Flexor
Superficial Digital Flexor

Homeopathy Arnica Montana 30c three times daily for 2 weeks.

Medications

- Polysulfated glycosaminoglycan (Adequan), which is given as an intramuscular injection, decreases inflammation in the joint. This product is available only through vets.
- Hyaluronate sodium (Legend). For chronic cases of soft tissue and cartilage inflammation, this drug works very effectively. Usually two or three injections are required 5 to 7 days apart. This is a drug that is available only from your vet.

Chiropractic Alleviates any pressure that is being put on the joints.

Magnetic Therapy Apply a magnet over the joint to increase circulation.

Herbs Add yucca to the diet. (NOTE: Yucca will sometimes test false-positive in a drug test).

Topical Apply arnica lotion, a topical form of arnica, on the affected area to help reduce inflammation.

Supplements

- Increase the vitamin C in the diet to 8 to 10 grams daily.
- Give chondroitin sulfates according to label directions.
- Give glucosamine HCL according to label directions.

Cold Treatment In acute cases of joint inflammation, where an injury has just occurred, apply ice over the affected joint.

Tendons

The two types of tendons that are most often injured are: the *flexor tendons*, which run down the back of the cannon bone and flex—bringing the leg back towards the body—during movement; and the *extensor tendons*, which run

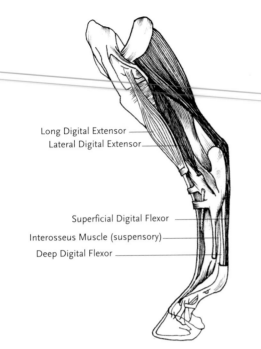

III-13 A lateral view of the tendons of the hind leg.

Long Digital Extensor

Lateral Digital Extensor

Superficial Digital Flexor

Interosseus Muscle (suspensory)

Deep Digital Flexor

down the front area of the cannon bone and move the leg forward.

There are three main flexor tendons that run down the back of the cannon bone. The one nearest to the cannon bone is the interosseus muscle, which is made up mostly of tendonous tissue. It is commonly referred to as the suspensory or superior sesamoidean ligament. The suspensory carries much of the horse's weight and fits tightly against the cannon bone. The middle tendon is the deep digital flexor, and the outer tendon is the superficial digital flexor.

The main extensor tendon runs down the front of the cannon bone. It is called the common digital extensor in the front leg and the long digital extensor in the hind leg. The lateral digital extensor lies on the outside or lateral aspect of the cannon bone.

Tendons can be injured in a variety of ways, leading to lameness. The tendons themselves can be sprained or torn, and the sheath covering the tendon can be torn also. Ultrasound has be-

come a wonderful diagnostic tool to help us assess tendon injuries. Now we can tell if there is a tear or just a strain. We can also monitor the healing process of the tendon with ultrasound. "Bowed tendon" is a term used to describe a tendon that is bulging outward (see fig. III-14, p. 230). A true bowed tendon can involve tearing of the sheath surrounding the tendon, tearing of the tendon itself, or both. Bulging of the tendon sheath without tears is often the result of a trauma such as a kick that causes subsequent swelling of the tendon and the surrounding tissue.

Any injury to a tendon is serious. Do not ignore even a strain to the tendon area, since it could turn into a more serious injury if stressed or left untreated. When a tendon is injured, the horse often limps as a result. If the limping is severe, excessive weight may be placed on the opposite leg, possibly overstressing it as well. Do not underestimate what a little excess weight can do to the good leg. Remember, the average weight of a horse is about 1,000 lbs (approx. 450 kgs) and a horse is designed to evenly distribute that weight over four legs—not three.

When a tendon is injured, it may be necessary to support it with a bandage. You will need to support the opposite good leg as well. However, be sure to check with your vet before applying a bandage to support the leg with the injured tendon because a bandage is not always the correct treatment. It takes a special technique to bandage an injured tendon, so if you don't know how to bandage a leg to support a tendon, consult someone who does. An improperly applied bandage can cause further harm.

If tendon injuries recur frequently, have your horse evaluated for possible liver disorders. Oriental medicine maintains that the liver nourishes the tendons and muscles. If the liver is stressed, diseased, or not functioning properly, the muscles and tendons may eventually be affected (see *Liver Disorders*, p. 254).

SYMPTOMS

- Lameness, with swelling, heat, or pain on palpation of a tendon

RECOMMENDATIONS

Vet Consult a vet to confirm the diagnosis.

Cold Treatment Apply ice for 20 minutes up to four times a day over the tendon area if the tendon is swollen and hot. You can also hose it with cold water for 20 minutes up to four times a day, but at least twice a day.

Acupuncture

- Check liver acupuncture points for tenderness. (See Point BL_{18} on the chart in the *Acupuncture/Acupressure Appendix I* on p. 291.) If the points are tender, consider having a blood chemistry workup to check the liver function.
- Acupuncture will help speed healing of tendon problems.

Acupressure Do on points SI_{16}, GV_{14} and TH_5 for the front leg or GV_3, GV_4, GB_{33}, GB_{34}, BL_{64}, and BL_{65} for the hind leg (see chart in *Acupuncture/Acupressure Appendix I*).

Magnetic Therapy Use a magnet over the affected tendon area. If a tendon injury has a great deal of heat after it first occurs, do not use a magnet immediately. Apply a magnet after the heat has gone—usually about 3 days in the case of a severe injury.

Homeopathy Choose one of the following remedies:

- Arnica 30C three times a day. Use if the condition is acute, with heat and pain present.
- Rhus toxicodendron 30C three times daily for 5 days. Use if inflammation, stiffness, and pain are present.
- Silica 30C. Use twice daily if fibrous adhesions have formed.

Topical/Herbs Use a comfrey compress over the affected tendon area. Make the compress using ground or whole comfrey leaves. If using ground

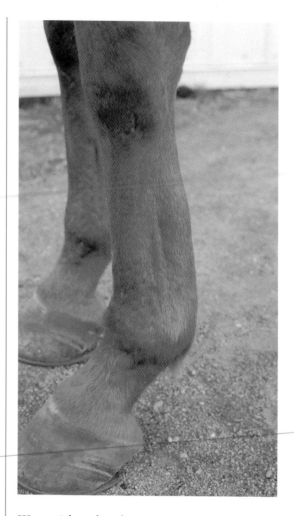

III–14 *A bowed tendon.*

comfrey, spread the ground leaves about 1/4 inch thick over a piece of cheesecloth or gauze that is large enough to cover the affected area on the tendon. Cover with another piece of cheesecloth or gauze and pour hot water over it. Cool slightly so the horse's skin will not be burned and place over the affected tendon. A soft polo wrap can be applied over the compress to hold it in place. If using whole leaves, place the leaves between pieces of cheesecloth and then soak for a few minutes in hot water and apply as above. Alternatively, you can soak the leaves without the

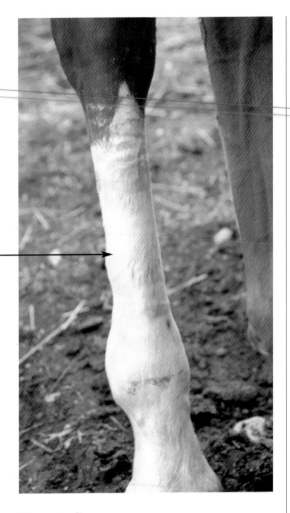

III–15 *A splint.*

cloth cover, apply the underside of the leaves directly against the skin once they have slightly cooled, and then hold them in place with a soft polo wrap. Leave the compress on the tendon for 20 minutes to 1 hour.

Splint Bone

A *splint* is an enlarged bony lump that can occur on the splint bones which are on the inside and outside of the cannon bone of all four legs (fig. III–15), and are most commonly seen on the inside of the leg a short distance below the knee. The splint bone is connected to the cannon bone by the interosseous ligament. If this ligament is torn the outer covering of the splint bone, the periosteum, becomes inflamed, and in the process of healing, the body forms new bone, causing a sometimes painful and unsightly lump. In the past splints were associated with poor conformation or traumatic injury, but we are now seeing them more in young horses who are worked before the connection between the cannon and splint bones has become strong.

SYMPTOMS
- An enlarged bony lump over the splint bone. Heat and swelling are present if the condition is acute, and the lump and the area around it are painful when palpated.
- Lameness may be present depending on the degree of inflammation. Lameness from an inflamed splint usually shows when a horse is worked on hard ground.

RECOMMENDATIONS

Exercise Rest from regular exercise since it may cause further concussion that will continue the inflammation. Return to exercise when the heat and inflammation around the splint has gone.

Cold Treatment Use ice packs on the splint when the inflammation is severe. Flexible cool packs, or frozen vegetables such as peas or corn that come in plastic bags, can be applied over the splint and bandaged in place. Leave ice packs in place for at least 20 to 30 minutes twice a day for 3 days.

Hydrotherapy Hose the affected area with cold water 15 to 20 minutes twice a day.

Test Get an X-ray or ultrasound. If the inflammation does not subside, or the lump becomes larger, ask your vet to determine the extent of the interosseous ligament injury, or if the splint bone is damaged.

Poultice Twice a day with comfrey to reduce inflammation (see remedy for a comfrey poultice in the *Herb Appendix IV*).

Topical Apply arnica lotion three times a day as an alternative if you are unable to poultice the area.

Homeopathy

Initial Treatment

Combine arnica montana 30C, three times daily for 7 to 10 days, until inflammation decreases, with hypericum 3C, or 6C, given three times daily for 5 days.

Follow-up Treatment

Ruta graveolens 3C, or 6C, twice a day for 14 days.

Acupuncture Treat only after initial inflammation has gone—usually 7 to 14 days. It will help the healing process and may decrease the size of the lump.

Moxibustion Use indirect moxibustion (see p. 24) only after all inflammation has gone, to help reduce the size of the bony enlargement. You must wait at least 15 days after the initial onset of the splint appearing, and there should be no heat present in the area. Use "moxa" around the enlargement area, and on GV$_{14}$.

Chiropractic Occasionally a slighly subluxated shoulder on the same leg as the splint is a factor. Have your horse checked for this when a splint starts to develop.

Fetlocks and Sesamoids

Problems in the fetlock area or the sesamoid bones can also lead to lameness (see fig. III–16, p. 233). The fetlock can be subject to traumatic injury in the joint itself, around the joint, or on the tendons that travel over the fetlock. Trauma to the fetlock joint can be self-inflicted through interference—the horse hitting himself with his other hoof—or it could come from an outside source such as incorrect shoeing. For instance, a shoe with a long toe and a heel that is too low can cause the fetlock to be placed at an angle that causes stress on the front of the joint. This prob-

lem can lead to injury due to excessive unbalanced concussion on the fetlock joint.

The tendons that run over the fetlock are held tightly in place by a fibrous band of tissue, and they are also subject to trauma. Repeated or excessive trauma to these tendons or the bone itself can occasionally cause calcification or extra bone formation at the fetlock around the edges of the joint, in the tendons themselves, or on the joint's weight-bearing surfaces. Calcification in the tendons limits their ability to function so they hurt when moved or stretched, and around the joint edges, calcification can interfere with normal movement or rub soft tissue surfaces, also causing pain.

Another problem that can occur in the fetlocks is windpuffs, also known as windgalls. This condition is called synovitis by vets. A windpuff is an unsightly swollen area that occurs on the side area just above the fetlock joint and behind the cannon bone (see fig. III–17, p. 234). Windpuffs can affect the joint or tendon sheath and can occur on either the front or hind legs. A windpuff usually appears after excessive exercise, exercise on hard surfaces, or trauma. Sometimes when a windpuff first appears, the area is warm and painful and the horse may show a slight lameness. However, after the initial inflammatory phase is over—usually in about a week—the lameness usually abates altogether, even though the windpuff is still there.

Lameness can also be caused by a problem with the sesamoids—two small round bones located at the back of the fetlock joint. The sesamoid bones are surrounded by and attached to the distal sesamoidean ligament which attaches to the suspensory ligament, the ligament that lies next to the cannon bone and supports much of the horse's weight. When an injury occurs to the ligaments, the blood supply to the sesamoid bones can be impaired, and inflammation can occur in the ligaments and around the

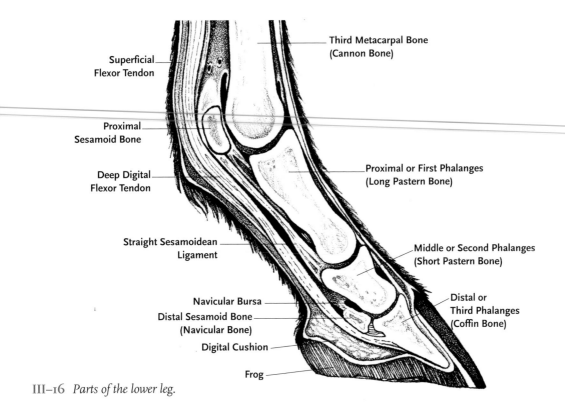

Superficial Flexor Tendon

Third Metacarpal Bone (Cannon Bone)

Proximal Sesamoid Bone

Deep Digital Flexor Tendon

Proximal or First Phalanges (Long Pastern Bone)

Straight Sesamoidean Ligament

Middle or Second Phalanges (Short Pastern Bone)

Navicular Bursa

Distal Sesamoid Bone (Navicular Bone)

Distal or Third Phalanges (Coffin Bone)

Digital Cushion

Frog

III–16   *Parts of the lower leg.*

sesamoids. Once inflamed, new bone growth called osteitis sometimes occurs around the sesamoids and this causes pain. If the blood supply is interrupted, the sesamoid bones may demineralize—a process in which the minerals in the bone become depleted. As a result, the bones become dry and brittle and may fracture.

Problems in the sesamoid area can also occur when the suspensory or distal sesamoidean ligaments become fatigued and can no longer properly support the sesamoids. When these ligaments are fatigued and the horse puts its weight on the hoof, the sesamoids on the back of the fetlock come closer to the ground. If there is a lot of pressure on the fetlock, and the fatigued sesamoids touch the ground with a great deal of impact, they can fracture. The sesamoids can be fractured in this way simply from riding on uneven ground or traveling at a faster gait such as a gallop. Severe bruising of the sesamoids can occur

also; this usually results in inflammation, a condition that can become chronic.

Most sesamoid fractures do not heal on their own because of the excessive movement of the tendons around them. They usually require surgical repair in order to heal. Chip fractures—tiny pieces of bone that break off—of sesamoids are less common but they may adhere to surrounding tissue forming fibrous adhesions or scar tissue and heal only after six to twelve months of confined rest.

SYMPTOMS
• Lameness
• Arthritic lesions of the fetlock can sometimes be felt by the owner. They feel like hard bumps and may be painful to the touch.
• Sesamoid fractures may produce swelling and heat. Horses affected with sesamoiditis or inflammation will show lameness when weight is placed on the hoof. Also, the horse may

stand with the foot slightly forward to avoid putting its full weight on the foot. If you touch the back area of the fetlock, the horse may indicate soreness.

- Swelling just above the fetlocks (windpuffs) on the back of the cannon bone.

RECOMMENDATIONS

Test X-ray the joint to confirm the diagnosis of arthritis of the fetlock joint or fracture of the sesamoid bone.

For arthritis of fetlocks:

Acupuncture

Homeopathy Arnica 30C two to three times daily *and* rhus toxicodendron 30C three times daily. (Unlike most other homeopathic recommendations, I suggest giving *both* of these remedies at the same time.)

Magnetic Therapy Place a magnet over the fetlock area or just above it.

For inflammation of the sesamoids:

Homeopathy Arnica 30C three times daily and apis 6C three times daily. (Unlike most other homeopathic recommendations, I suggest giving *both* of these remedies at the same time.)

Rest For two weeks to several months may be recommended by your vet depending on the severity of the inflammation.

Medication Hyaluronate sodium (Legend) can be given by the vet. Usually two or three injections are required 5 to 7 days apart.

For windpuffs newly formed:

Rest For several days.

Topical Apply arnica tincture over the affected area.

Bandage Apply a standing bandage to the affected leg.

Homeopathy Arnica 30C three times a day for 5 days and apis 30C three times daily for 5 days. (Unlike most other homeopathic recommenda-

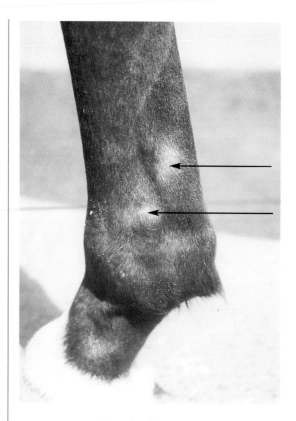

III–17 *A pair of windpuffs. The upper one is on the flexor tendon sheath, and the lower one, is on the fetlock joint capsule.*

tions, I suggest giving *both* of these remedies at the same time.)

Magnetic Therapy Place magnet over the affected area.

Herbs Use yucca. If 100 percent pure yucca is used, give 2 teaspoons (10ml) daily; if you don't have pure yucca, give according to label directions. (NOTE: You need to be aware that yucca may test false positive on a drug test).

For chronic windpuffs:

Shoeing Check feet to make sure they are well balanced since windpuffs can result from incorrect shoeing and trimming.

Herbs Use yucca (see above).

Magnetic Therapy Place magnets over the affected area.

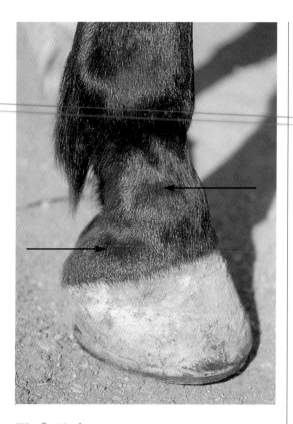

III–18 *Ringbone.*

Moxibustion Use a moxa stick over the swollen area for 2 minutes every other day for 2 weeks. (See *Indirect Moxibustion* on p. 24).

Acupressure Increases circulation and decreases any inflammation that is present.

Pasterns

The main lameness problem affecting the pastern is *ringbone* (also called "high ringbone"), and its diagnosis is especially unwelcome to horse owners, since it sometimes implies that a horse's usable time is limited. Ringbone is a type of arthritis that involves the occurrence of new bone growth on the bones in the pastern (see fig. III–18). There are two bones in the pastern—the third phalanx and the second phalanx. The third phalanx is between the fetlock and the second phalanx. The second phalanx is above the first phalanx, which is inside the hoof. When new bone growth occurs in this area, it can involve the weight-bearing joint surfaces or stay on the bone surface at the edge of the joint of either the first, second, or third phalanxes. This new bone growth eventually leads to a fusion of the phalangeal bones, but it can take many years to complete the process. Depending on the location of the growth, it can cause a great deal of pain.

Acupuncture is very helpful in relieving the symptoms of ringbone and in some cases slows its progression. The acupuncture must be repeated periodically, but most horses are able to compete free of pain if they are treated regularly. Homeopathy is also helpful in keeping the patient pain-free and able to continue working.

SYMPTOMS

- An enlarged hard area is sometimes palpable over the pastern bones near the joint.
- Lameness may or may not be present depending on the location of the ringbone.

RECOMMENDATIONS

Test Confirm the diagnosis with X-rays. This will also enable you to follow the progress of the bone growth.

Shoeing Discuss shoeing options with your farrier. Decreasing the concussion will slow the bone growth and give the horse greater comfort. High concussion absorption pads or the new neoprene shoes are both excellent options to consider.

Acupuncture

Homeopathy Choose *one* of the following:

- Arnica montana 30C given three times daily. Use arnica in the early stages of the disease when inflammation is severe, with heat and lameness present.
- Hekla lava 6C given three times daily. Use when ringbone is chronic, causing lameness, and the joint (or joints) involved is beginning to fuse.

Acupressure On points TH_I, SI_I, PC_9, LI_I on the front leg; ST_{45}, LIV_I, GB_{44} on the hind leg, and KI_I (see illustrations in *Acupuncture/Acupressure Appendix I*).

Magnetic Therapy Apply a magnet or magnetic wrap (commercially available from Norfields, see Appendix VI) or Magnetic Therapy Boots (from Natural Vibrations) and keep in place at least 8 hours a day.

Supplements

- A product containing chondroitin sulfates and glucosamine HCl can be very effective when ringbone involves the joint.
- MSM (methylsulfonylmethane), a naturally occurring nutrient which provides bio-available sulfur to the tissues, seems to help many cases of ringbone involving the bone surface. Use alone or in conjunction with other supplements. Give according to label directions.

Herbs Use yucca. If 100 percent pure, give 2 teaspoons (10ml) daily. If not pure, follow directions. Yucca contains saponin, a substance that is converted into a sterol-like compound in the body. Saponin increases production of substances produced by the endocrine system that help ease the pain of arthritis.

Hooves

For lameness problems relating to the hooves, see *Hoof Problems*, p. 217.

Other problems causing lameness in both the front and hind legs are discussed under their own headings: see *Arthritis* p. 187; *Fractures* p. 213; *Laminitis* p. 249; and *Navicular* (nearly always in the front legs) p. 257.

LAMENESS IN THE FRONT LEGS ONLY

Shoulder

Muscle Soreness in the Shoulder

Muscles surrounding the shoulder area can become strained and sore from overwork, leading to lameness. This problem can be difficult to diagnose since there are many shoulder muscles and the soreness can affect a number of them or just a few. The sore muscles could be on the outside or the inside of the shoulder. Sore muscles on the inside of the shoulder can only be palpated over the top of the shoulder blade or scapula and near the girth area between the foreleg and chest. Unfortunately, this limits the vet's ability to diagnose a problem in this area.

If a lameness or soreness problem has been narrowed down to the shoulder area and a specific diagnosis cannot be found, there are a few other potential causes to consider. A chiropractic evaluation may indicate an adjustment is necessary since ribs can become misaligned where they attach to the sternum. Additionally, the ribs—especially those under the shoulder areas—should be checked for sore areas that might indicate bruising, a crack, or a fracture. (Fractured ribs are sometimes surrounded by swelling and heat early on in the healing process). Although this can be difficult to do, it is best accomplished by lifting the front leg, carefully pulling it forward, and then feeling the ribs located beneath the leg. You may want your vet to perform this exam since great care must be taken. If the ribs are injured, they will be painful—and even pulling the front leg forward may cause pain. (Also see *Muscle Soreness*, p. 256.)

SYMPTOMS

- Heat and swelling over a muscle in the shoulder area.
- Muscle spasms may be present.
- The horse may not want to be brushed, touched, or tacked-up. Horses that become upset when the girth is tightened often have a rib or shoulder muscle injury.

RECOMMENDATIONS

Rest Rest the horse if the problem persists and have your vet examine him.

Homeopathy Choose *one* of the following:

- Arnica montana 6C, 12C, or 30C used two to three times a day if heat or swelling is present in the muscles.
- Magnesium phosphate 6C, 12C, or 30C used three times a day for muscle spasms.

Medications

- Hyaluronate sodium (Legend): For chronic, severe cases of muscle inflammation this drug works very effectively. Usually two or three injections are required 5 to 7 days apart. This drug must be obtained from your vet.
- Ketoprofen (Ketofen): This anti-inflammatory drug is similar to ibuprofen and is effective in relieving severe muscle soreness. One or two weeks of daily treatment are usually required. This drug is usually administered intravenously by your vet.

Caution: *Choose either hyaluronate sodium or ketoprofen. Do not use both.*

Acupuncture Stimulates the circulation.

Chiropractic An adjustment of the surrounding skeletal structure may be needed to allow the shoulder muscle to function at its optimum.

Aromatherapy Chamomile decreases muscular pain. Use as an inhalant or a compress.

Shoulder Joint, Bone, and Tendon Problems

Lameness that originates inside the shoulder area is quite common in horses, but it can be difficult to diagnose. A major portion of the shoulder area is inaccessible to palpation, X-rays, or ultrasound equipment. In addition, the shoulder joint itself is large and its joint surfaces are so close together that even if X-rays can be obtained, they may not be clear enough for the vet to make a definitive diagnosis.

The diagnostic process is further complicated by the fact that the natural shape of the shoulder bones varies among breeds. In some breeds, the bones are more flat or less round than in others, which gives each breed of horse its own distinct movement capabilities. However, these natural structural differences also make it even more challenging to determine what is "normal" for each particular breed of horse.

Since shoulder problems can be so difficult to diagnose, little research has been done into their specific causes and treatment. As technology improves and becomes more available to vets, we will develop greater knowledge and better techniques for treating the shoulder. For instance, in recent years some amazing advancements have been made in the treatment of shoulder lameness caused by nerve damage, particularly in the surgical repair of the nerves.

A horse can suffer a major dislocation in the shoulder joint as a result of a traumatic injury such as a bad fall or a kick from another horse. If a major dislocation is reduced (put back into place) quickly by a vet, it will usually heal well unless extensive muscle and tendon tearing has occurred.

Another shoulder problem that can cause lameness occurs when the biceps brachii tendon slips from its correct position on the shoulder joint. Sometimes the tendon is displaced because of a shoulder dislocation, but it may also slip as the result of a different type of injury. Ultrasound can be used to confirm that the tendon is not in its normal position. If there is any question about the correct location of the tendon as it passes over the shoulder, your vet will usually ultrasound the uninjured shoulder in order to determine what the normal placement should be.

For any sort of performance horse, it is vital that the biceps brachii tendon is in the correct position. It is essential as part of the combination of tendons, ligaments, and muscles that act as the "stay apparatus" of the front leg. This is a protection mechanism that prevents injuries from occurring to the lower tendons. So, if the lower tendons continually tear, or do not heal, check the biceps tendon position.

SYMPTOMS

- If the shoulder is dislocated the horse is usually in extreme pain. The affected leg will not be able to bear weight, and the horse may drag the leg.
- A horse with a biceps tendon problem may show a slight lameness because he is unable to lift the affected shoulder as high as the uninjured shoulder.

RECOMMENDATIONS

For a shoulder dislocation:

- Call your vet immediately. Ice the area and move the horse as little as possible until checked by your vet.

For a biceps tendon problem:

- If your vet suspects a problem with the biceps tendon, an ultrasound of the shoulder will have to be done to confirm the diagnosis. Depending on the location of the biceps tendon, the affected shoulder can usually be rotated or extended to allow the tendon to return to its correct position. The ultrasound will help to determine the exact location of the tendon and the direction in which the tendon needs to be moved. Once your vet has placed the tendon back in its normal position, the area can be rechecked with ultrasound to be sure the problem has been corrected.

Elbow

Capped Elbow

A capped elbow takes the form of a swelling over the point of the elbow and is usually caused by the horse hitting himself with the shoe on the same leg when lying down (see fig. III–19, p. 239). The constant trauma causes a bursa (fluid-filled sack) to develop. In its early stages it may appear as scar tissue but as the trauma continues the fluid starts to accumulate in the area and the bursa forms. It is usually painless, though an infection can develop and cause lameness.

SYMPTOMS

- Enlarged area in the form of a swelling on the elbow.
- Mild lameness occasionally.

RECOMMENDATIONS

Protection   Place a boot usually referred to as a "doughnut" or "sausage" boot around the pastern of the leg with the affected elbow.

Early stages when scar tissue only is present:

Acupuncture   Reduces the inflammation and scar tissue.

Topical   Between acupuncture treatments, use arnica lotion that will continue to reduce the inflammation.

Homeopathy

- Arnica 30C. Give twice a day for 10 days.
- Silica 30C. Give twice a day for 14 days.

Later stages when bursitis is present:

Acupuncture   Reduces inflammation and fluid.

Homeopathy

- Arnica 30C. Give twice a day for 10 days.
- Apis 6C. Give three times a day for 3 days to reduce swelling.

Vet   If necessary consult your vet for further treatment options which will vary according to the severity and duration of the bursitis.

Knee

A horse's front knees are made up of six to seven (the number varies with each horse) small bones arranged in two rows. These bones, known as carpal bones, enable the horse to have a very bendable joint, but so many working parts can also develop a variety of problems. Let's look at some of the more common ones:

Arthritis of the Knee

Arthritis of the knee joint that is caused by inflammation commonly results in lameness. However, arthritis can also be caused by a bony

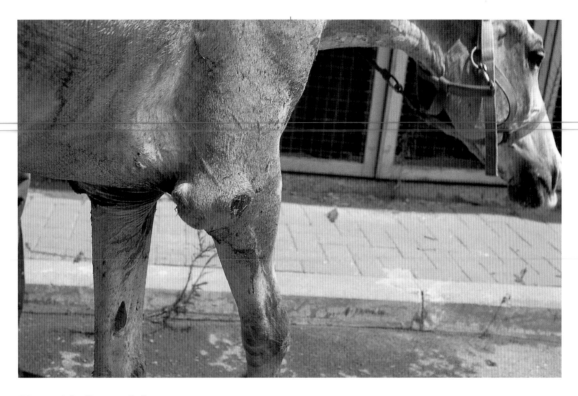

III–19 *A badly capped elbow.*

growth on one of the small carpal bones of the knee or joint surfaces. This extra bone formation, called exostosis, usually occurs as a result of trauma to the knee. If the extra bone formation is on an outer surface and not on one of the bone surfaces that bears weight, lameness does not usually occur. However, bone formation on the weight-bearing surfaces usually results in lameness. X-rays may be required to detect extra bone formation.

SYMPTOMS

• Advanced cases can be seen or felt as hard masses over the knee area.

• In some cases, the horse may be lame.

RECOMMENDATIONS

Test X-ray the knee to determine if the joint is involved. The X-ray will also serve as a baseline for tracking any further worsening of the knee problem.

Acupuncture Very helpful in relieving inflammation, swelling, and pain due to extra bone formation.

Magnetic Therapy Magnetic therapy works well in relieving stiffness caused by arthritis. Magnets that fit over the knee are available.

Homeopathy Choose *one* of the following:

• Apis 6C. Give apis if inflammation and swelling are present in the knee joint. In acute cases, give every 2 hours for the first day and then two to three times a day.

• Rhus toxicodendron 3C to 30C. Give rhus tox if excess bone formation is present and lameness or stiffness improves with exercise. Give two times a day for at least 5 days.

- Hekla lava 6C. Give hekla lava if the horse is suffering from a chronic case of arthritis that does not get better with exercise, particularly if there is extra bone formation on the joint surfaces.

Herbs Give the herb yucca. (NOTE: yucca may test false-positive in a drug test).

Carpal Bone Displacement

The two rows of carpal bones in a horse's knee allow the joint a wonderful range of motion. Unfortunately, this ability to move can also occasionally cause these small bones to move into an incorrect position. Even with X-rays, diagnosing displaced carpal bones is a challenge. Since the knee joint is round, it is difficult to see all the surfaces of these little bones and determine how they interface on a two dimensional surface. Your vet's best diagnostic method to determine if a carpal bone is out of position is to palpate the knee. The diagnosis of carpal bone displacement will be greatly advanced when magnetic resonance imaging (MRI) becomes more available to vets.

If one or more carpal bones are displaced, a vet trained in chiropractic medicine can use a variety of methods to coax the bones into their correct position. If you do not have a veterinary chiropractor in your area, rotate the knee gently by moving the lower leg in large slow circles both clockwise and counterclockwise. Swimming is another method that can help since the horse uses a great deal of force in the downward stroke of the leg. This force often puts the carpal bones back into their correct locations.

SYMPTOMS

- Symptoms vary depending on how many carpal bones are involved and where they are positioned. A minor displacement will cause soreness when the knee is palpated, cause the horse to shift his balance, and promote uneven hoof growth. When more than one carpal bone

is involved or the carpal bone is severely mispositioned, the signs can include lameness, sore tendons, or chronic tendinitis with heat and swelling over the affected area.

RECOMMENDATIONS

Chiropractic

Acupuncture Helps reduce inflammation and swelling.

Homeopathy Give arnica montana 30C: two or three times daily for 3 days.

Magnetic Therapy There are magnets made specifically for knees to help with circulation and inflammation.

Chip Fractures

Chip fractures of the knee occur all too often and can result in lameness that may be constant or occasional. Common in racehorses, chip fractures of the carpal bones can vary in size from a tiny piece to a large major part of the bone. In some cases when the bone chips are very small, they are reabsorbed into the body. However, there is also a risk that a tiny floating bone chip might lodge on a weight-bearing area of the joint, making matters worse. The development of modern surgical techniques has made it possible for most minor chips to be repaired using arthroscopic surgery. Horses that undergo arthroscopic surgery often have no further problems once the chip is removed. (See fig. III–20 on p. 241).

SYMPTOMS

- Occasional swelling can occur.
- Heat may or may not be present, and may appear following exercise.
- Lameness can be intermittent or constant.

RECOMMENDATIONS

Test X-ray the knee to confirm the diagnosis.

Surgery An arthroscopic procedure to remove the chip if necessary.

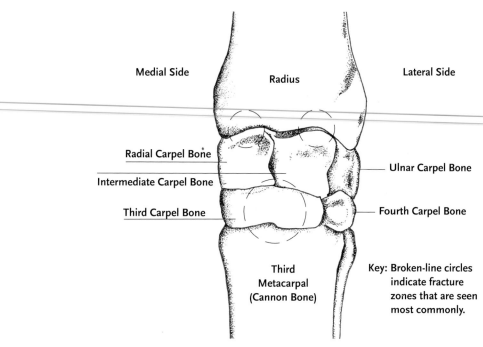

Medial Side

Radius

Lateral Side

Radial Carpel Bone

Intermediate Carpel Bone

Third Carpel Bone

Ulnar Carpel Bone

Fourth Carpel Bone

Third Metacarpal (Cannon Bone)

Key: Broken-line circles indicate fracture zones that are seen most commonly.

III–20 *Parts of the knee and common sites of chip fractures.*

Swollen and Bruised Knee

A horse's knee can become swollen and bruised due to a kick from another horse or a fall. I have also seen cases where this type of injury was self-inflicted by banging the knee against the stall wall or door at feeding time.

SYMPTOMS

• Swollen, hot, painful knee.

RECOMMENDATIONS

Evaluate Examine for cuts, abrasions, or puncture wounds.

Cold Treatments

• Apply an ice pack on the knee. Hold it in place with a leg wrap.
• Hose with cold water for 10 to 20 minutes. This can be repeated every 2 to 3 hours.

Topical Apply arnica tincture to the knee area and rub it in well.

Homeopathy Give arnica montana 6C, 12C, or 30C once every 2 hours the first day, and then three times a day until the swelling and bruising subsides.

Magnetic Therapy Apply a magnet over the swollen and bruised area for 4 to 8 hours daily. If the injured area is hot, do not start magnetic therapy until area is cool, and not until 48 hours after the injury took place.

LAMENESS IN THE HIND LEGS ONLY

Upper Leg Area

The upper area of the hind leg includes the hip joint (known as the coxofemeral joint), the muscles, and all internal structures. For the purposes of this discussion, I will also include lameness related to problems with the pelvis and the rear of the spine.

Lameness can result from inflammation, arthritis, or an injury that affects the hip joint itself or the ligaments that keep it in position. It is difficult to diagnose problems involving the hip joint itself because the joint is located so deep in the body. Often a hip joint problem is diagnosed by ruling out possible problems with the lower joints. However, as diagnostic techniques improve through the use of new medical technology, we will be able to better understand this complex area and the problems related to it.

Once the hip joint has been isolated as the cause of a lameness problem, the specific cause must be determined. The problem might involve just the joint itself, or it might be traced to a muscle or nerve or another internal problem. In some cases it is not possible to make a precise diagnosis and the vet has to try various treatments. Following are the common problems associated with lameness in the upper leg area. (Arthritis is addressed separately; see p. 187.)

Fibrotic Myopathy

The muscles, tendons, and ligaments in the hind leg can be torn or strained by excessive exercise or by trauma. When a muscle is injured, the fascia, a fibrous membrane of connective tissue that supports and separates muscles from body organs, can also be injured. As an injured muscle heals, fibrous adhesions are formed between the injured area and the surrounding fascia. These fibrous adhesions remain as a permanent part of the muscle and are called a fibrotic myopathy. Although these adhesions are very strong, they do not contract like normal muscle tissue; therefore the muscle may no longer function correctly when the horse moves.

The muscles most commonly affected by fibrotic myopathies are the ones that run down the back of the leg—the semitendonosus, semimembranosus, and biceps femoris muscles. Even a small tear in one of these muscles can cause a fibrotic myopathy and affect a horse's movement. Fibrotic myopathies can often be felt on palpation and confirmed by comparing the muscles on either side of the leg. However, some muscle tears may occur in the internal area of the muscle and can only be diagnosed by ultrasound.

SYMPTOMS

- Lameness is most noticeable at the walk. During the forward swing of the stride, the foot is suddenly pulled backward just before it contacts the ground.
- A hardened area can often be felt on the back of the leg.

RECOMMENDATIONS

Stretching Exercise Use the following stretching exercise designed to help loosen up the leg muscles: Pick up the hind leg. Your horse usually pulls his hock up himself before relaxing it. Once he has relaxed, hold the leg up with your hand supporting his cannon bone or hoof, not the pastern. (Holding his leg up from his pastern will cause the horse to pull back and flex his leg). Gently stretch his leg forward and backward. Be careful when doing this exercise so you don't get kicked. If your horse is reluctant to let you do this stretch, you may be asking for too much, so start with just a little forward and backward motion until he gains confidence.

Acupuncture

Massage Do over the hardened area as well as the surrounding muscles.

Moxibustion Do over the hardened area of the affected muscles.

Hip Joint Inflammation

Inflammation of the coxofemoral (hip) joint may be difficult to diagnose because the joint is covered by many layers of muscle. The deep location of the joint and thickness of the bone also make it difficult to X-ray clearly, so X-rays are rarely used to diagnose problems in this area. Often diagnosis is made by ruling out other possible causes of lameness. With the rapid advances in technology, it is possible that a

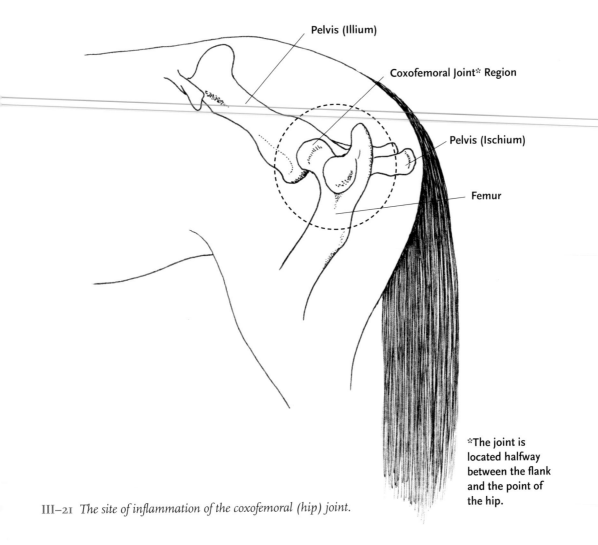

Pelvis (Illium)

Coxofemoral Joint* Region

Pelvis (Ischium)

Femur

*The joint is
located halfway
between the flank
and the point of
the hip.

III–21 *The site of inflammation of the coxofemoral (hip) joint.*

technique will become available in the near future to enable a clear viewing of the joint area.

If you suspect your horse's lameness is coming from the coxofemoral joint, feel over the horse's hind leg in the area illustrated (fig. III–21). Pain or inflammation in the joint can also develop when a problem occurring in another joint of the leg, causes the horse to alter the way he moves his hip joint. Whatever the cause, once the coxofemoral joint is sore, it will require diligence to successfully treat it since there is nothing external, such as bandaging, that can be done to alleviate stress on the joint.

Lameness from an inflamed coxofemoral joint will vary, but most commonly results in a shortened forward stride. When extreme soreness is present, the horse will rest the affected leg—often by lifting his heel in the air and shifting his weight to the other leg.

SYMPTOMS
• Lameness, or shortened forward phase of the stride.

RECOMMENDATIONS

Evaluate Check the horse for possible predisposing causes—such as shoeing—that may have altered the stride and affected the hip joint. Carefully inspect the opposing front leg for a problem since a horse often compensates by shifting his weight off a sore front leg to the opposing diagonal leg. For example, if the right hip looks sore, check the left front leg for a painful area—possibly his hoof, sesamoid, or fetlock joint.

Acupuncture

Homeopathy Give *both* of the following:

- Arnica montana 30C. Give every hour for a total of 6 doses the first day, then 3 times a day for as long as pain and inflammation are present.
- Ruta graveolens 30C. Give three times a day to help prevent formation of extra bone in the joint as a result of the inflammation.

Supplements

- Give chondroitin sulfates according to label directions. Any horse in hard work should subsequently be kept on this product to help prevent a recurrence.
- Give glucosamines according to label directions. Any horse in hard work should subsequently be kept on this product to help prevent a recurrence.

Medication Give Polysulfated Glycosaminoglycan (Adequan) by intramuscular injection for chronic cases. This drug is available from your vet.

Misalignment of the Hip or Pelvis

Lameness can also be caused by a misalignment of the hip (coxofemoral) joint or the pelvis, both of which can be corrected by chiropractic adjustments. The pelvis is the bony structure that supports part of the spine and connects the spine to the hind legs. A misalignment of the pelvis can be difficult to diagnose since the signs will vary depending on the specific area in which the misalignment is located, but lameness is usually present.

SYMPTOMS

- If the hip (coxofemoral) joint is misaligned, the affected leg may be shorter than the other leg, causing the forward stride to be shortened. When you view your horse from behind, one of his hips may appear lower than the other, or one hip may drop lower when the horse is moving forward. A fully dislocated hip joint is a serious injury and requires immediate veterinary treatment.

RECOMMENDATIONS

First Aid

- Do not allow the horse to move if you suspect a major dislocation of the hip joint. Call your vet immediately.
- If one of your horse's hips is lower than the other, call your vet immediately for a lameness examination.

Homeopathy Give both of the following when a misalignment has just occurred:

- Arnica montana 30C. Give every 15 minutes for a total of 5 doses, followed by a dose every hour to reduce inflammation.
- Magnesia phosphorica 30C. Give every 15 minutes for 4 doses to reduce muscle spasms.

Pelvic Fractures

Lameness can also be caused by an undiagnosed pelvic fracture. Although a fracture in the pelvis usually produces critical symptoms such as swelling, heat, and severe hind-leg lameness, this is not always the case. The type of lameness caused by a pelvic fracture varies depending on the severity of the fracture and exactly where it occurs. Cases in which the fracture is deep inside the horse's body are more difficult to diagnose because the massive amount of muscles (large and small) surrounding the pelvis often holds the bones in place well enough for the horse to bear weight and walk. Sometimes these cases can be diagnosed by the sensations of movement and grinding you may feel when you hold your hand against the horse's pelvic area as he walks forward.

Veterinarians who suspect an internal pelvic fracture sometimes palpate the horse rectally to check the bone structure, but the entire pelvis cannot be palpated in this manner. This method is also problematic because the muscles might be holding the pelvis in its proper position, so that it feels normal while the horse is standing still. For that reason, your vet may have the horse move forward a few steps while he is doing a rectal exam so any unusual movement of the pelvis can be detected.

SYMPTOMS
- Lameness is present.
- Swelling, heat, and pain on palpation of the affected area may be present depending on the location of the fracture.

RECOMMENDATIONS

Vet Call your vet if you suspect a pelvic fracture.

Homeopathy Give *both* of the following:
- Arnica montana 30C. Give three times a day for at least 10 days to help decrease inflammation and pain.
- Magnesia phosphorica 30C. Give every 15 minutes for 4 doses to reduce muscle spasms.

The prognosis varies depending on the severity of the fracture. Pelvic fractures require a minimum of four to six months of rest—sometimes up to a year for complete recovery. Most fractures heal with rest, and many horses can return to a productive life.

Sacroiliac Subluxation

A subluxation, a term for a misalignment of any area of the skeletal system, can occur in the pelvis at the area called the sacroiliac joint. This is the joint that attaches the pelvis to the spine. When the ilium (part of the pelvis) attachment to the sacrum (part of the spine) is broken and the three ligaments that surround and help stabilize this joint are stretched or torn, the ilium

slips upward. The result is a bump that can be seen along the top of the horse's back at the highest point of the hip. These bumps are called *jumper bumps* or *hunter bumps* because they are often noticed on jumpers and hunters. When a sacroiliac is first subluxated, lameness may be present. In most cases, the area then stabilizes with fibrous adhesions.

SYMPTOMS
- Lameness is sometimes present.
- There will be a pain reaction when the horse is palpated with fingertips around the affected raised area on the top of the hip if the subluxation has recently occurred.

RECOMMENDATIONS

Vet Call your vet immediately if you suspect a sacroiliac subluxation.

First Aid/Rest Confine the horse to a stall.

Cold Treatment Ice over the area if it is hot and painful.

Chiropractic Get an adjustment of the sacroiliac joint.

Acupuncture

Magnetic Therapy Use a magnetic blanket over the top of the hip.

Supplements Give 15 grams of vitamin C for the first 3 days, then reduce to 10 grams for an additional 10 days.

Homeopathy
- Arnica montana 30C. Give four times daily for 3 days, then three times daily for 3 more days.
- Apis 6C. Give every 2 to 3 hours the first day only (in addition to arnica).
- If swelling is hot and painful over the hip area, also give Rhus toxicodendron 30C three times daily for as long as the area is hot and painful.

Thrombus

A severe problem caused by parasitic thrombosis occurs at the posterior aorta or its branches into the internal and external iliac arteries. When this happens, blood flow to a hindquarter of the horse is impeded, or blocked, resulting in pain in the blood-starved muscles and lameness in that hind limb.

A thrombus is a blood clot, like a scab, which forms on the delicate inside wall of a blood vessel as a result of injury to that wall. The process of formation of a thrombus is called thrombosis. If the clot is not dissolved, it becomes firm and fibrous like a scar. The thrombus may obstruct blood flow by protruding into the pipeline of the blood vessel, or it may break off and be carried by the blood, in which case it is called an embolus. The embolus then lodges downstream at a fork or narrowing of the vessel.

Various injuries, large and small, to the arterial lining (epithelium) can cause thrombi, but in horses the most common cause is the attachment to the wall of the migrating larva of a bloodworm called *strongyles*. These worms migrate in their immature form, then return when mature to the stomach, intestine, or liver, according to the predilection of their species.

SYMPTOMS
- The lameness from a thrombus usually begins a little while after beginning exercise and may be accompanied by anxiety and by sweating on the hip area of the affected leg.

RECOMMENDATIONS

Review Discuss your current worming treatment and program with your vet.

Acupuncture Helps stimulate new blood vessel formation.

Homeopathy Give calcarea fluorica 30c twice daily for 10 days to help dissolve the thrombus.

Hip Abscess

Yet another cause of lameness in the hip area results most commonly from giving injections in this area. The hip is a poor injection site because,

if an abscess occurs, it is difficult to establish drainage there. If the abscess is not drained, the infection can spread throughout the surrounding tissue and cause extensive muscle damage. Many people still use the hip as an injection site and don't believe this problem will occur with their horses, but it's not worth taking the chance.

SYMPTOMS
- Extreme lameness. The horse may not be able to bear weight on the affected leg.
- The horse may have an increased pulse in the affected leg. Occasionally, laminitis may result from a hip abscess. See *Laminitis* on p. 249 for more information.

RECOMMENDATIONS

Vet Have your vet establish drainage.

Clean For follow-up care, keep the abscess flush out according to directions. An antimicrobial flush is usually used to keep it open so it heals from inside out.

Laser Treatment stimulates healing.

Medication Vet may suggest antibiotics as preventive measure.

Aromatherapy Tea tree: Stimulates immune system against infection.

Poultice If a poultice will stay on, poultice with hot linseed meal for one hour, then pack the area with cotton or gauze. Continue until abscess no longer drains, and the hole starts to fill in from the inside.

Stifle

The stifle is similar to the human knee, and—like our knees—it is somewhat prone to injury. This joint can be challenging to treat since it is large and complex in structure. Strained or sore stifles can occur due to overexertion, a quick lateral movement, or exercise on a deep surface, like sand. Inflammation of the stifle joint can involve bones and cartilage of the joint itself, the patella (the equivalent to the human knee cap), and the ligaments that hold the patella in place.

Inflammation of the stifle, called *gonitis*, can result in permanent lameness if left untreated. Gonitis can be caused by excessive exercise or by damage to another part of the affected leg that results in incorrect movement of the stifle. Among the specific types of injury that can cause inflammation of the stifle are a loose patella, a damaged medial meniscus (the pad inside the stifle that acts as a cushion between the femur and the tibia), or a damaged or ruptured anterior cruciate ligament or medial collateral femorotibial. If the inflammation is due to an injury to one of these structures, it may not subside until that injury has been treated.

It can be difficult to diagnose a meniscus or anterior cruciate ligament injury because it is hard to see inside the stifle joint. Sometimes these cases can be diagnosed using endoscopy, a technique similar to that used in human medicine where fiberoptics are used to look into a joint. Not all vets have access to this diagnostic procedure, however, so the case may be referred to a large clinic or veterinary school.

When a stifle is strained, when the patella ligaments are loose, or when the horse's conformation is poor, the patella can become loose or displaced. A conformation defect that lends itself to stifle problems is called "straight through the stifle." This means that the angle of the femur or the first major leg bone coming from the hip is too steep and does not create a prominent surface for the kneecap to maintain its proper position. When the patella ligaments are loose, the patella is displaced a tiny bit every time the horse uses his leg. The horse will automatically attempt to compensate in order to keep the patella in place. To do this, the next joint down, the hock, is swung outward. If you watch a horse with a loose stifle from behind, his hock swings in a definite outward motion with each stride.

Many treatments have been tried to tighten patella ligaments. However, the most effective one is to strengthen the stifle itself. This can be accomplished by trotting up hills. The horse should be lightly on the bit to engage the correct muscles to build the stifle. The trot should be a regular working trot, not a jog or fast trot. This is a controlled exercise and will yield results within three to four weeks. Start slowly, especially if your horse is out of shape. You can even start at a walk at first and build up to a trot. If you do not have any hills in your area, trot your horse over ground poles or cavaletti set on a large circle of about 20 meters. Work in both directions and once your horse gains some strength, you can raise the polls about six inches to continue building more muscle.

The term "locked stifle" refers to a condition that occurs when one of the three tendons that holds the stifle in place slips over a prominence on the bone and cannot go back. Horses naturally perform this locking-in of the stifle to enable them to sleep lightly while standing without falling over. Unfortunately, some horses have problems unlocking the stifle or are unable to control it when the tendon slips into the incorrect position. Again, a stifle conformation that is too straight is usually what leads to this problem.

There are two main treatments for a stifle that locks. The first is to strengthen the stifle through exercise as described above for displaced patellas. The second is used in severe cases of locking stifles and involves cutting the tendon that is slipping into the wrong position. Sometimes this surgery is necessary, but I prefer to use it only as a last resort as occasionally the horse's performance can be affected.

An injured stifle requires rest and treatment to speed recovery. Homeopathics and acupuncture can be very helpful in speeding the healing process. Osteochondritis Dissecans (OCD) can also appear in the stifle (see p. 225).

SYMPTOMS

- Stifle lameness is characterized by a shortened forward stride.
- Soreness or swelling can occur due to trauma.
- Locked stifle: The horse cannot move; the affected hind leg appears locked into a standing position. The horse will kick out to try to unlock the stifle.
- Displaced patellas: The stride will be short in the forward phase, and the hock will swing laterally to the outside.

RECOMMENDATIONS

Vet If the stifles are locked and the horse cannot kick outward to unlock them, call your vet immediately.

Strengthening Exercises Exercises described above to strengthen the stifle will help control locking stifles and displacing patellas. Perform these exercises three times a week.

Acupuncture Helps to decrease inflammation.

Homeopathy Give both of the following:

- Arnica montana 30C. Give three times a day.
- Ruta graveolens 6C. Give three times a day to help prevent extra bone formation following an injury to the joint.

Hock

The hocks are a source of concern since they are so prone to injury, but the hock joint has become more treatable in recent years with the advent of arthroscopic surgery and the improvement of joint injections. (Medications injected into the joint are hyaluronic acid and steroids.) We also have more advanced diagnostic tools to help us pinpoint the exact problem and avoid unnecessary treatment.

Let's look at some of the most common hock problems and how to treat them. A condition called *spavin* is a common ailment that affects hocks and it usually causes joint inflammation.

Spavin problems can be divided into two main categories: *bog spavin* and *bone spavin*. A bog spavin is an inflammatory process in the hock; bone spavin involves the formation of excess bone in the hock and is a degenerative joint disease.

Bog spavins can be caused by poor conformation or by excessive strain on the joint. They are characterized by swelling which is usually worse over the inside front area of the hock (see fig. III–22, p. 250). There may or may not be heat associated with a bog spavin. The swelling is soft and can easily be pushed inward. Once present, bog spavins rarely go away, but they generally do not cause lameness unless associated with inflammation.

Bone spavins usually cause lameness and sometimes progress to joint fusion. Most commonly, the lower part of the hock joint is involved and gradually the excessive bone formation spreads (see fig. III–23, p. 250). There are a variety of ways to treat bone spavin, and I recommend trying several to see what gives your horse the greatest relief. Acupuncture is very helpful and often allows horses to perform pain-free for long periods. Magnetic therapy is also very helpful. Indirect moxibustion used between acupuncture treatments can help to maintain the hocks in a pain-free state.

In advanced conditions, injecting the hock joint may be the only way to achieve a pain-free status. Even in these cases, acupuncture, magnets, and moxibustion will help maintain the joint, provide additional pain relief, and can allow greater time between injections.

Capped hock is caused by severe trauma to the point of the hock. The result is a distention of the point of the hock and an unsightly looking hock (see fig. III–24, p. 251). Permanent lameness usually does not result. Capped hocks should be treated aggressively to decrease the swelling of the hock as much as possible. A combination of acupuncture, moxibustion, and magnetic therapy can be very helpful to reduce the swelling and shorten the healing process.

A *Curb* is another problem involving the hock. It is a swelling three to four inches below the point of the hock due to a strain in the plantar tarsal ligament. When a curb first occurs, it is painful and causes lameness because of the acute inflammation of the ligament (see see fig. III–25, p. 251). Once the inflammation and lameness have subsided, the thickened area often remains. The occurrence of a curb is usually due to poor conformation—cow-hocked and sickle-hocked horses are particularly prone to curb formation. Exertion such as bucking and kicking, or any continuous exercise that stresses the plantar ligament may also causes a curb to appear.

SYMPTOMS

- Lameness. Horses with hock problems usually have a shortened forward stride and do not lift the foot very far off the ground.
- Swelling can occur around the joint in a *bog spavin.*
- *Capped hock* shows an enlarged point of the hock.
- With a *curb* the horse may stand with his heel elevated to take stress off the ligament. There may be swelling and heat on the back of the leg a few inches below the hock.

RECOMMENDATIONS

Acupuncture Very effectively treats most hock problems.

Cold Treatment Use ice packs at the onset of any swelling for 3 days. Flexible cold packs, or frozen vegetables can be bandaged in place.

Hydrotherapy For any swelling, run cold water over the area for 15 to 20 minutes twice a day for 5 days.

Poultice Use comfrey once a day for 3 to 5 days until inflammation has disappeared.

Homeopathy Choose one of the following:

- Arnica montana 30C. Three times daily for pain and inflammation for at least 10 days.
- Apis mellifica 6C, 12C, or 30C. Three times daily for bog spavin or joint inflammation and swelling.
- Bryonia 6C, 12C, or 30C. Three times daily for bog spavin.
- Rhus toxicodendron 30C. Three times daily for bone spavin.
- Hypericum 3C, or 6C. Three times a day for 3 days.
- Kali bichromicum 3C, 6C, 12C, or 30C. Two or three times daily to reduce the pain and inflammation caused by a curb.

Follow-up treatment
Ruta Graveolens 6C, or 12C. Give twice a day for 7 days.

Magnetic Therapy

Acupuncture A regular schedule can help maintain a hock that requires injection.

Acupressure On points BL_{38}, GB_{34}, and BL_{60} (see *Acupuncture/Acupressure Appendix I*)

Laser Use twice a week when treating a curb or a bog spavin.

Moxibustion Do every other day.

Supplements Chondroitin sulfate and glucosamine for chronic inflammation given according to label directions.

Injection A joint injection should be considered when bone spavins are involved or when the horse is not responding to other treatments (except for a curb which is not helped by joint injections).

LAMINITIS (FOUNDER)

Laminitis, also known as founder, is characterized by a decrease in the amount of blood circulating in the hoof. It is a serious and extremely painful condition with multiple causes.

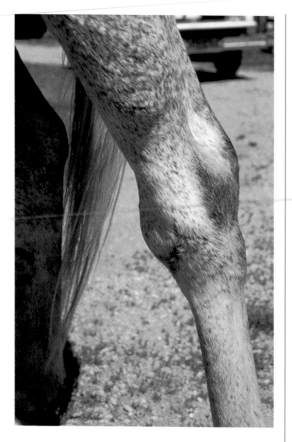

III–22 *A bog spavin.*

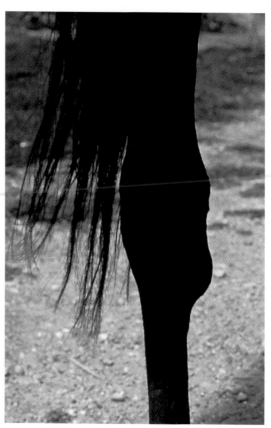

III–23 *A bone spavin.*

The horse's hoof is similar to your fingernail in structure, but the interior of the hoof is lined with two layers of tissue called laminae. The hard layer closest to the hoof wall is called the horny laminae, and the inner layer is called the sensitive laminae. When the blood supply to the sensitive laminae is decreased, they become inflamed. The union between the horny and sensitive laminae then begins to break down. In severe cases, the bone inside the hoof, called the coffin bone or third phalanx, rotates downward. In advanced cases, the coffin bone may even perforate the sole.

In addition, the inflammation of the sensitive laminae causes swelling inside the hoof. Because the external walls of the hoof are rigid and cannot expand to accommodate the swelling, the pressure that builds up inside the hoof exacerbates the horse's pain.

Laminitis may involve one or all four feet. Commonly known causes include eating excessive amounts of grain; eating too lush a pasture grass; drinking cold water while overheated; and being overworked when not in fit condition. Corticosteroids and certain antibiotics can also induce laminitis. A more recently recognized cause for laminitis, particularly in chronic cases, is a hypothyroid (underactive thyroid) condition. Ponies are often susceptible to laminitis, perhaps because many of them are overweight.

Signs of laminitis include refusing to move, hot hooves, increased pulse in the area just above the hoof (see fig. III–26 on p. 252), and occasionally a separation of hoof and coronary band. The

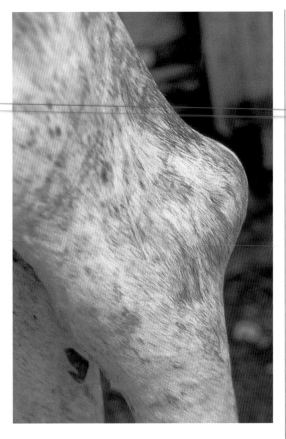

III–24 *A capped hock*

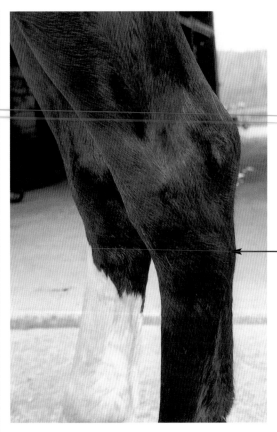

III–25 *Curb.*

horse may also try to stand in a way that puts more of his weight on his heels since the pain is often more intense in the toe area. The effects of laminitis can be devastating, so treatment must be initiated immediately. Call your vet at the first signs of laminitis, and do your best to keep your horse comfortable until the vet arrives.

Acute Laminitis

SYMPTOMS

- Refusal to move, standing with the front legs stretched forward.
- Hooves are hot.
- Increased digital pulse.
- Occasionally, a separation of hoof and coronary band.

RECOMMENDATIONS

Vet Call vet immediately and remove any feed, and access to grass. Do not remove existing hay—keep available to prevent added stress on the horse.

Stable Area Make the horse as comfortable as possible, preferably on a soft surface. Use peat for bedding to help prevent pressure ulcers on the hips, provide a firm footing for getting up, and good support for standing. Coarse sand may be used if peat is not available.

Hydrotherapy While waiting for the vet to arrive, cold hose the affected legs at ten-minute intervals for 30 minutes each time.

Cold Treatment If legs and feet are extremely hot, apply ice over the area until your vet arrives.

Magnetic Therapy Apply magnets to cannon bone area and hoof after the other treatments have all been completed. (Ignore my previous recommendation in earlier discussions on magnets to wait 48 hours after heat has gone. In this case use magnets as soon as possible.)

Acupuncture Get treatment as soon as possible. Treatment while the laminitis is in progress is very effective and sometimes stops the progression of the laminitis.

Homeopathy

- Aconitum napellus 30C every 30 minutes. Give as soon as laminitis is noticed. (May be given along with Belladonna in cases of acute laminitis.)
- Belladonna 30C every 30 minutes. Works well when pulse is increased, temperature is elevated, and the horse is sweating. (May be given along with aconitum in cases of acute laminitis.)
- Nux vomica 30C every 2 hours. Good in cases of decreased circulation.

Acupressure On points TH_3, TH_I, TH_5, SI_I, LI_I, GV_{14}, LU_{II}, and HT_9 (see *Acupuncture/Acupressure Appendix I*).

Aromatherapy

- Lemon. Dilute the essential oil to massage into coronary band to promote circulation.
- Juniper. Decreases toxins.
- Geranium. Heals damaged areas of the hoof.
- Thyme. Increases circulation.

Bach Flowers Gorse may relieve depression in horses with long-term founder.

Chronic Laminitis

Once laminitis has occurred and the emergency care complete, follow-up care begins. Each case must be assessed on an individual basis so a care plan can be initiated. X-rays should be taken to

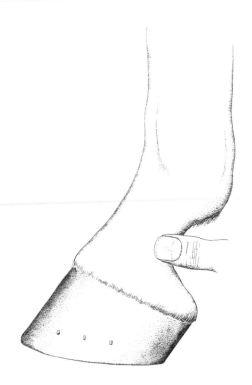

III–26 *The location of the digital pulse.*

determine the position of the coffin bone and your vet and farrier will decide how to reshape the hoof. Generally the toe of the hoof wall is rasped back and the heel lowered to achieve realignment. Heel-lowering must be carried out gradually, possibly over several shoeings, to guard against a sudden increase in tension on the deep digital flexor tendon which could cause further rotation of the coffin bone. Use of pads, bar shoes, or wide-web shoes must be decided on a case-by-case basis, according to X-rays, to decide which will make the horse most comfortable.

Alternative treatments are very effective in treating chronic laminitis, though since every case is different there is no specific treatment that will work for all horses.

SYMPTOMS

Look for these signs to occur after an acute case, and on and off throughout the horse's life after a case of laminitis:

- Lameness that is worse on hard ground.
- Horse landing on the heel of an affected hoof.
- Hoof wall grows differently, with a longer toe, higher heel, and concave front of the hoof wall.
- Rings on the hoof wall appear and the space between the rings is wider near the heel (unlike rings on the hoof wall due to other stress).
- The sole of the hoof may be dropped and very flaky in consistency.

RECOMMENDATIONS

Test Have your vet X-ray the foot.

Shoeing Consult your farrier as to the best way to reshape and shoe the hoof. Foundered horses often have rapid hoof growth so have your farrier visit as often as every four weeks.

Supplements

- Vitamin C. Give 8 grams per 1,000-pound horse, daily.
- Coenzyme Q-10. This antioxidant is very effective but dosage varies greatly according to symptoms. Consult a holistic vet for dosage best suited to your horse's needs. (See Appendix VI for *Product Suppliers.*)

Herbs All the herbs listed below can be helpful and a mixture of them all will give the horse needed benefits:

- Clivers. Use to promote lymphatic drainage. Effectively prevents a recurrence. Give 1/2 to 3/4 oz (15 to 20 grams) twice a day. You can make a compress (see p. 160) to help soothe swollen legs.
- Cat's claw. Helps to keep inflammation reduced and promotes circulation. Use 1/4 oz (5 to 10 grams). (***Caution***: See p. 323.)
- Comfrey. Helps with circulation, and promotes bone and soft tissue healing. Give 1 oz (30

grams) of the dried herb twice daily.
- Nettle. Stimulates circulation. It also contains vitamin C that has antioxidant properties. Feed 1/2 to 1 oz (15 to 30 grams) a day.
- Devil's claw. Has anti-inflammatory properties, and is particularly effective for pain associated with bone problems. Give 1/2 oz (15 grams) daily.

Homeopathy Chronic laminitis requires a very specific homeopathic workup that you should do in consultation with a holistic vet. To begin you can give Arnica 30C two to three times daily for inflammation and pain.

Aromatherapy Choose either one of the following, or alternate their use. If rosemary and thyme cannot be used (see ***Cautions*** on p. 308 and p. 310), use geranium, chamomile, juniper, or litsea cubeba as alternate choices:

- Rosemary. Improves circulation, decreases inflammation of the veins, acts as a diuretic, and reduces pain from arthritic type bone lesions.
- Thyme. Promotes circulation, and is one of the most helpful inhalants for treating laminitis.

Weight The horse should be kept slightly underweight to help prevent recurrence of laminitis. However, the horse should not be so thin that his ribs show.

Turnout Initially restrict it to areas without grass.

Acupuncture Helps to increase circulation and lymph drainage in the hooves. May also relieve pain.

Magnetic Therapy Use the small magnets that you glue onto the front of the hooves to help increase circulation (see p. 47). A magnet may also be applied over the cannon bone area to further stimulate circulation.

Acupressure

Front legs:

- LI_1; LU_{11}; PC_9; TH_1; SI_1; HT9: these points around the coronary band promote circulation.

- TH_3 aids with circulation, and helps detoxify the liver.
- TH_5 increases circulation.
- GV_{14}: stimulate this point last to help move the circulation, and Qi.

Hind legs:
- ST_{45}; SP_1; LIV_1; KI_1; BL_{67}; KI_1: these points around the coronary band promote circulation.
- GB_{34} increases circulation.
- GB_{44} increases circulation, and decreases fluid retention in the legs.
- Bai Hui: use this point last to help move the circulation and Qi throughout the hind legs.

LIVER DISORDERS

Most people don't give much thought to liver problems in horses since the symptoms usually aren't noticed until the condition is very advanced. The most well known sign of a liver problem is jaundice, a yellow coloring of the gums and the mucus membranes, such as those around the eye area. Jaundice is a sign that the liver is not functioning properly and is not converting the substance called bile. Jaundice is not indicative of a specific disease, only that the liver is unwell. Jaundice is not seen until a liver problem is advanced, and in some horses it may be difficult to notice the discoloration in the early stages. If you ever notice jaundice, call your vet immediately.

In Eastern medicine, the liver plays a major role in maintaining the health of the muscles and tendons. If the liver is stressed—or, as expressed in Oriental medical terms, deficient in energy, which is referred to as Qi—the muscles and tendons will not be properly supported. When this occurs, the horse may experience muscle or tendon problems, such as tendinitis or sprains.

How does the liver become deficient in Qi? Since the liver is the main organ that processes toxins, it can become overworked if the toxin load becomes too high. High toxin loads in a horse's body can be caused by the same stresses as those that affect people—poor diet, insecticides, inconsistent exercises, and emotional stress. (See Chapters One and Five for information on toxins in feeds and a general discussion of diet.)

Inconsistent exercise produces a high toxin load in several ways. When the horse is exercised—or over-exercised—if his muscle tone is poor, his body responds through a series of chemical reactions to meet the demands made on it. Once the exercise period is over, the liver must detoxify the body by processing all the extra by-products produced by the muscles during exercise. One of these products is lactic acid. Although lactic acid doesn't sound like a toxin, it acts like one because it must be broken down by the body and its components processed through the liver. When a horse is exercised only occasionally, the lactic acid produced during exercise can be high, and processing this high level of lactic acid requires lots of extra effort by the liver.

Stress also plays a role in liver disorders. When stressed, the body does not function as efficiently, and the liver has a heavier load to process in order to help deal with the stress. Each horse will interpret stress differently: some are more sensitive than others. Long distance travel, horse shows, and new environments all create stress in a horse's life. The smells are new, the horse rests less, and the food and water may be different. In addition, temperatures may change to either hot or cold and require the already stressed body to cope with yet one more thing. Evaluating your horse's stress level can be an important step in managing it.

Silver, a horse I owned before Charlie, disliked other horses and was difficult to manage when stabled in strange places. His liver frequently became stressed at horse shows or right after them. To help Silver cope with stress, I gave him a homeopathic remedy during the show and after it.

While taking the homeopathic, his appetite remained normal and he was calmer, with less nervous sweating and no muscle or tendon problems.

Once, I examined an Arabian mare that was shown extensively throughout the year. She held many championships and traveled long distances. When I saw her she had anhidrosis (inability to sweat) and, despite efforts to breed her, was not able to settle. A complete medical checkup, including hormone analysis and blood work, revealed nothing. When I examined her using Eastern medical techniques, I found that the mare's main problem was a deficiency in liver Qi. (Unless it is severe, a deficiency in Qi is not diagnosable by traditional allopathic methods.) Following a series of acupuncture treatments and homeopathy, the mare began sweating and cycling normally. Her overall condition improved so much that the owner, who had not seen the mare during the time of the treatment, did not recognize the mare when she returned home.

Liver problems can also be caused by nutritional supplements if they are not carefully balanced in the diet. Iron supplements are often given to horses to treat anemia and to help increase energy. However, iron supplements can lead to problems if there is not sufficient copper in the diet, since copper is necessary for the efficient utilization of iron. When this happens, the iron is absorbed and stored in the liver instead of being used by the horse's body as was intended. The excess can decrease the liver Qi, cause inflammation, and sometimes elevate the liver enzymes. Do not feed supplemental iron unless your horse specifically needs it. If he does, be sure he gets 70mg of copper in his diet along with the iron supplement.

There are few conventional methods to treat the liver, so Oriental medicine is the most effective. To evaluate the liver, consult the acupuncture/acupressure chart on p. 293, and locate Bladder 18 on the horse's back (labeled BL_{18} on the chart). Soreness over this point when palpated may indicate a liver Qi deficiency. If you suspect your horse may have a liver problem, no matter how minor, or if your horse is subject to a lot of stress, consult a holistic vet about treatment.

SYMPTOMS

- Muscle and tendon injuries, especially those that seem to recur often.
- Soreness over Bladder 18 acupuncture point (BL_{18} on chart).
- Change in attitude; seems irritable or angry.

RECOMMENDATIONS

Rest Reduce stress load until the horse is treated.

Test If signs of severe liver problems, such as jaundice, are present, have a vet do a complete exam.

Homeopathy Choose one of the following:

- Nux vomica 6C, 12C, or 30C three times daily. Use if the horse has a poor appetite or displays nervousness or irritability. If the liver points at BL18 are sore but the liver enzymes on a blood test are not elevated, use this remedy.
- Phosphorus 6C, 12C, or 30C three times daily. Use when liver enzymes are elevated on blood work or when jaundice (yellowing of the mucus membranes such as those around the eyes and in the mouth) is present. Other signs for this remedy include bleeding from the nose or around the gums, or blood in the urine or manure.
- Bryonia 6C, 12C, or 30C three times daily. Use when liver enzymes are elevated. Other possible indications that this is the remedy to choose include: stiff joints, a greasy coat, and the presence of any respiratory symptoms.

Acupuncture

Chiropractic Get an adjustment.

Acupressure On point BL_{18} (see chart in *Acupuncture/Acupressure Appendix I*).

M

MUSCLE SORENESS

(See also *Lameness and Leg Problems* Hind Leg: Upper Leg Area, *Fibrotic Myopathy*)

Muscle soreness is one of the most common problems affecting horses, but the more fit the horse, the less likely he is to suffer from it. During exercise, a continuous series of alternating chemical exchanges takes place within the horse's muscles. The first of these exchanges causes the muscle to contract, and the second causes it to relax. The by-products of these chemical exchanges are flushed from the muscles by the circulatory system, but it takes more time to remove all of the by-products than it does for the muscle to contract and relax. The level of by-products, therefore, builds up in the muscles and produces the effect called muscle soreness. As the muscles are exercised more, the exchange reaction becomes more efficient, and the blood vessels enlarge to help remove the by-products more swiftly. This effect is known as conditioning.

Muscle soreness is most often noticed following exercise. It can result from excessive exercise or from performing a type of exercise that the muscles have not done before. You may notice this soreness when you wash your horse and he is very sensitive to water on his back. Sometimes, a horse may seem sensitive about being touched while being groomed or tacked-up. This is another common sign of muscle soreness.

There are several things you can do to help prevent--at least minimize--muscle soreness. First, cool out your horse thoroughly following exercise. During the cool-down period, keep him walking while his respiration and heart rates gradually decrease. You can either hand walk your horse, or you can add a ten-to-fifteen minute relaxed walk under saddle at the end of your ride. This step is important because most horses won't move around enough on their own after exercise to keep their circulation at an optimum level for by-product removal.

This cool-down regimen will be most effective in decreasing muscle soreness if you walk your horse *before* you rinse him off with water, even in warm weather. Cold water can cause the blood vessels to constrict and reduce the rate at which by-products are removed from the muscles. If your horse is very hot and requires a rinse with water immediately after exercise to help him cool down, use lukewarm water. When the weather is hot and you do not have access to warm water, fill a bucket before you start your ride and set it in the sun to warm up. Another alternative if you have only cold water is to sponge the horse in spots under his chest, on his neck, and between his hind legs.

You should always follow the cool-down steps suggested above. Sometimes, however, when a horse has performed sustained or vigorous exercise, such as endurance training or a long gallop, walking at the end of the exercise may not be enough to completely remove all the by-products from the muscles. In these situations, the horse's body will try to expedite the process by increasing blood circulation which, in turn, can cause swelling, most noticeably in the lower legs. One way to relieve the excess fluid is to apply a poultice to the cannon bone area of the leg after the exercise. Another effective method is to use magnets applied on the cannon bone area. The magnets will maintain the circulation in the legs and speed up removal of by-products from the muscles while the horse stands still and rests.

Swelling can also develop over the back, hips, shoulders, and neck, but it may be less noticeable. Magnetic therapy in the form of a magnetic blanket can be used to maintain circulation and expedite removal of by-products from the muscles in these areas. If you don't have a magnetic blanket, a massage over these areas of the body can be helpful. (See *Massage Therapy*, p. 47).

Electrolytes are required for the body to carry out the chemical exchanges involved in contracting and relaxing the muscles. Many owners add electrolytes to their horses' feed or water in the summer only, since horses sweat more then and need to replace the electrolytes lost through sweating. But, if you exercise your horse on a regular basis during most of the year, giving him an electrolyte supplement year-round will help ensure that he maintains the correct level of electrolytes needed for efficient muscle function.

SYMPTOMS

- Heat and swelling over a muscle area.
- Muscle spasms may be present.
- The horse may not want to be brushed, touched, or tacked-up. Horses that become upset when the girth is tightened often have a rib or shoulder muscle injury.

RECOMMENDATIONS

Rest/Vet Rest the horse, and if the problem persists have your vet examine him.

Homeopathy Choose from one of the following:

- Arnica montana 6C, 12C, or 30C: Two to three times a day if heat or swelling is present in the muscles.
- Magnesium phosphate 6C, 12C or 30C: Three times a day for muscle spasms.

Medications

- Hyaluronate sodium (Legend): For chronic cases of muscle inflammation this drug works very effectively. Usually two or three injections are required 5 to 7 days apart. This drug must be obtained from your vet.
- Ketoprofen (Ketofen): This anti-inflammatory drug is similar to ibuprofen and is effective in relieving muscle soreness. One or two weeks of daily treatment is usually required. This drug needs to be given intravenously by vet,

since intramuscular injection of it can cause sore muscles, and even an abscess.

Acupuncture Treatment to stimulate the circulation.

Chiropractic An adjustment of the surrounding skeletal structure may be needed to allow the muscle to function at its optimum.

Aromatherapy

- Chamomile. Soothes muscles and decreases inflammation.
- Juniper. Decreases accumulation of toxins. Add a few drops of pure essential oil to a bucket of water to use as a rinse after strenuous exercise.
- Lavender. Relieves pain from sprains and muscle aches.

N

NAVICULAR DISEASE

The navicular bone is a small bone located inside the hoof directly behind the coffin joint (see diagram on p. 233). Navicular disease is the term used to describe lameness associated with the navicular bone or surrounding structures. It almost always affects only the front feet. The lameness can be caused by a wide variety of conditions, and the exact nature of navicular disease is not completely understood.

A horse suffering from navicular disease may be in pain most of the time, although it may not always be possible to determine precisely what is causing the pain. Sometimes navicular disease is brought on by arthritic changes to the navicular bone itself, but it can also be the result of an inflammation in the navicular bursa, a condition known as navicular bursitis. Given all of these factors, it can be a challenge to successfully diagnose and treat navicular disease.

First, let's review some of the most common causes of navicular bursitis. The flexor tendons that run down the back of the cannon bone can

but review recent changes in feed, supplements, or pasture management. Other sources of poisoning become apparent only by a process of elimination.

SYMPTOMS

- Convulsions.
- Gum color: extremely pale, yellow, dark, or bright cherry red.
- Staggering.
- Breathing difficulties.
- Collapse.
- Blood in manure, urine, or out of the nose.
- Illness that has no determined cause.

POTOMAC HORSE FEVER

See Chapter Four, p.72.

PUNCTURE WOUNDS

See *Cuts and Puncture Wounds*, p. 202, and *Hoof Problems: Puncture Wounds*, p. 220.

RABIES

See Chapter Four, p. 71.

RESPIRATORY PROBLEMS

The most common respiratory problems that afflict horses are pulmonary emphysema, viruses, and pulmonary hemorrhage (bleeders).

Chronic Obstructive Pulmonary Disease (Heaves)

Chronic obstructive pulmonary disease (COPD), also referred to as pulmonary emphysema, is commonly known as heaves and is a widespread problem in horses. Most horses develop this illness due to an allergic reaction to inhaled substances such as dust and molds. Constant coughing, difficulty breathing, and weight loss are signs usually associated with COPD. Horses suffering from this ill-

ness often have a visible line along their side where their ribs end (the point where the cartilage and bony part of the ribs meet), starting near the girth area extending up toward the hipbone. This is caused by stressed breathing. If you suspect your horse has COPD, contact your vet for a thorough checkup to rule out any other respiratory illness such as pneumonia.

SYMPTOMS

- Difficulty breathing; breathing from abdomen rather than chest area; development of a heave line.
- Wheezing sound with breathing.
- Weight loss.
- Coughing that is worse when the horse is in dusty conditions.
- Lack of stamina.

RECOMMENDATIONS

Test/Vet
- Have your vet do an examination to rule out pneumonia or other respiratory disease.

Feed
- Wet down all hay to keep dust to a minimum while the horse is eating.
- Decrease dust and molds by feeding extruded grain instead of whole grains.

Stable Area
- Reevaluate the type of bedding you use. Most horses with heaves do best with shavings as long as they are not dusty. (See Chapter Six for more information on the pros and cons of various types of bedding.)
- Keep the dirt surrounding the stall damp to keep dust down.

Exercise In as dust-free an area as possible.

Acupuncture Treatments can greatly reduce or eliminate heaves.

Homeopathy Remedies can assist in reducing coughing and allergic reactions. Each case is unique, however, and a specific history and complete workup are necessary to determine which of the many possibilities is best for your horse. The following are some homeopathics to consider trying (choose only one):

- Phosphorous 30C three times a day. If a homeopathic vet is available, ask about using a higher potency of phosphorous such as 200C. This remedy works well when coughing starts or breathing worsens during physical exertion. It is also indicated if symptoms worsen when a change of weather occurs, particularly thunderstorms.
- Sulfur 12C or 30C three times a day. Use sulfur when first treating a long-term chronic case of COPD with a homeopathic. Other guiding signs for this remedy are worsening of symptoms in the morning and the presence of heat or sweat on the skin, particularly the skin over the chest area. Use also with horses who seem to have stiff legs and a sore back in addition to the COPD symptoms.
- Bryonia 6C, 12C, or 30C three times a day. Use bryonia when the horse is irritable and tends to keep his head in a lowered position. This remedy works well when symptoms are worse at night, particularly after eating or drinking. Horses for whom this remedy is suitable become worse during warm weather and may display stifle problems as well as stocking up (swelling of lower legs). The hair coat may appear greasy.

NAET

Acupressure Do on points BL_{13}; SP_{21}; LU_1; LU_5; and LU_8 (see *Acupuncture/Acupressure Appendix I*).

Herbs Commercial mixes of herbs such as Cough Free (available at feed stores and from horse supply catalogs) have been formulated for this problem. They help to decrease coughing in some cases.

Aromatherapy

- Eucalyptus. Soothes respiratory tract.
- Hops. Decreases symptoms, makes breathing easier.
- Lemon and Litsea cubeba. Stimulate immune system.
- Peppermint. Relieves symptoms temporarily. (See **Caution** note on p. 308).

Supplement Tahitian Noni (available in health food stores). Use 5 tbsp (about 70ml) for every 1000 lbs (approx. 450 kgs) the horse weighs.

Respiratory Viruses

Respiratory viruses are a common problem and can be challenging to treat. They range from those that cause upper respiratory symptoms, such as nasal discharge and coughing, to more serious viruses that affect the lungs. *Equine influenza* and *rhinopneumonitis* (see Chapter Four for vaccination information) are very common examples. Although more prevalent during the autumn, viruses are a year-round problem. It is unclear why one horse is susceptible to a particular virus and other horses are not, but stress is often a major contributing factor. Traveling to horse shows, changes in environment, and even a sudden change in temperature can be enough to stress a horse's immune system and allow a virus to take hold.

Not every respiratory infection is caused by a virus, and unfortunately, it can be difficult to determine whether a respiratory infection is viral or non-viral. Conventional vets usually treat non-viral respiratory infections with antibiotics, but these medications are not effective against viruses. The diagnosis is often made by process of elimination: if the infection does not respond to treatment with antibiotics, it is most likely viral in origin. Blood work can also determine if a virus is present. Once the infection has been identified as viral, your vet will establish a treatment plan and advise you as to the best way to monitor your horse's progress. Among the signs that the treatment is working are an absence of nasal discharge, a return to normal breathing, and no coughing. If the infection involves the lungs, regular checks by the vet may be necessary to confirm that the infection has been eradicated.

There are several immune system stimulants on the market that help activate the immune system to fight off viral infections. These products have proven to be effective and are also given as a preventive before stressful events such as traveling. An injectable pharmaceutical available from your vet called Equi-Stim works well, but should be limited to two doses per year. Overuse of this drug can be harmful.

Many horses become ill with a respiratory virus like influenza even though they have been vaccinated. Viruses are constantly mutating into new strains. If your horse is exposed to a new strain of virus that was not covered by the vaccination, his body may be unable to overcome the infection on its own. At this point, an immune system stimulant, homeopathics, and acupuncture can help your horse combat the virus.

SYMPTOMS

- Coughing, nasal discharge, depression, lethargy, poor appetite.

RECOMMENDATIONS

Vet Ask your vet to recommend an immune system stimulant.

Acupuncture Treatments can help to stimulate the system to fight viral infections.

Chiropractic Adjustments of back vertebrae and ribs out of alignment due to coughing or viruses affecting the lung or spleen are very useful.

Homeopathy Choose one of the following:

- Phosphorus 12C or 30C three times daily. Use this remedy when there is a dry cough. Congestion may also be present in the lungs. Other guiding signs are an increase in hunger and a decrease in water consumption, an increase in gas accompanied by foul-smelling manure, and

gums that are ulcerated or bleeding.

- Aconitum napellus 6C, 12C, or 30C three times daily. Use when in the first stages of disease, particularly when fever is present. Do not use this remedy when symptoms have been present for more than 24 hours. Stop use of aconitum after 2 days. Other signs that may accompany respiratory symptoms are restlessness, such as stall-pacing, over-sensitivity to stimuli such as sounds, and colic.

- Lycopodium 30C three times daily. Use this remedy when a cough is involved or when pneumonia is present and breathing is difficult. If a blood workup has been performed, the liver enzymes are often elevated. The horse may show increased sweating, increased movement of his head from side-to-side, and pain in the lumbo-sacral area. If this remedy seems correct for your horse and the disease is severe, consult a homeopathic vet about using a higher potency such as 200C or 1M.

Herbs These can be used to treat the symptoms of the virus, as well as stimulate the immune system and strengthen the body. I have listed some herbs that are very effective. These can be mixed together, used separately, or work well when combined with acupuncture and/or homeopathy.

- Boneset. Use when the horse has a fever. This herb also acts as a mild stimulant to the immune system.

- Comfrey. This soothing herb reduces bronchial irritation and works as an expectorant.

- Echinacea. A good choice to boost the immune system to help fight a viral infection. When one horse in a herd becomes ill, give this herb to the sick horse and all the other horses in the herd, to prevent spread of the infection.

- Garlic. Add the powdered form to feed to help protect a horse from contracting a respiratory infection. Garlic also works as an expectorant and the sulfur it contains can assist the body in fighting off secondary bacterial infections. **Caution:** *Do not give to nursing mares.*

- Licorice. Boosts the immune system against viral and bacterial infections. Licorice also breaks up mucus and acts as an expectorant.

Acupressure Do on points LU_1, LU_5, LU_7, LU_8, and PC_6 (see *Acupuncture/Acupressure Appendix I*).

Supplement Vitamin C. Give 8 to 10 grams daily.

Aromatherapy

- Eucalyptus and Lavender. Make a vapor from these two essential oils to soothe the respiratory tract.
- Geranium. Soothes throat irritation.
- Lemon. Use as a disinfectant in its vaporized form to help reduce spread of infection to others.
- Marjoram. An excellent, effective immune system booster for respiratory disease. See **Caution** on p. 307.
- Peppermint. Relieves symptoms such as mucus in the respiratory tract. See **Caution** on p. 308.
- Tea tree. Stimulates immune system to fight bacterial and viral infections.
- Thyme. Acts as a decongestant. **Caution:** *See p. 310 for contraindications.*
- Sandalwood. Relieves dry cough and sore, irritated throat. Massage some diluted essential oil around throat area.

Pulmonary Hemorrhage

Pulmonary hemorrhage occurs when one or more blood vessels in the lungs rupture, usually during exercise, allowing blood to flow into the bronchioles, the lowermost portion of the lungs. In severe cases, the bronchioles will become partially filled with blood, thus decreasing the room for oxygen flow. When this happens, the horse's breathing becomes more and more labored as the air flow and oxygen exchange is reduced. In some cases, blood will eventually be seen coming from the nose, but it is the presence of blood in the lungs that causes damage. Recurrent bleeding in the lungs damages blood vessels and may create fibrous adhesions that will result in a chronic decrease in oxygen exchange.

Horses that are prone to pulmonary hemorrhage are often referred to as "bleeders." Over time, the effects of this condition cause a reduction in performance level, and many bleeders are eventually forced to retire from competition because of it. Although pulmonary hemorrhage is most often associated with horses on the racetrack, it seems to be on the rise in the rest of the horse population as well, especially among horses that are galloped frequently. Research is currently underway to try to determine what causes pulmonary hemorrhage and why it is becoming more common. Among the possible causes being investigated are insecticides in hay and grain, herbicides, and reactions to vaccines.

Racehorses that are bleeders are often given a drug called furosimide (Lasix) before a race or workout. Lasix can help to control pulmonary hemorrhage, but some horses bleed even when they are on this medication. In addition, as with most pharmaceutical drugs, Lasix has side effects, the most serious being damage to the kidneys after long-term use.

If you have, or are thinking about buying, a horse that was raced, be sure to find out if he was given Lasix, indicating a past bleeding or respiratory problem. The effects of bleeding can stay with a horse for years even if he no longer actually bleeds during exercise. Some bleeders, or former bleeders, stay relatively thin and have a dull, dry coat. These horses will not gain weight readily despite excellent diets. Sometimes former bleeders have a cranky disposition and demonstrate a poor attitude that does not seem to improve even with extra care. Occasionally, they exhibit a lack of stamina.

Bleeding in the lungs usually happens after exertion. If you notice that your horse experiences sudden fatigue, has trouble breathing, has blood coming out of his nose, or seems to have a desire to stop working during exercise, have him checked by your vet. Remember too that in many cases, the pulmonary hemorrhage may not be severe enough to cause bleeding from the nose, so you shouldn't disregard the symptoms of fatigue and breathing problems just because you can't see any blood.

Bleeding in the lungs can be detected by an examination with an endoscope, a fiberoptic device that allows the vet to view the inside of the horse's upper respiratory area and lungs. Although bleeding from the nose may indicate pulmonary hemorrhage, it can also have other causes such as a broken nasal blood vessel. If you notice blood coming from your horse's nose, before you panic, have an endoscopic examination performed to determine what is really happening.

Once a horse has bled, he may have a tendency toward recurrences, particularly when stressed with exercise. Extenuating circumstances such as allergies or illness can also precipitate bleeding in some horses. On the other hand, many former racehorses with a history of bleeding may never have a recurrence because they probably will never be stressed to the extent they were on the track.

Bleeders can usually be managed with proper treatment, although the possibility will always exist that the bleeding could recur given the right set of circumstances. I have had great success improving the condition of bleeders and preventing bleeding by using acupuncture, homeopathy, and herbs.

SYMPTOMS

- Slowing down or seeming fatigued during exercise.
- Weight loss.
- Dry, dull hair coat.

- Blood coming from the nose following exercise.

RECOMMENDATIONS

Acupuncture As soon as possible after a bleeding episode.

Homeopathy Can be very effective in controlling and preventing future bleeding. Choose one of the following remedies:

- Phosphorus 30C three times daily. If bleeding is severe, consult a homeopathic vet concerning the use of higher potencies such as 1M or 10M. Use this remedy when the bleeding occurs on a regular basis.
- Bryonia 6C, 12C, or 30C three times daily. Use bryonia when a horse affected with bleeding problems takes deep breaths; keeps his head down most of the time, especially when exercised; and may have an associated dry cough. Bryonia works well on bleeders who sweat excessively and are irritable.
- Aconitum napellus 6C, 12C, or 30C three times daily. Use when bleeding is first noticed.

Herbs Yunnan Paiyao, a Chinese herb, is very effective in controlling bleeding. However limit the use because it can cause severe side effects if used repeatedly. I recommend using it a maximum of twice a month.

RHINOPNEUMONITIS

See Chapter Four, p. 69.

S

SADDLE SORES AND GIRTH GALLS

Saddle sores and girth (cinch) galls are areas of skin inflammation under tack that if left untreated can become open sores. The areas affected by the saddle usually occur around the withers, though the skin over the horse's back and sides can also be involved. Girth galls are commonly found where the girth is attached to the saddle (see fig. III–27, p. 266). Both types are caused by tack rubbing the skin enough to cause abrasions. Examples are:

Saddle Sores

- Saddle that does not fit the horse.
- Dirt underneath the saddle.
- Unevenly stuffed English saddle, and loss of the sheepskin padding on a Western saddle.
- Low withers allow a saddle to move around and not stay in place.
- Poor riding.
- Fat horse. Saddle moves around easily.
- Horse in a fitness program. The muscle and fat over the back, sides, and withers shift and change as the horse becomes more fit, and the saddle often becomes looser as it does not fit as well.

Girth Galls

- A dirty girth or cinch. Dirt, mud, and sweat can irritate.
- A partially broken, or cracked, girth.
- Girth too loose, or too tight.
- Allergy to material in the girth or cinch.
- Dirty, muddy, or sweaty hair under the girth.

SYMPTOMS

- Sore, inflamed areas of skin around and under the saddle and girth areas.
- After healing, white patches of hair may be seen where the sores or galls appeared.

RECOMMENDATIONS

Saddle sores: healing

Rest Until the area is healed.

Topical Ointments to decrease inflammation: Use calendula ointment, aloe vera, or vitamin E (break open capsules and apply topically).

Clean Clean open sores with Betadine mixed with water (1/4 Betadine to 3/4 water). Allow the area to dry then apply one of the ointments mentioned above twice a day. Keep the sores clean. If a severe infection is present, you should call your vet.

Moxibustion Use indirect moxibustion every other day to increase the rate of healing. Moxibustion treatments increase the blood supply to the area. NOTE: Do not use moxibustion if infection is present.

Saddle sores: prevention

Protection When starting up, do not use a pad directly on the sore area. Take a therapeutic pad, made of stiff foam, make a hole in it so it does not touch the sore area when placed on the horse's back. Put a thin pad on top of this, and then the saddle. This system works by keeping the saddle pressure off the sore area and allowing it to heal underneath.

Review

- Grooming products and particularly new products that might leave a residue on the horse's skin that when mixed with sweat causes skin inflammation.
- Check (or have an expert check) the saddle fit and the condition of its padding.
- Check your saddle pad for worn or uneven padding. If the saddle pad is new perhaps the horse is reacting to the material.
- If saddle and pad are in good condition, have a knowledgeable person observe the rider. Riders who lean to one side, bounce excessively, or shift their weight frequently, may cause saddle sores.

Girth galls: healing

- Use the same recommendations as for Saddle Sores: Healing, above.

Girth galls: prevention

Review Check the girth for cracks or tears. It should be soft and flexible, never hard or stiff.

Protection

- Use a girth cover to prevent chafing. They are made of synthetic fleece, neoprene, or sheepskin—all easily washable after use—and provide padding.

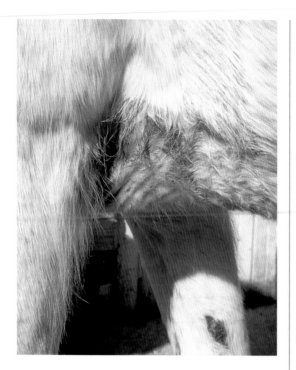

III–27 *A girth gall.*

exposure to allergens as well, since some horses affected with sarcoids experience increased tumor growth when exposed to allergens. Medical researchers have not yet been able to determine why allergens interact with sarcoids in this way. How can you tell if an allergic response is causing the sarcoids to grow faster? Unfortunately, it's mostly guess work or deduction. An example would be a horse affected with sarcoids that experiences an increase in the growth or number of sarcoids when turned out only in a particular pasture. Obviously there is something in the pasture that the horse is reacting to which is affecting his immune system.

Sarcoids do not usually disappear spontaneously, so a variety of treatments have been tried. Surgical removal of sarcoids often results in a recurrence. Cold cautery, which involves the

• Groom the girth area thoroughly before tacking-up.

SARCOIDS

(See also *Cancer*, p. 196)

A sarcoid tumor or skin lesion is most often found on the skin of the legs, lower abdominal area, around the top of the tail, or head (see figs. III–28 and 29). Sarcoids can be elevated and tumor-like in appearance or look like a roughened patch of skin. Some gradually get larger, while others may remain inactive for long periods of time. These tumors are not usually life threatening; but sarcoids become a problem when they become unsightly or uncomfortable or interfere with tack.

While it is believed that this common tumor is caused by a virus, it seems to be related to an

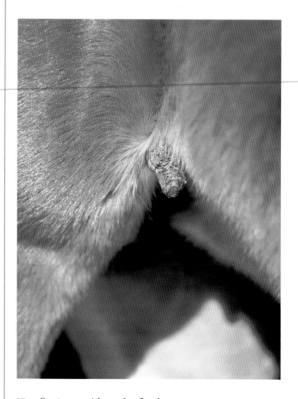

II–28 *A sarcoid on the flank.*

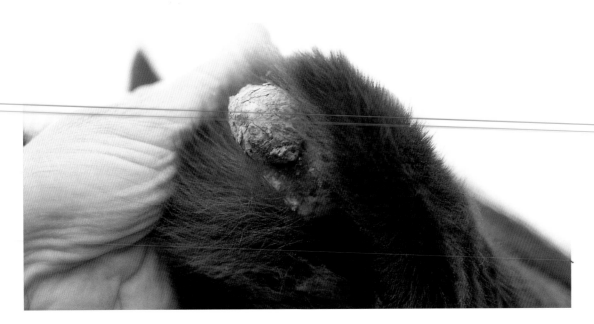

III–29 *An ear sarcoid.*

use of liquid nitrogen to freeze the sarcoids, is most often used when the sarcoids are found on the head. More recently, immune stimulants have been successfully used to treat sarcoids. There are a variety of immune stimulants on the market today, some more successful than others. Acupuncture and homeopathy can also help to stimulate the immune system and balance the body as an aid to the treatment program, but neither of these approaches alone leads to remission.

SYMPTOMS

- One type of sarcoid is found on the surface of the skin and feels smooth, crusty, and/or looks like a wart. Growth is usually very slow. It may remain unchanged for long periods, or suddenly disappear.
- Another type of sarcoid appears as an enlarged area, similar to a tumor. The skin over this enlargement may stay intact, or be a scabby area that doesn't heal. This type of sarcoid can have episodes of growth. It can also be present in multiple places.

RECOMMENDATIONS

Medication Discuss the use of immune stimulants with your vet.

Review Watch the growth of the sarcoid carefully. If there is an increase in the size of the tumor or more tumors appear, an allergen may be affecting the horse. Consider the horse's entire environment and note any recent changes in the feed, the stall, or the pasture that might be affecting the horse. (Also see *Allergies*, p. 182).

Refer to Recommendations *For All Types of Cancer* on p. 198.

SHOCK

A horse can go into shock due to any trauma, from an injury or reaction to a medication, vaccination, a fire or other emergency situation. Shock can be very serious and even lead to death. Rapid assessment and treatment of shock could save your horse's life.

SYMPTOMS

- Sweating, trembling, a decrease in pulse, pale gums.

RECOMMENDATIONS

Caution: *Call the vet immediately.*

Bach Flowers Give Rescue Remedy and repeat every 5 minutes until the condition improves. Use Star of Bethlehem for a few weeks after horse is stabilized.

Acupressure Do on point GV$_{26}$ (see *Acupuncture/Acupressure Appendix I*).

SKIN PROBLEMS

There are many conditions that can affect the health of your horse's skin, including lice, sunburn, sweet itch, scratches, reactions to diet, bacterial and fungal infections such as rain rot and ringworm, stress, hives, warts, and insect bites. The challenge in treating skin problems is determining which influence or combination of influences is the culprit. This section will help you narrow down the possible cause for a skin problem and lists steps you can take to improve the condition.

Bacterial Infections

Bacterial infections can have an appearance similar to fungal infections (see p.ooo) and the two are often confused. The main signs of a bacterial infection that are noticeable on the skin are hair loss and itching, with occasional areas of crusty or scaly skin. Symptoms differ depending on the type of bacteria causing the infection. Your vet will be able to determine whether the infection is bacterial or fungal by scraping the skin and then looking at it under a microscope or actually growing the bacteria or fungus in the lab.

Whenever a bacterial skin infection is present, it's important to investigate the problem thoroughly, particularly if the horse does not have a history of skin disorders. When the body is not able to fight off the skin infection, the root cause may be stress or a physical problem elsewhere in the body. Think about your horse's history just prior to the appearance of the skin infection. Were there any dietary changes, behavioral changes, or changes in environment? Any excessive stress—or what your horse interprets as stress—can influence his immune system and allow a bacterial infection to proliferate. Don't ignore other changes and simply treat the skin infection.

I was once asked to treat a mare with a persistent bacterial skin infection. The owner had heard that acupuncture could boost the immune system and get rid of the skin infection. An examination of the acupuncture points indicated that those associated with equine protozoal myeloencephalitis (EPM) were reactive. Combined with the mare's recent history of having a sore back, these reactions seemed to be an indication of EPM. I advised the owner that a blood test and a spinal fluid test could be done to check for this disease. Although reluctant because of the expense, the owner followed my recommendation and learned that the tests were positive for EPM. After the EPM was treated, the skin infection disappeared.

In this example the skin infection was caused by stress from a medical problem. However, stress from the environment can also weaken the immune system, allowing an infection to occur. Environmental stress can include the stabling or pasture situation, a reaction to seasonal weather changes, or changes in the horse's routine care. Each horse will react differently to stress in his environment; some are more sensitive than others, each interpreting his environment in a different way. There are some environmental stresses that are unavoidable, particularly when a horse is introduced into a new stabling situation that he must adapt to or when the weather changes. If you think that his environment might be a significant contributing factor to your horse's stress and the resulting skin problem, try to make whatever changes you can to improve it. You can also reduce the effects of stress by using a homeopathic or Bach Flower remedy.

SYMPTOMS

- Hair loss, itching, areas of dry or scaly skin.
- In severe cases, areas of pus may be present.

RECOMMENDATIONS

Review/Vet A complete physical exam to rule out an underlying medical problem.

Acupuncture Boosts the immune system and balances the body.

NAET

Homeopathy Nosodes for the specific bacteria, work very well. If you do not know which bacteria are causing the problem and cannot test, begin with a staphylococcus nosode because staphylococcus is one of the primary bacteria found in skin infections.

Herbs Use herbs to stimulate the immune system, in a tonic form to support the entire horse, or applied on skin directly to treat bacterial and fungal infections, and as an anti-inflammatory:

To stimulate immune system:

- Cat's claw and echinacea. These herbs may be used individually, or combined.

General "body tonic":

- Clivers, dandelion, fenugreek, garlic, kelp, nettle, and pau d'arco. These herbs may be used individually, or combined.

Applied directly on skin for an anti-inflammatory effect:

- St. John's Wort Oil, calendula, aloe vera, and chamomile.

Aromatherapy

- Chamomile. Can be inhaled, or as a poultice or compress directly on the affected area.
- Rosemary. Reduces dry and irritated skin.
- Sandalwood. Moisturizes and softens skin.
- Tea tree. Stimulates immune systems against bacterial and fungal infections.
- Thyme. Discourages hair loss.
- Ylang Ylang. Soothes irritated skin.

Antibiotic If the above holistic remedies don't work, your vet may prescribe antibiotic therapy (oral or topical depending on the case).

Fungal Diseases

Fungal diseases are a chronic problem in warm moist climates and can be very challenging to treat. There are a wide variety of fungal infections that can affect horses, and some are difficult to diagnose. The most common diagnostic methods used by vets are a skin scrape of the affected area or examining the skin under a "woods light" (ultraviolet light). The skin scraping can be examined directly under the microscope or applied to a growing medium to try to grow the fungus. If a fungus is present, there will be a color change as it grows, but growing fungus is sometimes a slow process. The woods light can help diagnose those varieties of fungus that fluoresce, most commonly some forms of ringworm. Not all fungus is fluorescent, however, so don't rely on a woods light as the only test.

A fungus can appear as a dry, flaky area or as a red, irritated area. It may also show no signs at all. It can stay in one location or spread to different areas on the skin. Fungal infections can also resemble bacterial skin infections, making diagnosis and treatment difficult. Some types of fungi are contagious even to humans, so be careful when treating them. When multiple infections or re-infection occurs, a depressed immune system may be the cause.

The most common type of fungus in horses, referred to as *rain rot* or *rain scald*, occurs due to moisture building up under the hair and providing a favorable environment for fungal growth (see fig. III–30, p. 270). There are a variety of fungi that can cause rain rot depending on the conditions present.

Another common fungus is *ringworm*. Though its name makes it sound like a type of

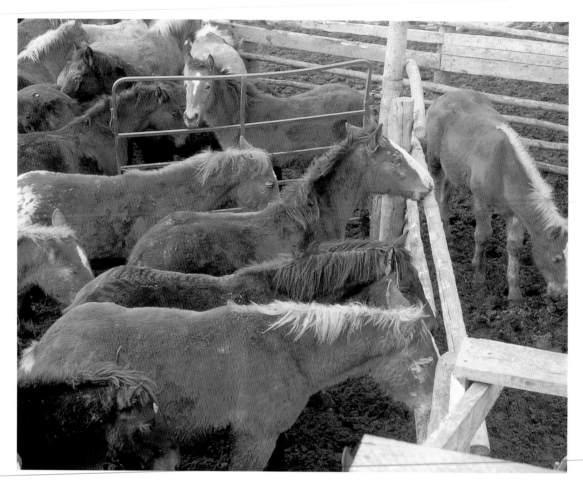

III–30 *A herd of young stock, many with cases of rain rot.*

parasite, ringworm is actually a fungal infection. Its name is derived from the fact that as it grows, ringworm fungus spreads in a circular shape (see fig. III–31, p. 271).

Fungal infections also commonly occur in horse's ears. These infections give a whitish, flaky appearance to the inside of the ear and cause discomfort.

Treatment must be strictly adhered to since a fungus can be very difficult to kill. Sunlight is an important part of treatment, because fungi thrive in dark, warm, and moist areas. Therefore it can be helpful to leave brushes, saddle blankets, and other tack items in the sun to help kill

a fungus. It also helps to stand a horse in the sun for an hour or so, particularly if an affected horse is usually confined to a stall.

SYMPTOMS

- Hair loss, flaky skin, itching.

RECOMMENDATIONS

Topical

- Betadine or other brand of tamed iodine solution, diluted percent with water applied on affected areas. (This type of iodine does not stain.)
- Use of a topical antifungal medication available without prescription may be effective against many types of fungus affecting horses.

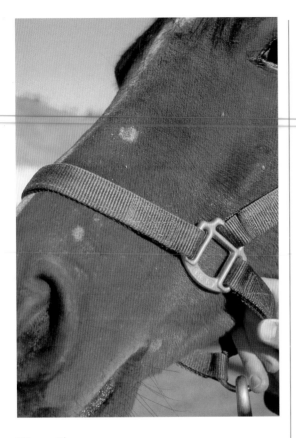

III–31 *Ringworm.*

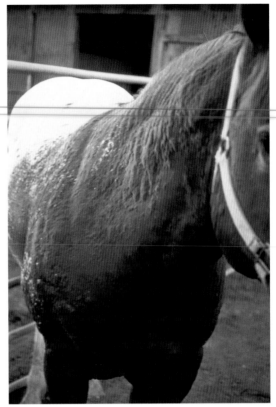

III–32 *An outbreak of hives.*

Clean Bathe with Betadine shampoo (or other tamed-iodine shampoo) or antifungal shampoo after exercise.

Turnout Be sure your horse gets lots of sunlight.

Acupuncture Helps stimulate the immune system.

Herbs See list under *Allergies* on p. 185.

Aromatherapy

- Lavender. Stimulates healing in some types of fungus.
- Lemon and litsea cubeba. Stimulates the immune system.
- Tea tree. Stimulates immune system, and can also be used topically directly onto the fungus areas.

Protection To prevent spread of the fungus do not use the affected horse's brushes, blankets, or tack on other horses. Wear latex gloves to avoid contact with your own skin and be sure to rinse the gloves in an antifungal solution (one-part bleach to three-parts water) if you do not throw them away after use.

Vet Consult if the condition does not improve.

Hives

Hives are raised spots of varying sizes on the body which sometimes cause itching (see fig. III–32). They are usually the result of the horse being exposed to something to which he is allergic or reactive. The source of the problem can be something that the horse has eaten or something that has touched him externally. If you find hives, immediately check for symptoms of shock such as pale gums, trembling, and sweating since the horse may be having a serious reaction to something. If any of these symptoms are seen, the reaction could be life threatening and a vet should be called immediately. Hives that are caused by shock are the exception rather than the rule. Most cases of hives are not serious and often go away without treatment. However, I have treated cases that were life threatening so always check your horse carefully if hives appear.

One such case that I treated was a three-year-old Morgan that had staggered in from the pasture with huge hives across one side. There were also scratches on the horse, with the swelling worse around the scratched areas. I was able to get to the horse immediately since he was only five minutes from my office and found that he was in shock when I got there. The scratches were from a toxic thorn bush common to the area. Since the owner was new to the area, she was unaware of the danger from the bush and had not checked the pasture before turning out her horse. The horse responded to immediate treatment for shock, and the hives disappeared.

SYMPTOMS

- Raised areas on the skin, usually round, and most commonly found on the neck and sides.
- Shock, indicated by pale gums, trembling, and sweating, may accompany this reaction.

RECOMMENDATIONS

Homeopathy Works well in minor cases. Unless otherwise stated, choose one of the following:

- Apis mellifica 6C three times a day. Can be used in conjunction with urtica urens. Use when hives are large and painful to the touch.
- Antimonium crudum 6C three times a day or, in an emergency, give hourly. Use when hives are small.

- Urtica urens 6C, 12C, or 30C three times a day. Use when swollen areas are warm to the touch.

Acupuncture Can be helpful in persistent cases.

Medication Diphenhydramine hydrochloride, available as an over-the-counter antihistamine, may be temporarily effective. Consult a vet before giving to your horse.

Aromatherapy Lemon and litsea cubeba: Use one to stimulate immune system.

Supplement Protease, a digestive enzyme (available in health food stores) is very effective in treating hives. Many allergens are identified as "foreign" proteins by the body, and protease helps the body handle these proteins. It comes in a powdered form which you can add to the horse's feed. Give twice a day in a dose about 10 times the amount recommended for an adult human for an average-sized horse (1000 lbs or approx. 450 kgs).

Lice

Lice infestation generally occurs during winter months. These tiny (2-3 mm long) cream-colored parasites hide under the long winter coat and frequently congregate in the mane, along the top of the back, and in the top of the tail (see figs. III–33 and 34, p. 274). Horses may be infected by two different types: *haematopinus asini,* a biting louse, and *Damalinia equi,* a blood-sucking louse. The biting lice are more active and can be seen moving around on the horse, while the blood-sucking lice either move slowly or not at all.

Lice can spread throughout a herd of horses through contact, or if the same grooming tools are used. Lice also lay eggs that are extremely difficult to brush off.

SYMPTOMS

- Horse scratches, rubs and bites himself, sometimes resulting in patches of hair loss, scabs, and sores.
- Hair appears dry and dull.
- Horse will be irritable and restless.

- Signs of lice are obvious when horse's coat is examined and hair is parted.

RECOMMENDATIONS

Vet

- Alternative treatments have not been totally effective in treating lice, but ask about new options which are being developed as I write this. Traditionally insecticides and worming preparations have been used as remedies.
- If only one horse is affected, have your vet give him a complete health checkup.

Protection Do not share grooming equipment, saddle pads, or blankets when lice are present in a barn or stable.

NOTE: Lice eggs attached to hair may not be affected by a treatment, so most horses will need to be treated again in three to four weeks.

Reactions to Diet

Diet can adversely affect your horse's health in a couple of ways. Sometimes the basic diet does not supply the correct nutrients, but there are also cases where the horse is fed a diet that does not agree with his system. Dietary reactions are some of the most difficult to assess, but they should be investigated if a skin problem is present because they are so prevalent for horses. The signs of a reaction to diet can vary greatly. Horses reacting to feed often have a dull coat and frequently experience a lightening or fading of their normal coat color. The acupuncture points corresponding to the immune system and liver are often sensitive to touch. Some horses in strenuous exercise programs, such as event horses, polo horses, and racehorses, don't seem to get as fit and muscled as they could be.

If you suspect a dietary imbalance or allergy is influencing the health of your horse's skin, start with a review of his entire diet. Consult your vet to find a laboratory that can run a complete nutritional test on all feed that is given to your horse. If the grain is a mixture of grains, test each individual type of grain in the mix. As discussed in Chapter Five corn (maize in the UK) is often a problem for horses due to rancidity, mycotoxins, and loss of nutrients. Don't forget to test the hay. Remember, many hay fields are fertilized and this may influence the level of the nutrients in the hay. You may be surprised at what you find.

Some horses are fed a vitamin and mineral supplement to make sure they are receiving all the nutrients they need in their diet. It's best to know the feed value of your horse's diet before adding supplements so you don't feed too much or too little of the nutrients your horse needs. Many horse's diets are deficient in calcium, particularly across the southern areas of the US where less alfalfa hay is fed. (The importance of maintaining the correct balance of calcium in the ration is discussed in detail in Chapter Five.) The level of calcium in the horse's system can influence the body's ability to use minerals such as magnesium, iron, and zinc, all of which are important to the health of the skin.

Individual horses may have sensitivities to very specific ingredients, such as molasses or an iron supplement. Once the problem substances are identified, remove these ingredients from your horse's diet and replace them with other feeds or supplements that your horse does not react to. If you are not sure about how to balance the diet properly, consult an expert such as an equine nutritionist. Many large feed companies provide this consultation service.

Specific supplements are available on the market to improve the coat. They usually contain the three essential fatty acids necessary to maintain coat condition. These products are a better choice than feeding vegetable oils such as corn (maize), canola, or olive. Individual vegetable oils do not contain a balance of all the essential fatty acids but are usually highest in one or another. Therefore, your horse is not receiv-

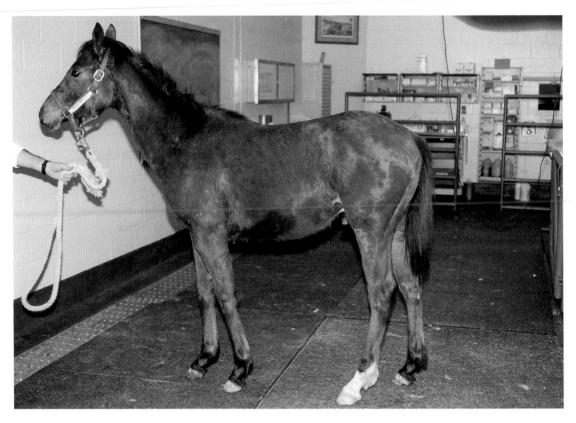

III–33 *An unthrifty looking young horse with lice.*

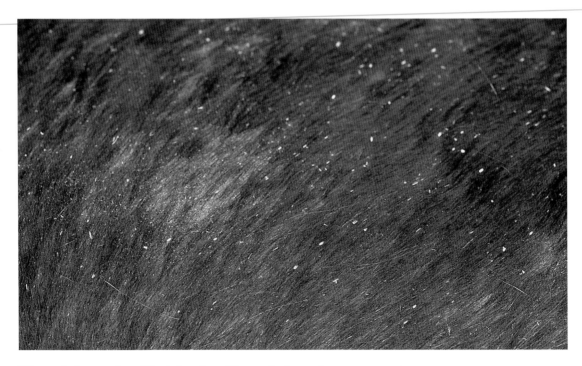

III–34 *A close-up shot of the infestation of lice on the horse above.*

ing the benefit of all the fatty acids that could help his coat. In addition, vegetable oils can be detrimental to health because of the chemicals used in processing them and because they can become rancid very quickly.

RECOMMENDATIONS

Supplement Use an oil with a balanced mix of essential fatty acids. One suggestion is DAC oil (see *Product Suppliers, Appendix VI*).

Reactions to Insect Bites

For immediate treatment see *Insect Bites* on p. 194. Longer-term reactions to insect bites form a raised bump and then gradually become hardened. Unfortunately, these bumps seem to occur most in places where they interfere with the saddle or girth. Some of the hardened areas can progress to calcification and may cause irritation in addition to appearing unsightly. Many treatments exist for insect bites but few are very successful. The most common conventional treatment is a mixture of DMSO and a steroid to paint over the affected area, but in many cases it is not very effective and the steroid can have negative side effects on other body systems. Also, if you show your horse, the steroid may show up in a drug test.

SYMPTOMS

- A raised bump that becomes hardened; may progress to calcification and cause irritation.

RECOMMENDATIONS

Topical

- The best treatment I've found for insect bites is to put cider vinegar on the bitten areas daily.
- If the cider vinegar is not effective, make a homemade mixture recommended by Juliette de Bairacli Levy in the book *Herbal Handbook for Farm and Stable*:

> *1 cup (225ml) castor oil*
> *1/2 cup (110ml) vinegar*
> *1 teaspoon (5ml) spirits of camphor*

Apply this mixture hot, morning and evening. Massage deeply into the bitten areas. ***Caution:*** *Sometimes castor oil can cause swelling so do not use this mixture on a horse you know has sensitive skin.*

- Witch hazel, available in pharmacies or from an herbalist, is effective in some cases when applied daily on the area.

Acupuncture Around the enlarged area followed by indirect moxibustion often decreases the size and softens the affected skin.

Aromatherapy

- Eucalyptus. Use *undiluted* essential oil directly on the bite to help ease irritation.
- Lavender. Promotes healing.
- Ylang Ylang. Soothes irritated skin around the bite.

Scratches (Mud Fever)

Referred to as *scratches* in the US, and *mud fever* in the UK, this is an infection of the skin at the back of the heel and pastern area (see fig. III–35, p. 278). It is also known as "grease heel", and "cracked heels." It is associated with horses who stand in wet or muddy conditions. Scratches, or breaks in the skin, become infected by bacteria or a fungus, and the legs become itchy, warm, and painful to your touch. If left untreated, the legs can swell up, the skin cracks and becomes ulcerated.

SYMPTOMS

- Skin around the heel, pastern, and occasionally extending up the leg and on the abdomen, can be itchy, warm, sensitive, swollen, and possibly covered in sores.
- Lameness is often present on the affected leg.

RECOMMENDATIONS

Stable Area Put your horse in a dry stable during the healing process.

Clean

- Clip the hair of the affected area.
- Gently clean the area using an antibacterial

cleanser. Remove any loose, dead skin, and scabs, and pat the area dry with a soft cloth or towel.

Aromatherapy

- Tea tree oil, diluted half-in-half with rubbing oil, can be applied topically. (See *Aromatherapy Appendix II* for instructions p. 301).
- Lavender and thyme used as an inhalant every 2 days will stimulate the immune system.

Herbs Use to stimulate the immune system, promote circulation, and increase lymphatic drainage. Refer to the list of herbs under the recommendations for Allergies, on p. 185.

Poultice Herbal poultices can be used. Comfrey, clivers, slippery elm, marshmallow, chamomile, and calendula are all helpful for this condition. Select 2 or 3 of these herbs and make the poultice according to instructions on pp. 157 and 160. Leave in place for 12 hours, then remove and dry the leg(s) thoroughly. If there is some decrease in the swelling, reapply and repeat process for 3 days or longer until inflammation is reduced. If there is no improvement after first application, try a different combination.

Acupuncture Consider using to stimulate the immune system if other treatments are ineffective.

Homeopathy Use to support the direct treatment, particularly if the case is severe or responding slowly. Choose one of the following, or consult your vet:

- Arsenicum album 6C or 12C, two times a day. Use when the itching is associated with dry, swollen areas, or there are open sores on the skin.
- Sulfur 6C, two times a day. Use when there is heat and itching. This remedy should be selected if the condition reoccurs seasonally.

Sunburn

Burns from the sun can be caused by direct sun exposure or reflected off the snow in winter. Horses with white skin—muzzle, around the eyes, and udder—are most commonly affected (see figs. III–36 and 37, p. 279). If your adult horse has not suffered from sunburn before and suddenly develops a symptom of sunburn, be aware that it may be from a condition called photosensitization which occurs when a horse eats a certain plant, St. John's Wort, for instance, which causes the horse's skin to absorb UV rays. A horse can also develop photosensitization from plant-induced or metabolic liver disease. In either case you should call your vet.

SYMPTOMS

- Light areas of skin become red, and in more advanced cases of sunburn, may peel, weep serum, and crack.

RECOMMENDATIONS

Protection

- If the eye area is affected use a fly mask to cover for shade and give some protection from the sun.
- Apply sun block to light areas of skin on sunny days. Do not use sun block on a mare's udder when she is nursing as it may be unsafe for the foal.

Vet In chronic, severe cases of sunburn around the eyes, check with your vet on a procedure where the areas around the eyes are tattooed to prevent recurrence.

Homeopathy Eyebright. Use twice a day to treat conjunctivitis that may accompany sunburn.

Herbs

- Aloe vera. Use the fresh juice, gel, or cream to soothe and promote healing. This can be used on a mare's udder when she is nursing.
- Calendula. Use the cream to soothe an affected area. Also safe to use on the udder.
- Poultices or compresses can be made from calendula, clivers, or marshmallow root, and may be used alone or altogether. Eyebright may be used around the eye.

Sweet Itch

Sweet itch is caused by an allergic reaction to the bite of the fly family, *Culicoides,* known as a midge. This condition often reoccurs each year to a sensitive horse and becomes progressively worse with each occurrence. It affects the horse in the mane and/or tail area and the itching can become so severe that complete loss of mane and tail hair may result (see fig. III–38, p. 282). Standard treatment for this condition—medicinal shampoos and lotions, fly control, and treatment with corticosteroid creams or oral medication—are frequently ineffective. A series of injections to desensitize the horse may be helpful initially, but usually do not provide a lasting cure. Alternative medicine combined with proper management can often control the allergic reaction and the best time to start treatment is just prior to the time of year the midges arrive and before the horse starts to show signs of the allergy. However, it is never too late to start the alternative treatments I've outlined below since improvement will be seen. Plan to start the treatments earlier the following year.

The allergic reaction to midges is also influenced by other factors including pasture, grain, hay, and minerals. Each horse must be treated individually to sort out which of these things might be involved, and how to control or change them. Keep a record of all treatments as well as the horse's diet and supplements.

SYMPTOMS

- Rubbing the mane and tail area, resulting in hair loss. Severe cases may progress to scabby, inflamed skin and open lesions.

RECOMMENDATIONS

Protection Control the flies. Use fly repellent (non-toxic varieties are available commercially), and fly sheets. Screened doors and windows can help to some degree.

Review Keep a record of when the allergic reaction begins and what the horse's diet consists of, and which supplements he is being fed.

NAET Treatment for allergies. Test for pasture grass, dirt, and other plants, feed, and supplements.

Diet

- Remove horse from pasture and confine him to a dry or non-grass paddock.
- Do not feed corn (maize) since toxins in corn can influence the immune system. Do not feed clover or alfalfa hay. Feed whole, crimped, or rolled grains, and not grain mixed with molasses or sweeteners.
- Add cider vinegar to feed. Give 2 tbsp (25ml) to a small horse, 3 tbsp (35ml) to a large horse daily. Start in the winter months at least 4 months before the start of the fly season. Vinegar helps to repel flies.

Supplements

- Give free choice minerals.
- Add sulfur to the diet. The most common source is MSM (available in most feed stores, or from mail order suppliers, see Appendix VI).
- Add a digestive enzyme like protease to the diet.

Acupuncture To "balance" the body, and help decrease the skin reaction.

NOTE: For more information and recommendations of herbs, aromatherapy, acupressure, and homeopathy, refer to the section on *Allergies* on p. 182.

Warts

Warts are commonly seen on young horses, foals to three-year-olds (see fig. III–39, p. 283). They are caused by a virus, *equine cutaneous papillomatosis,* which is not contagious to humans or other species. This virus, however, is very contagious to other young horses. Even though contagion has probably already occurred when you first see the warts, it is advisable to isolate a horse, and take care to isolate his grooming equipment and tack too. It is thought that once a horse is exposed and catches this virus, he will be immune in the future.

The warts develop on the muzzle, lips, and face, and occasionally occur inside the mouth and on the front legs. Although they are unsightly, it is best to leave them alone unless they interfere with eating and just wait for the virus to run its course (about eight weeks) since removing the warts may cause scars and even stimulate the area so more warts appear.

If the warts have not gone away after eight weeks, you need to stimulate the horse's immune system with acupuncture or administer a vaccine that is made of material from the horse's warts.

SYMPTOMS

- Cauliflower-like growths on the horse's muzzle, lips, or face. Seen occasionally in the mouth, and on the front legs.

RECOMMENDATIONS

Protection Isolate the affected horse to prevent the virus spreading.

Acupuncture Stimulates the immune system.

Homeopathy

NOTE: It takes a strong remedy to affect a wart virus so 200C potencies work best (available from vet).

- Thuja occidentalis 200C once a day for 2 weeks. This is the main remedy for warts, and in particular, for warts that bleed.
- Calcarea carbonica 200C once a day for 7 days. For small, firm warts that do not bleed.

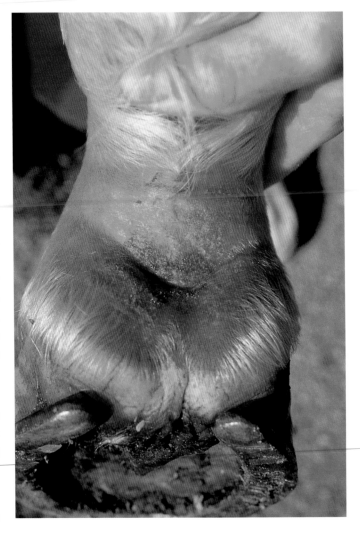

III–35 *Scratches, also known as mud fever or grease heel.*

Aromatherapy Refer to the lemon treatments detailed in the *Aromatherapy Appendix*, p. 305.

SORE BACK

A sore back is one of the most common problems that a horse experiences. It can indicate simple muscle soreness or a problem of a more complex nature. Back soreness is often first no-

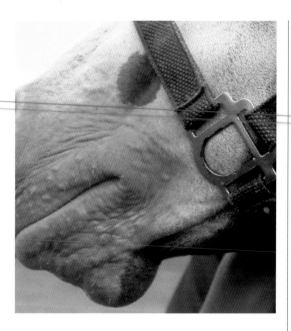

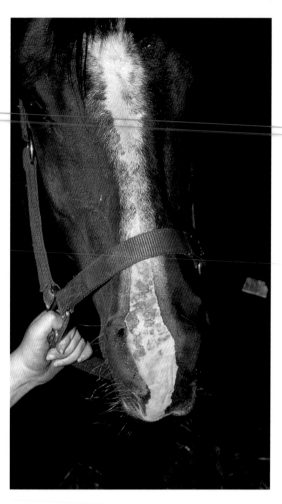

III–36–37 Two cases of sunburn. The first, immediately after occurrence, the second, a short time after exposure to the sun.

ticed during grooming when a horse flinches away from being brushed, or after exercise when a horse shows sensitivity to touch. He may also be lame or stiff in his movement. Sometimes a small area is involved; other times the entire back is sore. In most cases, it is necessary to have your vet treat this problem. The first step to take with a sore back is to evaluate the possible causes, which include, but are not limited to:

- Incorrect fitting tack
- Overwork during exercise
- New exercises
- Injury to the back
- Injury to a leg
- Misalignment of vertebrae in the spine
- Change in shoeing
- Illness

In this section, I will explain how each of these factors can cause a sore back and suggest ways that you can correct the problem.

Incorrect Fitting Tack

Whenever back soreness is noticed, be sure to evaluate your saddle and pad. Back soreness can develop due to a saddle that is incorrectly fitted. The area most often affected by incorrect saddle fit is on either side of the withers just behind the shoulder blade. Muscle spasms are frequently noticed there when the saddle's tree fits incorrectly or if there is a problem with the stuffing in the panels. (Also check your girth for proper fit and look at any areas that might rub.) Then check the saddle pad for any uneven or worn areas to make sure it fits properly under the saddle being used.

Look at any other pieces of tack such as a breast collar or crupper strap and make sure the fit is not too tight.

Problems with the saddle, pad, and other tack can sometimes be difficult to spot. I remember a gelding I was called to check for a possible sore back. When I was unable to find any other cause, I suggested checking the saddle, which had been used for a number of years. The owner didn't think the saddle was responsible because it was guaranteed not to cause back problems. The fit seemed to be okay, and, despite its age, the padding wasn't in bad shape. However, when I put the saddle on the ground for a closer look, I noticed a slight movement as I pushed on the front and back of the saddle. Further investigation revealed a broken tree. This seems like an obvious problem but it was not immediately noticeable because of the type of saddle and the particular way in which the tree was broken. Crooked or warped trees are more common than broken ones, so always check the saddle thoroughly or have an expert check it for you.

(*Also see *Proper Fitting Tack,* Chapter Eight.)

RECOMMENDATIONS

Review Replace saddle, pad, or other tack that doesn't fit properly.

Overwork During Exercise

The most common cause of a sore back is muscle soreness. If the problem is limited to muscles that have been overworked, a sore back is usually not difficult to treat. It can generally be cleared up by a few days of reduced exercise, along with some massage therapy and a homeopathic remedy to reduce the inflammation. For more, see Muscle Soreness on p. 256.

RECOMMENDATIONS

Exercise When a horse is excessively exercised and a sore back results, it's best to treat the condition as soon as possible. However, do not rest the horse completely since even sore muscles must be stretched. Also, a slight increase in circulation from walking or jogging helps to move out any leftover lactic acid or other by-products produced by the muscles during exertion. Immediately following a long or demanding period of exercise, cool the horse out slowly, protecting the back from cold with a cooler or blanket if necessary. A short walk or trail ride for 10 to 20 minutes works best to gradually cool out the horse and is sufficient to increase the circulation and stretch the muscles.

Topical/Massage
- Work directly with the muscles. Apply a liniment to the back muscles and massage it in. I prefer to use arnica lotion as a liniment since it serves as an excellent topical anti-inflammatory and it doesn't irritate the skin. If you use another type of liniment that acts as a counter-irritant, or that causes heat to occur, do not use more than twice since you can make the horse's skin sensitive or sore.
- If the weather is cold, cover the horse with a blanket after massaging.

Homeopathy Give homeopathic arnica 12C or 30C and magnesia phosphorica 6C together in oral form to further treat inflammation and help reduce muscle spasms.

Magnetic Therapy Use a magnetic blanket to keep the circulation going and continue the removal of lactic acid and other by-products.

Vet If the muscle soreness is severe, call your vet. He may decide to administer fluids to help rehydrate the horse and flush out any undesirable by-products left in the muscles.

New Exercises

The addition of a new form of exercise to the regimen often results in sore muscles, particularly those of the back. Think of how you react when asked to perform an exercise that you have never done before. Afterwards, you often hurt. It may not seem like you are asking much of your horse at the time, particularly if your horse responds enthusiastically and enjoys the exercise, but he may be using muscles that are not properly strengthened and doing so could result in a sore back. So whenever you add something new to your exercise program, do so gradually to avoid a sore back and check your horse's back the next day.

Examples of dressage exercises that can result in a sore back are pirouettes at the canter, flying changes, and lateral work. For a pleasure horse, riding over a different type of terrain, such as steep hills, can result in a sore back, particularly if the horse is used to riding on level ground. Examples of Western riding disciplines that can cause soreness are barrel racing, cutting, roping, and reining. This can happen even if your horse is very fit and ridden daily. Most often it is an excessive amount of a new type of work that causes back problems.

Moderation is the best guide to use when adding new exercises to your horse's program. As you gradually add new exercises, avoid the potential for back soreness by including preventive measures such as massage and anti-inflammatories such as arnica lotion (as a liniment) and homeopathic arnica given orally.

RECOMMENDATIONS

NOTE: Treatment of back soreness due to new exercises is the same as for *Overwork During Exercise* above.

Injury to the Back

When an injury occurs to the back it may first appear like a sore muscle or group of muscles, but it does not improve with basic treatment and rest. The most common injuries to the back are pulled or torn muscles, inflamed spinal discs, fractured vertebral spinous processes, and fractured vertebrae. One of the most under-estimat-ed injuries following a fall occurs to the tops of the vertebral spinous processes, most commonly over the withers. In the most severe form, the top of the vertebral spinous process can be crushed, although this injury may not be diagnosed until later when arthritis develops in the area. When any of these injuries occur, the horse usually gets up and seems a little sore but may not show any other major symptoms or problems with the back.

A serious injury to the back might be difficult to diagnose. Even if inflammation and heat are present in the back, the swelling which usually accompanies a serious injury may not be seen due to the effects of gravity pulling the fluid down into the back. Injury to the vertebral body where the spinal cord is located is difficult to diagnose because of the deep location of the vertebrae. X-rays cannot penetrate to this depth. Often it's impossible to diagnose a vertebral fracture or crack unless there are accompanying neurological signs. Due to an increase in necropsies (evaluations of animal cadavers) in order to study Equine Protozoal Myeloencephalitis (EPM), we now know that horses incur many more spinal injuries than we had been aware of—particularly damage to the vertebral bodies. This evidence indicates that some of the falls and accidents that horses have result in more serious injuries than previously thought.

RECOMMENDATIONS

Vet/Test If you suspect your horse may have a more serious injury than simple muscle soreness in the back, consult your vet. Do not exercise your horse further until a veterinary examination and diagnosis have been done and an exercise program developed. The vet may decide to use ultrasound to help diagnose muscle injuries and to monitor the progress of the healing.

Illness

When all other causes of back soreness have been eliminated, illness must be considered as a possibility. Since back soreness may be the only obvious sign, illnesses causing it often go undiagnosed. Examples of illnesses that can cause back soreness include Equine Protozoal Myeloencephalitis (EPM), liver disease, ovarian problems, gastric ulcers, and viral diseases. It is not possible to list all the diseases that can effect a horse's back. However, once all the other obvious causes of back soreness have been ruled out it is important to look at the possibility that an internal illness is the culprit.

RECOMMENDATIONS

Vet A thorough examination may be necessary so contact your vet for:
- Blood workup to check for liver, bacterial, or viral disease.
- Rectal palpation to check for a problem with the ovaries.
- Endoscopic examination of the stomach for an ulcer evaluation.

Review Compile a history of any "changes" in your horse. These might give your vet clues to help him with a diagnosis. Include any changes in behavior, training, diet and supplements.

STRANGLES

See Chapter Four, p. 70.

SWELLING (SEVERE)

Swelling can occur almost anywhere on the horse's body. It usually develops as part of the body's reaction to inflammation, but swelling can also be caused by a hematoma. Hematomas are formed when a blood vessel breaks internally and the blood forms a clot under the skin causing noticeable swelling. For a more detailed discussion, see *Hematomas* on p. 216. Often swollen areas are hot and painful to the touch. If the swelling is severe or develops suddenly or the horse seems uncomfortable or colicky, be sure to check with your vet since more extensive treatment than that outlined below may be necessary.

RECOMMENDATIONS

Vet If severe, call the vet while checking for signs of shock.

Cold Treatment Pack the area in ice for 10 minutes every 2 hours and/or hose with cold water three times a day for 20 minutes.

Homeopathy Choose one of the following:
- Apis mellifica 30C three times daily. Use when the swelling is due to an insect bite or involves itching.
- Bryonia 6C or 12C three times daily. Use when swelling involves the feet.
- Hypericum 6C three times daily. Use when the swelling involves great pain or bruising is involved.
- Arsenicum album 6C three times daily. Use when the swollen area seems hot and the horse is restless.

Topical Apply arnica lotion or gel over the swollen area, but be sure that you don't get it in any open wounds.

Herbs Make an herbal cold compress. Boil a liter of water and add a handful of either fresh comfrey leaves that have been slightly crushed, or dry chamomile. Allow to steep for at least 10 minutes. After the herbal tea has cooled, soak a towel in it and then place the towel on the swelling. As an alternative, remove the cooled herbs from the tea and wrap them in cheesecloth and apply to the affected area.

Aromatherapy Geranium. Improves circulation.

T

TEETH AND GUM PROBLEMS

Tooth problems are often overlooked until they are severe and have caused other difficulties. Regular dental checkups should be done every six months as a part of your horse's health care. See discussion on *Teeth* in Chapter Five, p. 93.

SYMPTOMS
- Uncomfortable with a bit in the mouth.
- Dropping grain out of the mouth when eating.
- Weight loss.
- Grinding teeth.

RECOMMENDATIONS

For infected teeth:

Clean Use a syringe to rinse the horse's mouth with a small amount of a mixture of one-part salt and three-parts water.

Supplement Increase vitamin C in the diet. Give 5 grams daily for small horses and 8 grams daily for large horses.

Surgery Have the tooth removed.

Antibiotics If tooth is abscessed, discuss using antibiotics with your vet.

For tooth removal:

Homeopathy Give homeopathic arnica montana 30c three times a day to relieve inflammation.

For irritated gums:

Topical Rub homeopathic psorium tincture over affected area of the gum.

Supplement Give additional vitamin C.

TETANUS

See Chapter Four, p. 68.

TUMORS

See *Cancer*, p. 196.

"TYING-UP" SYNDROME

There are two conditions referred to as "tying-up." One type is also known as azoturia or "Monday morning sickness," a condition caused by feeding grain, not exercising the horse for a day or two, then suddenly working the horse. It was commonly seen in workhorses years ago when they were given Sunday off with full feed, stood all day tied in a stall, then were returned to work on Monday morning.

I will focus on the other type of tying-up, referred to as myositis, which is associated with over exercise or a metabolic imbalance. Tying-up occurs when the horse is unable to move because the muscles stay contracted and will not relax. The most frequent cause of tying-up is loss of electrolytes from exercise and the resulting imbalance, but it may also be genetic. Recent research also suggests a vitamin or mineral deficiency may be responsible. Affected horses may have a need for a nutrient that is missing from their diet or the nutrient may be in their diet but the body is unable to assimilate it.

If your horse stops and is unable to move, do not try to persuade him, but call the vet immediately. If your horse ties up and is unable to move and you are unable to get immediate help, do not force the horse to move even if you are a long way from home, but seek help if possible. You will need to wait until the horse's muscles relax to attempt movement. This can take up to several hours.

SYMPTOMS
- Horse stops and is unable to move; may be in pain.
- Muscles may be hard or rigid.

RECOMMENDATIONS

First Aid Do not attempt to move horse.

Vet Call immediately.

Homeopathy   Give Magnesium phosphate 6C, 12C, or 30C every 15 minutes until the horse is able to move.

Supplements

- Discuss the feeding of vitamin E and selenium with your vet.
- Baking soda is a remedy often used on racehorses. Feed one teaspoon a day. While its effectiveness is questionable, it doesn't seem to cause any harm.
- Include an electrolyte supplement in your horse's diet.
- Offer a free-choice mineral system to the horse.

U

ULCERS (GASTRIC)

Veterinarians are increasingly recognizing the presence of ulcers in the stomach. Once thought of as occurring mainly in foals, it is now known that gastric ulcers are present in 60 percent or more of horses. The symptoms of gastric ulcers can be vague and many horses do not show any signs of illness or discomfort so the condition usually goes untreated.

Ginger was a mare I was called to examine because she had a recurring stiff neck and back. During the exam, the owner told me Ginger was experiencing bouts of colic following both horse shows and their one riding lesson a week. This case presented quite a challenge since she did not colic when ridden at home, seemed to be performing well, and had a good appetite. She had had colic surgery one year before, with no further colic problems until this time. The exam revealed incredibly tight neck muscles and several cervical (neck) and thoracic (attached to the ribs) vertebral misalignments. In addition, the acupuncture points along her back associated with the stomach and small intestine were also sore. I felt Ginger was suffering from either irri-

tation of the stomach lining or stomach ulcers, which probably involved the first part of the small intestine. The discomfort associated with the extra exercise and stress at a horse show or a riding lesson was enough to cause her to colic. Following treatment for stomach ulcers, the back and neck soreness disappeared, and a follow-up exam revealed that the vertebrae had gone back into place once she stopped trying to protect her stomach from painful movement.

Signs to look for are poor performance, colic, poor appetite, poor hair coat, and a bad attitude. Another clue is the recurrence of a lameness that you thought had been treated successfully—it may have been due to gastric ulcers. Some horses may try to avoid movements that cause them stomach discomfort, specifically changing their canter leads. You may notice a conformational change that occurs gradually whereby the muscles along the horse's backbone lose strength. Consequently horses who are required to elevate their backs during work, such as dressage horses, exhibit a decreased ability to do so. Because the affected horse may alter his gait to decrease discomfort, lameness can occur. Also you may see the back area just behind the withers become lower, or slightly swayed, with the abdomen also appearing lower down and lacking muscle tone. Foals affected with gastric ulcers may also grind their teeth, salivate, and lie on their backs with their legs in the air trying to relieve their discomfort.

The exact cause of gastric ulcers in horses is not known. Bacteria, as yet, have not been implicated as a factor, as they have in humans. No single cause has been identified, although feeding programs, stress, medications, and illness have all been associated with the formation of equine gastric ulcers. Therefore, when considering treatment and management of a horse with gastric ulcers, there are a number of considerations for long-term control of the problem.

The vet has several ways to diagnose gastric ulcers. An instrument called an endoscope can be used to see the interior of the stomach and examine it for ulcers; however, this requires an endoscope that is at least three meters long and few equine veterinary practices have these instruments. So, in many cases the vet will make the diagnosis and determine a treatment regimen based on the physical signs and symptoms, combined with a thorough examination and history.

A veterinary acupuncturist has another diagnostic tool because he can check the acupuncture points associated with the stomach. If gastric ulcers or a stomach problem in general is present these points will be very sore when touched. Two of the acupuncture points to check are located on either side of the back on the bladder meridian at BL_{21}, which is just behind the last rib. This point correlates to the area where the rear of the saddle rests, along with a great deal of the rider's weight. CV_{12}, another acupuncture point associated with the stomach, is found on the underline of the abdomen half way between the end of the sternum and the umbilicus (belly button). If you decide to check these points yourself, take great care. They can be extremely sore and the horse may react violently if they are pushed too hard.

In order to effectively deal with gastric ulcers you must not only treat them but also prevent recurrence. As of this writing there is a great deal of research being done on the cause and treatment of ulcers but only one medication is marketed as an equine gastric ulcer treatment. It contains the medication omeprazole and it comes in the form of a paste. Other less expensive treatment options can be very effective when they are combined with proper management (see Recommendations below.) It is important to work with your vet when treating gastric ulcers so you can benefit from the latest information available on the subject.

SYMPTOMS
- Poor appetite.
- Colic.
- Poor performance.
- Hair coat may become dull, rough, or change color.
- Muscle tone decreases despite exercise.

Symptoms most associated with a foal:
- Teeth grinding
- Lying on his back
- Inconsistent nursing
- Reoccurring colic
- Diarrhea
- Drooling saliva

RECOMMENDATIONS

Vet Consult your vet to confirm the diagnosis and develop a treatment plan.

Medications
- Coat the horse's stomach lining with 4 teaspoons (20ml) milk of magnesia, sucralfate (Carafate), or try other stomach coating products available, twice a day to diminish the discomfort. Best results are achieved when the stomach coater is given at least 5 minutes before a feeding and this schedule is continued for at least 30 days.
- Administer a stomach acid blocker such as cimetidine (Tagamet) or ranitidine hydrochloride (Zantac). Consult your vet for correct dosage.

Diet Make the following dietary changes:
- Soak hay with water to soften it before feeding.
- Discontinue feeding pellets which can irritate the stomach lining. If unable to discontinue pellets, soak them before feeding.
- Feed at exactly the same time every day.

Acupuncture

Homeopathy Choose *one* of the following:
- Nux vomica 6C, 12C or 30C. Give three times a day for 2 weeks. Use when the horse's appetite is decreased, his attitude is poor, and his

back is sore due to the ulcers.

- Phosphorus 12C or 30C. Give twice a day for 2 weeks. Use when the horse is the nervous type or a constant worrier. Very effective with Thoroughbreds.
- Kali Bichromicum 30C. Give three times a day for 2 weeks. Use when gastric ulcers are associated with a decrease in appetite or diarrhea. Particularly effective with foals.

Herbs

- Comfrey leaf. This herb has a high mucilaginous content that soothes the stomach lining and helps it to heal. It can be fed in the dried herb form 1/2 oz (15 grams) twice a day in the horse's food, or you can give a large handful of the crushed fresh comfrey leaves. For horses with severe pain from ulcers, make a comfrey leaf tea and administer it with a dose syringe to sooth the stomach. Make it by pouring 2 pints (1 liter) of boiling water over a handful of the fresh herb or 1/2 oz (15 grams) of the dried herb. Allow to steep for 20 minutes. Then strain and allow the liquid to cool.
- Licorice. When ingested, licorice produces mucus that helps reduce stomach acid and also acts as an anti-inflammatory agent to help heal the stomach lining. Give 1/2 oz (15 grams) per feeding.
- Marshmallow root. This herb is effective throughout the entire digestive tract, soothing the stomach, small and large intestines and the colon. Mix 1/2 oz (15 grams) of a powdered form of this herb with water, and dose syringe it to help relieve mild colic due to ulcerations of the digestive tract. Give twice a day. An alternative is to add 1/2 oz (15 grams) of the fresh cut root to your horse's feed twice a day.
- Meadowsweet. This herb helps to reduce inflammation in the entire digestive tract as well as decrease the stomach's acidity. It is particularly effective when treating ulcers that have been caused by overusing pharmaceutical drugs. NOTE: Do not use the tincture—liquid form—of this herb when treating stomach ulcers. Mix one handful of the cut fresh herb, or 1/2 oz (15 grams) of the dried herb, into the feed twice a day. Meadowsweet tea is also very soothing. Make it by pouring 2 pints (1 liter) of boiling water over a handful of the fresh herb. Allow to steep for 20 minutes, then strain and allow the liquid to cool before administering with a syringe.

- Commercial herbal mixtures, such as Hilton Herbs Phytotherapy Mix 2, are also specifically made for gastric ulcer management.

Aromatherapy Use as an inhalant once a day. The melissa and sandalwood work well between meals. During a meal it will help your horse if you get him to inhale a tiny amount of lavender oil. Apply a little oil to the horse's halter while he eats, then remove the halter when he finishes. Choose from:

- Lavender to relieve stomach discomfort.
- Melissa to decrease excess neural stimulation that can contribute to stomach ulcers.
- Sandalwood to relax the horse and decrease stress.

Bach Flowers Review the section on Bach Flower remedies on p. 34 and in the *Bach Flower Appendix III*. Choose from: Impatiens, mimulus, walnut, or one or more Bach Flower remedies that fit your horse's profile.

WEIGHT PROBLEMS

A horse that is overweight could be suffering from a metabolic disorder—or he might just be eating too much food and getting too little exercise. On the other hand, an underweight horse is not desirable either. If your horse begins to lose weight suddenly, a consultation with your vet is advisable since any number of health problems could be causing rapid weight loss.

If your horse is overweight, you should carefully consider the ramifications of this extra weight. Excessive weight places a burden on the body; it makes the heart work harder, puts additional stress on the muscles, and makes the liver and kidneys work harder when they detoxify the blood. What can you do if your horse is overweight? Many horses are overweight because of an imbalance of feed versus exercise. The following issues should be evaluated when weight gain occurs: What does the diet consist of? How much exercise is the horse getting? Is he turned out daily on good pasture?

Sometimes a weight gain is due to an imbalance that is influencing the horse's metabolism. If your horse has gradually picked up a few pounds and he has consistently had the same amount of exercise, ask your vet to do a blood test to make sure every function is normal. The thyroid should also be checked. This type of workup should also be done for a horse that is very obese. Also do a complete review of his diet and exercise program. (Review the section in Chapter Five on older horses since many of the same recommendations may help an obese horse.)

A horse that just eats too much or is an "easy keeper" that is fed very little and still gains weight is one whose weight needs to be carefully managed. If you have any questions concerning alternative choices in your horse's diet, review Chapter Five.

When starting a weight reduction program, weigh your horse so you can keep track of his progress. You can purchase a weight tape from many feed stores, but they are not very accurate. Some veterinary clinics have scales and occasionally you can find them at large Thoroughbred training facilities. Weigh him about once a month if possible. Begin the weight reduction program by decreasing the amount of grain you feed by one-quarter. Then gradually reduce the grain to one-half of the normal ration. If the horse doesn't lose weight on this regimen, you may have to reduce the hay and time out on pasture as well.

If you put your horse on a diet and find that the weight is coming off too quickly, increase his hay first to slow the process down. If he continues to lose weight too fast, increase the grain as well. I do not recommend a hay diet alone unless absolutely necessary since hay is not usually a balanced ration, but if he is reduced only to hay, be sure to add a vitamin and mineral supplement to prevent dietary deficiencies.

Exercise is an important factor in weight loss and regular exercise will help facilitate it. Pasture turnout is not a substitute for exercise. Try to exercise your horse at least every other day. Exercise can be in the form of longeing or riding, or even including your horse in your own exercise program. It amazes me that horses seem to enjoy walking or jogging alongside their owners for miles. One of my friends used to send her horse jogging with her husband to help the horse stay fit for eventing. Even when increases in distance and speed were made gradually, the horse could not out-jog the man. The horse tired first and required rest periods. However, if your horse is out of shape, be sure to start any exercise program slowly. Do not overdo it; horses can get sore muscles and suffer from exhaustion just like humans.

If your horse is underweight, start by reviewing the horse's medical condition. Many internal problems can affect the horse's weight. The worming history should also be reviewed to determine if parasites might be contributing to weight loss. (See Worms and Worming in Chapter Six, p. 101) It is possible that the horse is in good health but simply requires more food than others to maintain his weight. This is often the case with Thoroughbreds. Review both the amount of food you are feeding and the type. Since some horses just don't like all types of feed, it may take some trial and error to find the type of food that works best for your horse. Feeds that are extruded and are high in fat are often used to assist in weight gain. If a change of diet and regular worming have not improved your horse's weight, it's time to investigate further. Start by consulting your vet and having a thorough checkup. The checkup may reveal a problem or blood tests may be required for further diagnosis.

With most underweight horses I recommend adding acidophilus and lactobacillus to aid digestion. There are many products on the market that work well. Digestive enzymes can also be added to the diet to assist with the proper digestion of nutrients.

If your horse has a medical condition such as hypothyroidism that has lead to a weight problem, it's best to consider all the options for treatment. Medication for hypothyroidism works well. However, if the condition is not advanced, acupuncture, homeopathics, and nutritional supplements can be used to treat the problem. The levels of thyroid in the system, the exercise regimen, and the current medical condition must be evaluated before deciding whether it's better to use thyroid medications or holistic treatments.

RECOMMENDATIONS

Overweight:

Diet Decrease grain by one-quarter of normal ration at first and then by one-half until weight loss is achieved. Review diet chapter (see Chapter Five). Also decrease hay if necessary. If your horse is on pasture, time in the pasture may have to be limited.

Exercise Review exercise regimen (see Chapter Nine).

Tests

- Talk to vet about the possibility of metabolic problems and whether blood chemistry workup is advisable.
- Weigh the horse at least once a month so you can keep track of weight loss (or additional weight gain).

Medication If hypothyroidism is diagnosed, discuss thyroid medication with your vet. Not medicating a low-thyroid condition can result in heart problems, and occasionally, founder. If your horse must be maintained on thyroid medication, have the thyroid level rechecked after the first 30 days, then every 4 months for the first year to be sure the amount of medication is correct. The amount needed may differ from winter to summer.

Acupuncture

Supplements Check with your vet about nutritional supplements for a thyroid condition.

Homeopathy

- Thyroid 4C or 6C given twice a day. Use when thyroid levels are low or horse does not respond to thyroid medication.
- Adrenal 6C given twice a day. Use in conjunction with thyroid and pituitary homeopathics to stimulate this part of the endocrine system.
- Pituitary 6C given twice a day. Use with adrenal and thyroid homeopathics to stimulate endocrine system.

Underweight:

Tests

- Consult with vet to determine if a health problem is causing weight loss.
- Check the horse's teeth

Diet Consider a more digestible feed ration:

- Extruded feeds are easily digested by most horses. NOTE: These feeds usually contain sugar or molasses which some horses do not tolerate.
- Rolled barley in the feed helps horses to gain weight without becoming overly "hot." Barley is high in phosphorus, so if fed as the only grain, a source of calcium, such as alfalfa hay, will need to be added to the diet.

Supplements

- Give a product containing acidophilus and lactobacillus according to label directions.
- Give digestive enzymes according to label directions.

I Acupuncture and Acupressure

Acupuncture treatment should be performed by a qualified veterinary acupuncturist only. Acupressure, however, can be administered by the horse owner. Please review the general discussion on acupuncture and acupressure in Chapter Three, p. 21 before starting any acupressure treatments.

Information on which acupuncture and acupressure treatments should be used for specific health ailments can be found under the alphabetical listings of health ailments in Part Three, and/or in the indexed listing of the ailment.

Acupressure is not an alternative to proper medical care. If your horse is suffering from an illness or injury, obtain veterinary care as soon as possible. As I have already said, acupressure can be very helpful as an adjunct to a healing program, but if your horse is ill, do not depend on it for a cure. If a vet is treating your horse with a daily medication for a medical problem, check with the vet before starting acupressure treatments. The acupressure can alter the horse's response to the medication, and the dosage may have to be changed.

Acupressure should not be done on an area where the horse exhibits extreme sensitivity. If you inadvertently touch an area that is painful, release the pressure immediately. If your horse shies away from being touched in a certain area, an injury, a localized infection, or a behavioral problem could cause this sensitivity. The sensitive area may relate to a meridian line and sometimes to a specific organ associated with that meridian line. If you are able to pinpoint a specific area that is extremely uncomfortable when touched, consult a veterinary acupuncturist to have it checked.

If your horse refuses to allow touching anywhere on his body, the reason may be health-related. For instance, horses with Equine Protozoal Myeloencephalitis (EPM) can be extremely sensitive to touch. EPM primarily affects the muscles along the back, but some forms of the disease cause sensitivity throughout the entire body. Other horses that are sensitive to touch may not have bonded sufficiently with humans. If your horse is resistant to touching, and you have ruled out any medical reasons for his resistance, try to get him used to it gradually. If that doesn't work, consult a professional horse trainer who is experienced with starting young horses in a gentle manner. Eventually you may be able to progress to acupressure. But don't try to use acupressure on an unwilling patient; the stress of the situation will, in all likelihood, outweigh any potential benefits.

Some health problems can be aggravated by acupressure if you are treating an injured area. Do not apply acupressure directly to wounds, bruises, or cuts because you could damage tissue and increase pain. However, it can be helpful to press points that are near an injury in order to increase circulation in the area. Use only the points that are not painful. If your horse indicates he is in pain when you touch a point, you are too close to the injury.

PREPARATIONS FOR ADMINISTERING ACUPRESSURE

Before starting an acupressure treatment, wash your hands and dry them thoroughly. (If your hands are cold, run them under warm water.) As you are washing your hands, focus your mind on a healing attitude. A calm, reassuring, and positive attitude is important because your patient will sense and "pick up" on your feelings. Choose a time when you are not pressured and can devote yourself to your horse and his needs. Play soothing music to help create a healing environment.

PRESSING THE ACUPRESSURE POINTS

Acupressure is done by exerting pressure with one finger on precise places on the body. Most often, you will use either the middle finger or the thumb. Sometimes, you will find it easier to use one or the other, depending on the exact spot you are treating. To determine the amount of pressure to use, experiment on your own body, pressing your thumb or middle finger against various places on your face, chest, and on your other hand, for 10 to 15 seconds. The pressure should be firm enough so that you experience it as hard and steady, but it should not be painful or damaging to the skin. Bear in mind that you are going to do this to your horse. If your horse is ex-

tremely sensitive, exert less pressure. If he seems unaffected by a lighter touch, use more pressure for the treatment to be effective.

LOCATING THE ACUPRESSURE POINTS

When I teach my clients to do acupressure on their own animals, I give them charts like the ones in this book. They are usually concerned, however, that they will not find the correct points when I'm not around to guide them. I try to reassure them that unlike acupuncture, acupressure doesn't have to be totally "on target" to be effective. If you are near the acupressure point, you will be doing a lot of good whether you've hit the precise point or not. By pressing in the vicinity of the acupressure point, you will be increasing energy flow in the associated meridian line.

List of Acupressure Points

See charts throughout this Appendix.
(**Caution:** *If your mare is pregnant, avoid acupressure points BL_{60} and KI_3. Stimulating these points on a pregnant mare may cause abortion.*)

Bladder Meridian

BL_1: This point is located slightly above the inside corner of the eye. Acupressure on it assists in healing of eye problems. Stimulate this point with the side of your hand or with your fingers. If you use your fingers, do so carefully because a quick movement by the horse could cause you to accidentally stick a finger in his eye. Do not use moxibustion on this point.

BL_2: This point is located just above the eye at the inside point of the eyebrow. Stimulate BL_2 to assist in healing eye problems, head pain, or trauma.

BL_{10}: This point is located about 2 inches (5 cm) from the middle of the mane in a depression just behind the wing of the atlas (the large piece of bone that protrudes from the first cervical vertebrae). Stimulate BL_{10} to help with stiffness in

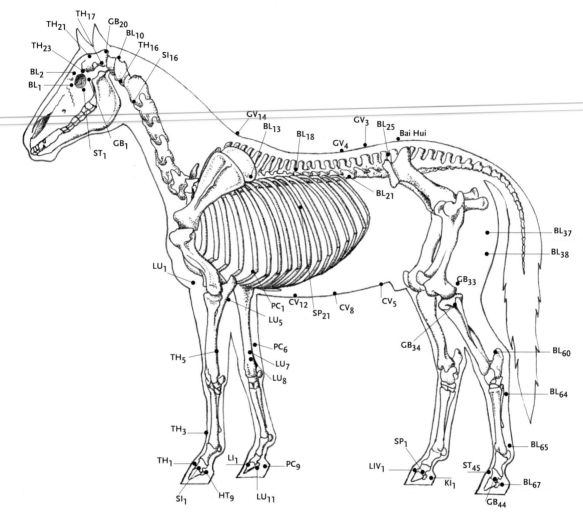

IV–1 *Commonly used acupuncture points on the horse's body.*

the neck, upper respiratory congestion, and problems associated with the head and neck. This can be a very sensitive point, so start by massaging it gently.

BL_{13}: This point is located two to 3 inches (5 to 8 cm) from the midline, just behind the scapula and between ribs eight and nine. Stimulate this point when treating problems associated with the lung, such as respiratory disease. This point also supports the immune system; stimulating it can help when treating cases of anemia.

BL_{18}: This point is located about 3 inches (8 cm) from the midline, in the middle area of the back, in the space between ribs thirteen and fourteen. BL_{18} is associated with the liver and can be used to help treat the liver when blood enzymes associated with the liver are elevated. Stimulation of this point will also help increase appetite in stressed horses.

BL_{21}: Located about 3 inches from the midline, just behind the last rib. BL_{21} is associated with the stomach, so if it is sore, suspect a digestive

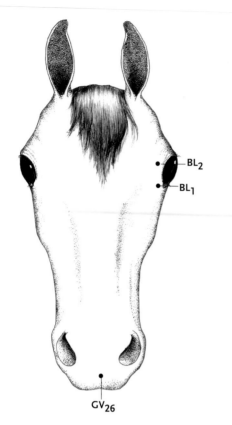

IV–2 Acupuncture points on the head, frontal view.

BL$_{37}$: This point is located about 5 inches (13 cm) below the tuber ischii, or point of the hip, in the crease on the side and toward the tail on the hind leg. Stimulating BL$_{37}$ is helpful when treating stifle and back pain. If this point is sore when touched, stifle problems are indicated.

BL38: This point is located about 3 inches (8 cm) below BL$_{37}$ in the same muscle crease as BL$_{37}$. Stimulating BL$_{38}$ is helpful when treating hock and stifle pain.

BL$_{60}$: This point is located on the outside of the hind leg, in the bottom of the depression near the point of the hock. Acupressure is used on this point to treat hock and back pain. Once a mare is in labor, it may be a useful point to stimulate if she is experiencing difficulty giving birth. Do not stimulate this point if the mare is pregnant; it may cause abortion to occur.

BL$_{64}$: Located just behind and below the head of the outside splint bone (fourth metatarsal bone). Stimulation primarily relieves hock pain, and sometimes helps back pain in the lumbar and sacral area.

BL$_{65}$: Located below the end of the outside splint bone (fourth metatarsal bone) and above the fetlock in the hind leg. This point can be stimulated to treat tendinitis and/or pain in the fetlock area in both hind legs. Also useful for treating any inflammation in the eye area.

BL$_{67}$: Located on the outside of the hind leg, just behind the lateral cartilage (the hard area on the side of the foot), just above the coronary band. Stimulation of this point will help with treatment of laminitis and foot problems. Acupressure on this point may also help a mare having difficulty giving birth.

Triple Heater Meridian

TH$_{I}$: This point is located just above the coronary band on the front leg, slightly to the outside of the midline. Acupressure on TH$_{I}$ is used to

upset or possibly gastric ulcers. Problems in the pancreas may also cause point sensitivity. Do not use moxibustion over this point if stomach ulcers are a possibility. Stimulation of this point calms digestive disorders and is helpful when treating pain related to the stifle.

BL$_{25}$: This point is located about 3 inches (8 cm) from the midline above the flank area and before the hip, in the space between lumbar vertebrae five and six. Acupressure on BL$_{25}$ is used to treat problems associated with the large intestine and can be very helpful when treating colic. It is also helpful to stimulate this point for back and hip pain. Moxibustion can be used over BL$_{25}$ to help relieve pain associated with gas colic. Always consult your vet for colic—do not rely on acupressure as the only treatment.

treat problems involving the hoof. Stimulation on this point is also helpful when treating gas colic, fever, and problems involving the throat.

TH$_3$: This point is located in the middle of the front leg immediately below the bottom of the cannon bone. Stimulate this point to treat laminitis, and fetlock and shoulder pain. Include this point when treating for liver disorders as it helps to stimulate the liver.

TH$_5$: This point is located on the outside of the front leg in the crease that runs down the middle of the leg (between the lateral and common digital extensor tendons), about 3 inches (8 cm) above the knee. Stimulate this point when treating laminitis, or tendinitis, and to stimulate circulation throughout the leg, which helps in treatment of navicular disease or when trying to heal an injury. Acupressure on TH$_5$ may be helpful in relieving neck and shoulder pain and in reducing a fever.

TH$_{17}$: This point is located in the depression about 1/2 inch (1 cm) below the ear. Stimulating TH$_{17}$ is useful when treating all problems affecting the ear.

TH$_{21}$: To locate this point, first find TH$_{17}$, then follow the slight ridge around the bottom of the ear toward the forehead approximately 1 inch (2 1/2 cm). Stimulate this point when treating ear problems.

TH$_{23}$: This point is located about 1/4 inch (1/2 cm) above the outer edge of the eye. Stimulate TH$_{23}$ when treating eye problems. Acupressure on this point may also be useful in relieving tension when a horse is stressed.

Lung Meridian

LU$_1$: This point is located on the front of the chest in a small depression in the pectoral muscle. Stimulate LU$_1$ to aid in the treatment of respiratory viruses, pulmonary emphysema (heaves), and chest and shoulder pain.

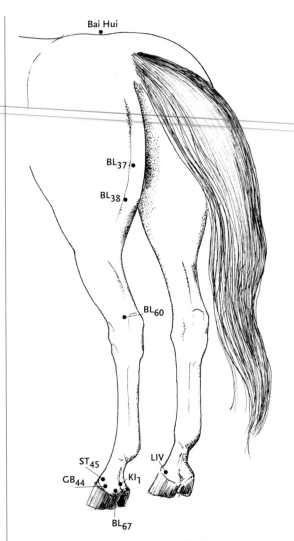

IV–3 *Acupuncture points on the hindquarters.*

LU$_5$: This point is located on the front leg to the inside (medial) of the biceps brachii tendon—the tendon that runs down over the front of the shoulder joint. Acupressure on LU$_5$ helps the treatment of respiratory infections involving coughing, fever, and congestion. This point also helps to regulate fluid retention in the body so use it to treat cases of edema or excessive swelling. It may also relieve some elbow pain.

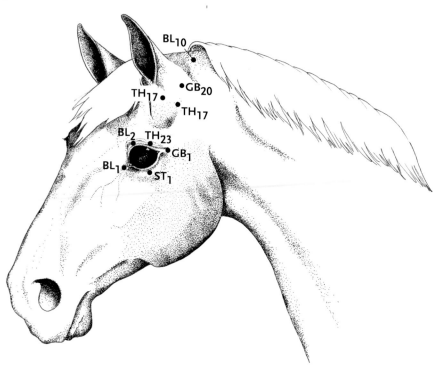

IV–4 *Acupuncture points on the head and neck, lateral view.*

LU$_7$: This point is located on the inside of the front leg just above the area where the radius bone flares outward (area of the radius called the medial styloid process), and just behind the tendon (extensor carpi radialis) that runs down the side of the knee (carpus). This is an important point that has many applications in treatment. Acupressure on this point is used for knee, neck, and tooth pain, or when facial paralysis is present. It is a helpful point to use when treating coughs or pulmonary emphysema. Since LU$_7$ communicates with the large intestine meridian it may also be used to support treatment of large intestine problems, particularly constipation.

LU$_8$: This point is just below LU$_7$ on the inside of the leg on the part of the radius bone that flares outward (medial styloid process) just above the knee. Stimulation of LU$_8$ is helpful for chronic lung problems such as pulmonary emphysema and lingering viruses. It also can be used to treat local knee pain.

LU$_{11}$: This point is located on the inside of the front leg about 1/2 inch (1 cm) above the coronary band just in front of the hard area (medial collateral cartilage) located on the side of the foot just above the coronary band. Acupressure on LU$_{11}$ is used to treat laminitis and is helpful when treating ringbone. It is also helpful to stimulate lung energy to help treat respiratory infections.

Pericardium Meridian

PC$_1$: This point is located behind the elbow in the space behind rib 6. Stimulate PC$_1$ when treating problems of the hoof and elbow. It is also helpful for treating chest pain.

PC_6: This point is located on the inside of the front leg just above the chestnut. This is a master point for the chest and heart and should be included in treatments that involve them. It is helpful when treating pulmonary emphysema. Acupressure on PC_6 can also be calming and soothing to an upset horse.

PC_9: This point is located on the back of the front leg in the middle of the depression at the bottom of the pastern between the bulbs of the heel. Stimulation of this point is helpful in relieving pain in the hoof such as that associated with navicular disease and ringbone. May help with treatment of pain in joints of the front leg as well as stimulating circulation and energy flow throughout the leg.

Kidney Meridian

KI_1: This point is located on the back of the hind leg in the depression at the bottom of the pastern between the bulbs of the heel. Stimulation of KI_1 is helpful in relieving pain involving the hoof or hock. It is also helpful when treating heat stroke or anxiety.

Liver Meridian

LIV_1: This point is located on the inside of the hind leg just above the coronary band. Acupressure on this point is helpful when treating laminitis, fluid retention, and some problems associated with the uterus, such as prolapse and hemorrhage.

Gall Bladder Meridian

GB_1: This point is located about 1/4 inch (1/2 cm) from the outer corner of the eye. Stimulate this point to treat eye problems such as conjunctivitis. Stimulation of this point may also help in treatment of facial paralysis and heat stroke.

GB_{20}: This point is located above TH_{17} in the depression behind the ear. GB_{20} has many uses and is closely linked to problems with the liver meridian. It is an important point to use when treating eye problems, particularly those associated with an illness affecting the liver. An ear problem can also be helped by stimulation of GB_{20}. Neck problems such as stiffness and pain also may be helped by stimulation of this point.

GB_{33}: Located 2 to 3 inches above GB_{34} and level with the stifle joint. Stimulate when treating a stifle problem, especially if tendons and ligaments are involved.

$GB34$: This point is located in the top area of the middle of the gaskin on the outside of the hind leg near the top of the fibula bone. This point can be stimulated to treat pain in the hind leg, particularly in the stifle and hock. Stimulation of GB_{34} also increases circulation in the hind leg and assists in the treatment of tendinitis.

GB_{44}: This point is located on the outside of the hind leg just above the coronary band. Stimulate GB_{44} to treat hoof problems such as ringbone and laminitis. It may also be helpful when treating pain in the hind leg.

Heart Meridian

HT_9: This point is located on the outside of the front leg just behind the lateral cartilage, (the hard area on the side of the foot), just above the coronary band. Stimulation of HT_9 will help when treating laminitis and local foot problems. Stimulate this point if shock or coma is present.

Small Intestine Meridian

SI_1: This point is located on the outside of the front foot just above the coronary band. Stimulate SI_1 to treat laminitis and ringbone.

SI_{16}: This point is located in the middle about one-third of the way down the side of the neck, between the second and third vertebrae of the neck. This point can be used to treat tendinitis as well as local neck pain.

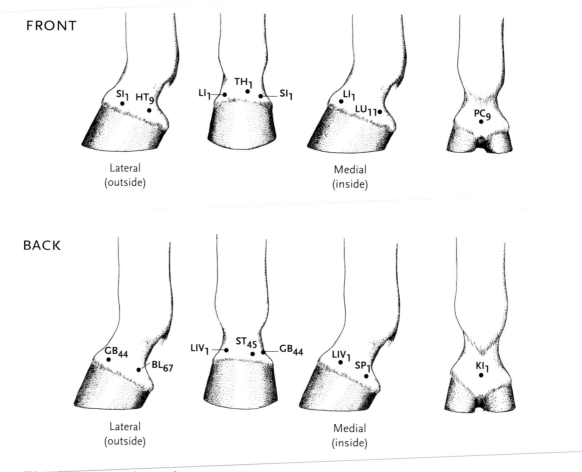

IV–5 *Acupuncture points on the pastern and coronary band.*

Large Intestine Meridian

LI$_1$: This point is located on the inside of the front foot just above the coronary band. Stimulate LI$_1$ when treating laminitis and ringbone. It may also help in treatment of upper respiratory illness.

Stomach Meridian

ST$_1$: This point is located just below the eye at about the midpoint. Stimulate ST$_1$ when treating eye problems.

ST$_{45}$: This point is located just slightly to the outside of the midline of the front of the hind foot about 1/4 inch (1/2 cm) above the coronary band. Stimulate ST$_{45}$ when treating ringbone and local foot pain.

Spleen Meridian

SP$_1$: This point is located on the inside of the hind leg just behind the lateral cartilage (the hard area on the side of the foot) and about 1/4 inch (1/2 cm) above the coronary band. Stimulating SP$_1$ is useful when treating laminitis.

SP$_{21}$: This point is found in the middle of the side at the level of the shoulder joint and just behind rib ten. Stimulation of this point is helpful when treating pulmonary emphysema, as well as problems associated with the liver.

Governing Vessel

GV_3: This point is located on the top of the back just in the middle of the lumbar area between the third and fourth lumbar vertebrae. Stimulation of GV_3 is helpful when treating lumbar pain.

GV4: This point is located on top of the back just in front of GV_3, between the second and third lumbar vertebrae. Stimulation of this point helps to relieve pain associated with the hind leg. It can also be used to help with treatment of kidney and bladder problems, particularly if moxibustion is used. It also may be a helpful point when treating fertility problems.

Bai Hui: This point is located in the space between the lumbar and sacral vertebrae. This is considered a master point for treatment of the hind legs. Acupressure on Bai Hui is also helpful when treating gastro-intestinal and reproductive problems.

GV_{14}: This point is located at the space where the neck meets the withers (between the seventh cervical vertebrae and the first thoracic vertebrae). Stimulate GV_{14} to treat neck and back pain.

GV_{26}: This point is located at the center of the upper lip, midway between the nostrils. Stimulate GV_{26} for a general calming effect, and to treat shock and facial paralysis.

Conception Vessel

CV_{12}: Located halfway between the umbilicus and xiphoid process at the end of the sternum (the bone that runs between the horse's front legs) on the midline. This point is also called an alarm or mu point since it can be used to help diagnose a problem with the associated organ—the stomach. If it is excessively sore the horse may have a digestive upset, or gastric ulcers. Stimulate this point for any stomach or spleen problems.

II Aromatherapy & Essential Oils

For more on Aromatherapy and Essential Oils see the general discussion in Chapter Three, and throughout Part Three: Common Horse Ailments, *where individual essential oil remedies are recommended for specific problems.*

Essential oils can be obtained from health-food stores, specialist mail order catalogs, and from companies who have their product listed on the Internet. Bear in mind that you cannot check the quality of the oils when ordering by mail, so try to purchase from well-known companies. (See Appendix VI for a list of suppliers).

QUALITY OF ESSENTIAL OILS

Essential oils are taken from plants or parts of plants by expression, pressure, steam, water, or dry distillation. Once removed, the resulting oil may require further purification until eventually liquid oil is left. There are a few essential oils that exist in solid or semi-solid states, depending on the room temperature. It is important that you use the highest quality essential oil to decrease the possibility of contaminants and increase the medicinal results. Unlike ordinary plant oils, such as corn oil, essential oils evaporate when exposed to air. To be sure that the oil you are using is of good quality, put a drop on a piece of paper; this drop should evaporate leaving no oily residue.

HOW TO USE ESSENTIAL OILS

Essential oils can be purchased 100 percent pure, or in a diluted form. The pure oils are extremely potent and must be handled carefully. Avoid contact with your skin.

Essential oils must never be given orally. The aroma should be inhaled through a vaporizer, diffuser, or from the aroma on a cloth that is permeated with the oil. When diluted, the essential oils may be applied directly on the horse's skin in the form of a poultice or compress, and occasionally rubbed on a small area.

You can treat with aromatherapy once a day, unless treatment for a specific problem requires more frequent exposure. Do not mix essential oils except where specified otherwise—treat with a single oil at a time for best results and safety. Aromatherapy is most effective when used consistently for one to two weeks, discontinued for a week, then resumed for a few more weeks. I suggest that if you see no improvement after the initial two- week treatment, discontinue that oil, and try another one. Regular therapies for any health problem or condition should be continued in conjunction with aromatherapy treatment.

ADMINISTERING ESSENTIAL OILS BY DIFFUSION

In many cases, essential oils are administered by allowing the patient to either smell or inhale the oil. As a general rule I recommend that you continue the diffusion treatments for one hour.

Aromatic Diffuser Put 5 drops of the essential oil into an electric aromatic diffuser, which can be purchased in most health food stores. Caution: Do not use aroma pots that are powered by a candle since they represent a major fire hazard in the stable area.

Vaporizer When a concentrated steam is desired, for instance for respiratory problems, put 5 drops in a warm vaporizer (available in drug stores and chemists). NOTE: Cold vaporizers are not as effective.

Oily Cloth Essential oils can also be administered by putting a little amount (3 drops or so) of the oil on a cotton cloth. You hang it in a horse's stall (out of his reach), or attach to the bottom ring of his halter where there is no possibility of the cloth having prolonged contact with his head.

Caution: *When using essential oils, do not be tempted to use a nebulizer (an apparatus that is made to fit directly over the horse's nose and administer medications such as antibiotics directly into the nose). Nebulizers may concentrate the oils too much and cause an irritation of the mucus membranes, the sensitive tissue that lines the nasal passages.*

ADMINISTERING ESSENTIAL OILS DIRECTLY ON THE SKIN

Some essential oils can be administered directly on the skin as a "rub" or massage after being diluted with another oil such as sweet almond oil, grapeseed oil, or extra virgin olive oil. It is important to select as the dilutant oil that has been cold pressed (available in health food sections of stores), and not oil that has been chemically extracted like most commercial vegetable oils, since the diluting oil will also be absorbed by the horse's skin. Many commercial vegetable oil manufacturers use chemicals in the extracting process that may be harmful.

Dilute your essential oil so that it represents about 2 percent of the oil you use. Following is a simple dilution chart. (20 drops of an essential oil equals about 1/4 teaspoon, or 1ml)

ESSENTIAL OIL	DILUTING OIL
40 drops	*1/2 cup (100ml)*
20 drops	*1/4 cup (50ml)*
5 drops	*2 teaspoons (10ml)*

Use about 1 tablespoon (14ml) at a time. Dip your fingers in the oil mixture and rub it in on the area. If your skin is sensitive to essential oil, wear rubber gloves.

ADMINISTERING ESSENTIAL OILS BY COMPRESS OR POULTICE

If you want to use an essential oil to soothe an irritated or painful area, mix about 5 drops of essential oil with 2 1/2 cups, (1 liter), of water in a large bowl. Either hot or cold water can be used. It depends on the problem being treated. Use hot water when treating problems such as chronic back pain or arthritis. Use cold water for acute injuries such as sprains or swellings. For a compress (on an area you cannot bandage successfully) soak a cotton cloth, a wash cloth or flannel, rolled cotton, or cotton balls, then apply the mixture to the affected area and hold there as long as possible—at least 15 minutes. Poultice, where possible, for up to four hours so the essential oil is absorbed thoroughly.

Caution: *Due to the potential for toxic effects, do not administer essential oils orally, or administer topically without dilution. Try to avoid* *prolonged contact with undiluted oil yourself and use gloves where necessary.*

I am listing below the plants used for aromatherapy and essential oils in alphabetical order. (You will notice that I am discouraging the use of the essential oils from some of the plants mentioned, but since they are available in shops I want to bring their potential for harm to your attention.) All of the oils are sold either with an eyedropper, or in a bottle that allows one drop out at a time. As a general guideline use 5 drops of oil in a diffuser or vaporizer, but less—3 drops—on an oily cloth you hang in the stall or attach to your horse's halter. If applying directly on the skin in the form of a salve for insect bites as an example, dilute the essential oil according to the chart above. With a compress or poultice, use 5 drops of essential oil then dilute with hot or cold water as outlined above.

List of Essential Oils

Chamomile, (Chamaemelum nobile or Matricaria recutica)

The essential oil version of chamomile is obtained primarily by steam distillation from the flower heads, which produces a pale liquid that becomes yellow over time.

USES OF OIL OF CHAMOMILE:

- Reduces inflammation, particularly arthritis and muscular pain.
- Treats dermatitis, including sensitive skin, and cuts and burns.
- Helps treat colic (usually associated with gas colic).
- Improves appetite.
- Helps balance a mare's hormones.
- Treats depression, particularly when associated with separation.

Eucalyptus (Eucalyptus globulus)

A native of Australia and Tasmania, the eucalyptus tree is now found throughout the world. Its distinctive odor is easy to recognize and it is considered stimulating and helpful to concentration. The fresh or dried leaves and twigs are steam dis-

tilled to obtain an essential oil. When used externally or inhaled, this oil rarely causes a problem, however it is very toxic, so be aware that it should never be used internally. The oil is clear when first made and yellows as it grows older.

USES OF OIL OF EUCALYPTUS

- Treats lesions from insect bites, cuts, or infections.
- Soothes the respiratory system when dealing with influenza, sinusitis, bronchitis, and coughs. An excellent remedy using a mixture of oils to treat respiratory problems, is to place a container containing the recipe below near your horse. The strong eucalyptus vapors will permeate the area even after the mixture cools down.

> *Oil of lavender 5 drops*
> *Oil of thyme 5 drops*
> *Oil of eucalyptus 10 drops*
> *Rubbing alcohol 1/2 cup (100ml)*
>
> Mix together. Use 15 drops of the solution to 1 quart (1 liter) of boiling water. Leave near the horse so he can inhale for about 30 minutes.

Geranium (Pelargonium graveolens)

This plant has a long history as a medicinal herb. There are about 700 varieties; however, pelargonium graveolens is the main one which is commercially cultivated and harvested for oil. The entire plant is processed for oil through a steam distillation process, resulting in a green liquid. There are ancient herbal references concerning the use of geranium for healing fractures and treating cancer; however, no recent research has been done in this area for horses.

USES OF OIL OF GERANIUM

- Helps the healing process of burns and bruises.
- Repels mosquitoes and lice.

- Decreases pain and reduces inflammation due to nerve inflammation. Particularly effective for facial nerves.
- Helps relieve cellulitis by improving circulation, particularly when associated with a leg.
- Eases discomfort associated with engorgement of the mammary glands which may be helpful to heavy milk-producing mares at weaning time.
- Helps the respiratory system by soothing irritation of the throat.
- Quiets the nervous system.

Hops (Humulus lupulus)

The most widely known use of hops is for beer production; however, it is also used as aromatherapy to treat a variety of ailments. The essential oil of hops is derived by steam distillation from the part of the hop plant called the cone. The yellow liquid is highly valued as a treatment for nervousness and to stimulate female hormonal activity. Different cultures developed different uses for hops as aromatherapy—the Europeans as a calmer and a remedy for headaches and indigestion and the Chinese for treating pulmonary (lung) and bladder problems. It is also a common component of commercial fragrances, tobacco, and spice products.

USES OF OIL OF HOPS

- Helps to calm nervous tension and treat neuralgia (pain caused by a nerve).
- Supports female estrogens and helps activate a mare's reproductive cycle.
- Helps reduce sexual over activity in mares and geldings.
- Reduces symptoms of asthma and decreases coughing.
- Reduces indigestion, particularly when associated with nervousness.

NOTE: Do not treat horses suffering from depression with hops.

Caution: *Some horses may react badly to long-term use of the essential oil of hops.*

Jasmine (Jasminum)

Widely known as a tea and component of perfumes, jasmine oil has been used for healing purposes for thousands of years. Specific varieties of jasmine are recommended for certain uses. The oil comes from a solvent extraction process that first produces a form called a concrete. It is then separated with alcohol to make an absolute. The absolute is distilled with steam to obtain the resultant brownish-orange oil. Due to the amount of processing involved, jasmine oil is sometimes more expensive than other essential oils. If a specific variety of jasmine is desired, the expense may be increased.

JASMINUM GRANDIFLORUM

- Helps treat liver problems such as hepatitis.

JASMINUM SAMBAC

- Heals skin lesions or "pressure" ulcers (bed sores).

JASMINUM OFFICINALE

- Assists with a difficult birthing process.
- Relaxes contracted tendons.
- Produces a feeling of well-being and confidence that may be useful when a horse seems depressed, or is exhausted.

Juniper (Juniperus communis)

The oil distilled by steam from juniper berries is used medicinally. It is important to use the oil that has been distilled from the berries rather than the wood, since the wood oil does not have the same properties, and often has turpentine oil added to it. Do not use juniper oil if using iodine, since some of the effects of iodine will be negated.

Juniper oil is sometimes considered to be toxic to the kidneys, though studies have shown no indication that juniper oil can cause kidney disease. Other medical studies have found that there is a possibility that juniper oil causes abortion.

USES OF OIL OF JUNIPER:

- Treats cystitis (bladder infection or irritation).
- Treats arthritis.
- Helps to deal with the accumulation of toxins in muscles and joints. For this purpose, a few drops of juniper oil can also be added to rinse water after a strenuous workout.

True Lavender (Lavandula angustifolia)

True lavender has a long history of medicinal use for humans and is still used in some medications today—especially in skin treatment creams. Although found throughout the world, the oldest and most valuable varieties of lavender are found in France and Italy.

In the Alps, True lavender is still used by some hunters as an immediate treatment for dogs bitten by venomous adders. The crushed lavender rubbed on the bite is said to neutralize the venom. Another type of lavender from the same family, Spike lavender (lavandula latifolia), possesses different characteristics and is not recommended for horses since it contains camphor that can be neurotoxic and sometimes lead to convulsions.

Lavandin (lavandula x intermedia) is a hybrid in the lavender family and is thought to first have been created by insects cross pollinating True lavender and Spike lavender. The effects of lavandin are similar to True lavender; however, caution should be taken when using the oil since it tends to be stronger and produce a more intensified effect. The oil from all the plants in the lavender family is obtained by steam distillation from the flowering tops and is a pale yellow or colorless.

USES OF OIL OF LAVENDER

- Treats skin to heal abscesses, inflammations, insect bites, and some types of fungi.
- Use on muscles to help relieve pain from sprains and aches.
- Relieves stomach cramping and colic-like symptoms.
- Assists the respiratory system deal with bronchitis symptoms and respiratory conditions resulting from nervous tension or stress.
- Effective against many types of bacteria, but unfortunately only in strengths greater than those considered safe for aromatherapy. However, even though the horse cannot be safely treated with pure oil of lavender for this purpose, it can be used to help rid a contaminated area, such as a stall, of bacteria. Many types of staphylococcus and streptococcus are killed by lavender. Use a mixture of 5 percent pure oil of lavender and 95 percent water in a vaporizer, or apply to surfaces with a cloth. Take all animals out of the area before treating it and do not bring them back into the treated environment for 12 hours.

Caution: *Lavender cotton (santolina chamaecyparissus) is not a member of the same botanical family as True or Spike lavender; it contains a high amount of artemisia ketone which can be neurotoxic or cause abortions.*

Lemon (Citrus limon)

The use of lemon oil for medicinal purposes is extensive and very effective. It is one of the essential oils that has been well researched and documented. There are many uses for lemon oil; I will mention only those most applicable to horses.

Two types of lemon oil are available—the essential oil of lemon, which is used for aromatherapy, and another type of lemon oil, which is manufactured as a food flavoring. The essential oil of lemon is made by cold expression of the outer part of the fresh lemon peel. Even though some people apply fresh lemon onto their skin, I emphasize that essential oil of lemon should never be applied directly to the skin of people or horses, since it can cause the skin to become sensitive to light (phototoxic) and burn easily. Therefore, always limit the use to a mixture that has been diluted according to the directions at the beginning of this appendix.

USES OF OIL OF LEMON:

- Stimulates the immune system and appetite.
- Calms during fevers and digestive upsets.
- Hardens hooves: Add 5 drops of lemon oil to 1/2 cup (110ml) cider vinegar and paint the hooves with this mixture twice a day.
- Promotes circulation to a swollen area. Gently massage or rub in some diluted lemon oil as directed at the beginning of this section.
- As a disinfectant, lemon oil is very effective in the vaporized form. Use in the stable area if you suspect a bacterial respiratory disease outbreak and want to prevent further spread to other horses. It works well combined with lavender oil for this purpose. Add 5 drops of both oils to the water in the vaporizer and treat the area twice a day for three days.

In addition to using the essential oil of lemon, there are also several ways to use fresh lemons as a treatment for horses. There are two types of treatments for warts in which some successes have been documented. Therefore, given the noninvasive nature of these treatments, they are worth trying:

First Wart Treatment: Apply pure lemon oil on each wart twice a day. The treated horse must not be allowed in sunlight for 12 hours afterward. Consequently, this treatment should not be used on horses that are going to be turned out, or exercised in the sun.

Second Wart Treatment: Mash the rind of two fresh lemons in 1 cup (220ml) strong cider vinegar, cover the mixture and allow it to sit for 8 days. Then apply the mixture directly on the warts twice a day. Take the same precautions concerning sunlight as mentioned above.

Fresh lemon juice can be used to treat water when the only water available may be contaminated with bacteria. Add the juice of 1 lemon to 2 pints (1 liter) of water. However if your horse objects to the strong lemon flavor and doesn't drink, add more water. Allow the water to stand for 3 hours before using.

Lemongrass (Cymbopogon citratus)

While lemongrass may be given to horses, the essential oil form of lemongrass is not recommended because it can lead to health problems. Lemongrass oil can cause complications when pressure in the eye (ocular tension) is increased. It can also affect hormonal balance, and possibly, reproductive glands. The research available on lemongrass essential oil was conducted primarily by using it internally; however, due to the reactions of similar compounds it is possible that if used as aromatherapy, it might produce similar unpleasant results if used over a long period of time. The effects of lemongrass are dangerous to people as well, particularly those with glaucoma, and men with enlarged prostate glands.

Lemon Balm (Melissa officinalis)

Lemon Balm is also referred to as melissa. I will use the term lemon balm but be aware that these terms are used interchangeably where it is sold. The use of oil of lemon balm is associated with disorders originating from the nervous system. The oil is very effective in calming and is an antidepressant as well. The essential oil is distilled with steam and should be pale yellow. Unfortunately, it is difficult to find lemon balm since much of the oil sold as lemon balm or melissa, does not actually contain lemon balm at all but is a mixture containing lemon, lemongrass, and/or citronella. Since very little real lemon balm oil is sold, it is important to check your sources carefully when purchasing this oil. Excessive, or constant, aromatherapy using oil of lemon balm should be avoided, especially if horses or people in the area have any eye problems, hormonal imbalances, or prostate enlargement.

USES OF OIL OF LEMON BALM

- Treat with lemon balm when a horse is nervous or depressed. This oil is particularly useful when dealing with abused horses by helping to relax them.

- Can be used when a health problem is caused by excessive neural stimulation—a nervous horse colicking, for example. The colic must be treated in the usual way, with the essential oil of lemon balm helping to calm the horse.

Litsea cubeba (Litsea cubeba)

This plant is native to East Asia, mainly China, where much of the oil is made by steam distillation of the fruit. The herb form of litsea cubeba is made from the root and stem and used in Chinese medicine to treat aches and pains as well as indigestion. Litsea cubeba may also be useful when treating a fluctuating heartbeat, also known as cardiac arrhythmia.

USES OF OIL OF LITSEA CUBEBA

- Increases the body's immune system response.
- Decreases flatulence (gas) production in the digestive tract.
- Aids in the treatment of indigestion.
- Helps decrease stress.
- May help to reduce blood pressure; regulate the heartbeat; increase concentration; assist the endocrine system by stimulating the parathyroid gland.

Marjoram (Origanum marjorana)

The use of marjoram dates back thousands of years, so its uses are well documented. Oil of marjoram is obtained by steam distillation. Its color ranges from yellow to amber. Although marjoram has many useful properties, there are also instances when its use should be avoided. **Caution:** *Do not use marjoram in foals less than six months old; when a horse has a fever; with any horse that has a history of seizures. Never use marjoram on a pregnant mare.*

USES OF OIL OF MARJORAM

- Stimulates the immune system against upper respiratory diseases.

- Acts to calm the nervous system. May relax the horse enough to cause sleep.
- Stimulates intestinal motility (movement) in the digestive system. *Caution: Marjoram should not be used when excessive intestinal motility is occurring. Do not use when colic is present unless your vet knows the type of colic and suggests otherwise.*

Parsley (Petroselinum sativum)

Parsley is not recommended for use in horses due to the potential toxic effects. Use of parsley oil has not been well documented, however the effect may be cumulative over time. *Caution: The oil can cause abortion, as well as liver, kidney, and possibly heart damage when given orally.*

Patchouli (Pogostemon cablin)

The scent of this oil was very popular during the 1960s as a perfume. In aromatherapy, it is used for its distinctive scent as well as its medicinal qualities. The leaves are first dried, fermented, then put through a steam distillation process to produce thick amber oil. The oil itself is often used to treat minor burns as it has antiseptic and anti-inflammatory properties. The oil is also used in Japan and Malaysia to treat some types of venomous snakebites.

USES OF OIL OF PATCHOULI

- Very calming to the nervous system.
- Helps mares who resist being bred. Also helps to stimulate stallions.
- Acts as a mild diuretic.

Peppermint (Mentha piperita)

One of the most well known scents, peppermint has been used for thousands of years as aromatherapy. Its use is safe in moderation; however, oral ingestion of the pure oil can be toxic. Oil of peppermint should not be used at strengths greater than 3 percent. Even when used as aromatherapy, if the oil is concentrated at a strength greater than 3 percent, it can irritate the mucus membranes, the tissues that line the nasal passages, and the mouth.

Caution: Do not use peppermint as aromatherapy when these situations may be present (in humans as well as horses):

- A fever.
- Anyone in the stable has a history of seizures.
- If any people or horses in the stable have a history of heart problems.
- If horses or humans in the area are less than 6 months old.
- If the horse does not tolerate the sulfonamide (sulfa) family of antibiotics.
- If the horse is currently being given a homeopathic remedy.

USES OF OIL OF PEPPERMINT:

- Relieves systems of asthma, upper respiratory infections, and bronchitis. Peppermint has a mild, antispasmodic effect and temporarily clears mucus.
- Assists the digestive system, by calming the stomach and decreasing intestinal cramping and excessive gas production. Works well as a supportive therapy to help in the treatment of gas colic.

Rosemary (Rosmarinus officinalis)

This well-known seasoning herb has been extensively used for medicinal purposes for thousands of years. The quality of oil of rosemary varies according to the amount of the plant being used in the process. The best essential oil is made with only the fresh flowering tops that are steam distilled. This processing leads to the smallest amount of camphor in the final product. Oil from Tunisia is generally made in this way and is therefore the best quality. In comparison, much of the oil of rosemary that comes from Spain is made from the whole plant. It has much higher camphor content and, therefore, a greater potential for toxicity.

NOTE: Because of its very powerful aroma, rosemary can be overdosed when used as aromatherapy, resulting in adverse affects. Also, rosemary can cause horses to become easily frightened or difficult to handle.

Caution: Do not use rosemary if any horses in the stable area have a history of seizures, if mares are pregnant, or if any horses have a fever.

USES OF OIL OF ROSEMARY:

- Soothes and improves irritated or dry skin. Stimulates hair growth.
- Improves circulation in general and decreases inflammation associated with veins.
- Is helpful as a diuretic.
- Helps horses suffering from nervous exhaustion or depression.
- Helps to relieve symptoms of hepatitis.
- Reduces pain from arthritis when used as a compress or massaged over the arthritic area. For massage, mix rubbing alcohol with oil of rosemary and dilute according to the directions at the beginning of this appendix, or make a liniment of rosemary, juniper oil, and ginger oil using the formula below. You can also make a compress with fresh rosemary (see Rosemary in the *Herbs Appendix IV* p. 321).

EXTERNAL LINIMENT FOR SORE MUSCLES AND ARTHRITIC AREAS

Rubbing alcohol	1 pint (500ml)
Rosemary oil	30 drops
Juniper oil	40 drops
Ginger oil	20 drops

Sage (Salvia officinalis)

Caution: The use of salvia officinalis (sometimes referred to as common, garden, or dalmation sage) as an essential oil is not recommended due to its toxic effects. This sage contains thujone, which, when used over time leads to degeneration of the liver. As with some other essential oils there is also camphor in sage oil, a component that can produce seizures or convulsions.

However, clary sage oil (Salvia pratensis) is not the same as the above mentioned sage oil and is considered non-toxic. It is useful for soothing throat inflammation and aids in the treatment of respiratory infections. *Caution: Do not use around pregnant mares, or in conjunction with a treatment or medication, containing alcohol.*

Sandalwood (Santalum album)

Use of sandalwood dates back about 4,000 years and has roots in both Chinese and Ayurvedic medicine. It is widely used in perfumes and burned as incense, and in ancient times this parasite-resistant wood was used as a building material, particularly in temples. True sandalwood oil comes from the water or steam distillation of the powdered dried roots and heartwood. A tree must be thirty years old before it is ready to be used for oil production. An Australian sandalwood, S. spicata, produces oil that gives similar results, however the West Indian sandalwood tree, Amyris balsamifera, is not related and the oil does not produce the same results.

USES OF OIL OF SANDALWOOD:

- Moisturizes and softens the skin.
- Assists the respiratory system by helping to clear dry coughs and is very effective in relieving sore, irritated throats.
- Eases the pain of bladder infections (cystitis).
- Aids in the treatment of diarrhea.
- Helps relieve depression, and relaxes tense, stressed horses.
- A few drops of the diluted essential oil massaged onto the skin around the throat area can help relieve internal irritation of the throat and act as a deterrent for dry coughs.

Tea Tree (Melaluca alternifolia)

This Australian plant has been researched extensively by modern methods as well as used for a long time by aborigines. The original use was as a tea prepared from the leaves, which is how the plant came by its name. The oil from the plant is derived from steam or water distillation of the leaves and twigs, and it is the oil that is most effective for medicinal use. Scientific study has shown that tea tree oil can effectively fight bacteria, viruses, and fungi. It has also been found to actively stimulate the body's immune system. More often tea tree oil is found in topically applied products such as creams, shampoos, or soaps. However, the essential oil can be useful in aromatherapy.

USES OF TEA TREE OIL

- Stimulates the immune system to respond to bacterial, viral, or fungal infections.
- Topical application: Use the diluted essential oil directly on the affected area. Unlike most essential oils where you use only a few drops mixed into the diluting oil, you can use as much as 50 percent tea tree oil with 50 percent diluting oil.

Thyme (Thymus vulgaris)

Thyme is used extensively, from medicinal purposes to cooking, as an ingredient in perfumes, and even as the main ingredient in love potions. The oil is made by steam distillation, with the best oil produced only from the flowering tops of the plant. This oil requires a two-stage process. The first distillation results in red-brown oil; after another distillation white or clear oil is produced. After the second distillation process some of the working components of the oil may be decreased or lost entirely. Because of this, thyme oil often has other oils or constituents added to it.

Thyme is a very useful essential oil if certain precautions are followed. ***Caution:*** *Do not use thyme oil on or around pregnant mares. And, when preparing thyme for aromatherapy oil use only 1 percent of the oil in the final diluted mix since higher concentrations can irritate skin and mucus membranes.* Oil from lemon thyme is less irritating and will produce the same results as oil made from common thyme.

USES OF OIL OF THYME:

- Promotes general circulation. This heals wounds and helps to treat founder.
- Acts as a decongestant—most effective when vaporized.
- Helpful with dermatitis.
- Stimulates the immune system when combined in equal amounts with oil of lavender.
- To stop hair loss, prepare the fresh herb as an infusion (detailed below). Make a compress from the liquid and use once a day on the affected area of the skin.
- Works as a strong bactericidal to help cleanse wounds. Prepare the fresh herb as an infusion.

INFUSION USING FRESH THYME

Boil 1/4 cup (2 tablespoons) of thyme leaves and flowers in 4 cups (1 liter) of water until half the water is gone. Strain the leaves and flowers out and reserve the liquid.

Caution: *People with high blood pressure should not be present when thyme oil is used as aromatherapy.*

Ylang-Ylang (Cananga odorata var. genuina)

In addition to its medicinal uses, this essential oil is used in cosmetics, hair care products and perfumes. Freshly picked flowers are steam distilled to a form of essential oil called "ylang-ylang extra," which is considered the highest grade of this type of oil. This is the best for aromatherapy purposes.

USES OF OIL OF YLANG-YLANG:

- Reduces the breathing rate when it is too high (a condition called hyperpnea).
- Decreases the heart rate when it is too fast (a condition called tachycardia).
- Helps mares or stallions that are reluctant or difficult to breed.
- Decreases nervous tension and stress and can help a horse relax into sleep.
- Quiets angry and frustrated horses.
- Soothes irritated skin and insect bites. (Use a few drops of essential oil diluted in water and spread directly on the skin.)

NOTE: Excessive use of ylang-ylang may cause nausea and headaches in humans.

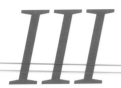

Bach Flower Remedies

I discussed the origin of the Bach Flower remedies at some length in Chapter Three. Please review before you proceed with any treatments.

TO SELECT THE PROPER BACH FLOWER REMEDY

Review your horse's personality, mental state, recent or past traumas, and changes in his environment. Take notes if necessary.

Then, consult the list of Bach Flower remedies below and select the appropriate remedy that fits your horse. Some remedies have similar descriptions, so it is important to review them carefully.

TO PREPARE AND USE BACH FLOWER REMEDIES

- Buy a 1 ounce (2 tbsp/28ml) glass dropper bottle. It should be dark in color to protect the liquid from sunlight.
- Put 2 or 3 drops of the selected Bach Flower remedy into the 1-ounce dropper bottle. If you are using more than one remedy put 3 drops of each remedy in the bottle. Horses respond best to one or two remedies; however, up to five remedies can be used at one time. Add 1 teaspoon (5ml) of brandy. (The brandy is used as

a preservative—it is not required for the remedy to be effective).
- Fill the bottle to the top with distilled or spring water.
- Shake the bottle vigorously. To stay consistent with homeopathic principles (which you will learn in the *Homeopathic Appendix V,*) I suggest you shake (or succuss) the bottle 108 times, though it is not a strict requirement here with Bach Flowers.
- Put a label on the bottle so you will know which specific Bach Flower remedy (or combination of remedies) it contains.
- Two or three times a day—or more often for acute problems—put a dropperful of the liquid into your horse's water or food, or directly into his mouth. Give the remedy until the bottle is used up. If no improvement is noticed by this time, review the list of Bach Flower remedies and determine if a different remedy or combination of remedies should be selected. If you feel the remedy you have been giving is the correct one, but the condition has not improved,

prepare another bottle of that remedy and continue giving it.

Bach Flowers are a very useful adjunct to holistic therapy, opening the door to a whole new form of treatment. They are readily available at many health food stores and a number of books are available describing their use. While these books refer to human use, an astute owner can translate a horse's behavior and mental state to the descriptions in the book. You can also order Bach Flowers, and books on methods, through the mail from companies listed in Appendix VII.

List of Bach Flower Remedies

Rescue Remedy (also known as Calming Essence)

This is a combination Bach Flower remedy and is made of equal parts of five other remedies: Star Of Bethlehem, Rock Rose, Impatiens, Cherry Plum and Clematis. (Each of these remedies is described in detail below.) You can purchase this combination remedy under the brand names Rescue Remedy and Calming Essence, or you can mix these five remedies together yourself. (For brevity in this book, I refer to this remedy as Rescue Remedy.)

Rescue Remedy was formulated by Dr. Bach specifically for use in emergencies. It can calm, and return a person or animal's mental state to normal after an upset. Rescue Remedy is one of the most remarkable remedies because it acts very quickly and the effects are lasting. Dr. Bach felt that Rescue Remedy could save lives in emergency situations by giving you a little extra time until you can get appropriate help. In my experience, this remedy does exactly what Dr. Bach designed it to do, and more. Numerous times, Rescue Remedy has helped to stabilize a horse in shock until the vet arrives. Often, a horse comes completely "out of shock" after Rescue Remedy is administered.

Rescue Remedy can also be used by an owner herself (taken according to package directions) when an emotional upset occurs. I have often recommended that people take it when they are confronted with traumatic situations, and I've found that most people respond well and are better able to cope.

Another use for Rescue Remedy is to help calm a horse who is frightened, confused, or upset, whether at a horse show, traveling, struggling with a new training challenge, or encountering any other situation that causes the horse's behavior to change. The horse who is showing fear in new surroundings may require just a few doses to help him settle in, while the horse who is having a training problem may need repeated doses.

An example of the use in training of Rescue Remedy is a case I treated several years ago. An aged gelding was involved in a trailer accident and, although not seriously hurt, was badly bruised and shaken. For the year following this accident whenever trailering bandages were put on, he would develop profuse diarrhea that continued for several days. I suggested that the owner give Rescue Remedy: before the wraps were brought out, again before the horse was loaded in the trailer, and again after arrival at the destination. After one month on this regimen, the diarrhea no longer occurred.

Of the 38 Bach Flower remedies, I have listed below the 32 that are most commonly prescribed for horses. I have organized the list by:

1. Personality Type. I describe how each remedy is associated with a horse's type of personality—particularly relating to the horse's behavior and emotional makeup.

2. Key Characteristics. I outline the key characteristics of that personality type.

3. When to Use. I list the health conditions or behavioral problems you can treat with that specific Bach Flower.

Bach Flowers

Agrimony (Agrimonia eupatoria)

PERSONALITY TYPE

The Agrimony horse is kind, and enjoys whatever type of work he performs. But he doesn't like to be alone and tries to make friends with other horses. When left alone, he frequently becomes restless and may walk around in circles in his stall for instance. He also tries hard to please people in order to avoid any upsets in his life, becoming distressed when he does something wrong—particularly if he doesn't understand what is being asked of him.

KEY CHARACTERISTICS

Restless, worried, but with normal behavior when with other horses, or being schooled.

WHEN TO USE AGRIMONY:

- A horse is a stall walker, restless, or unable to settle down—especially at night.
- A horse that fits this Agrimony type has difficulty understanding, or not making progress, with his training.
- The Agrimony horse who is diagnosed with stress-related illnesses such as gastric (stomach) ulcers, or equine protozoal myelytis (EPM).

Aspen (Populus tremula)

PERSONALITY TYPE

An Aspen horse is fearful of the unknown. In extreme cases, he breaks out in a sweat and shakes when fear takes over his mind. The best example of an Aspen horse is one who spooks at objects that he cannot see behind or around, such as large mounting blocks, bushes and trees, or rocks. Another example of an Aspen horse is one who shies at holes in a fence, especially if they are at the bottom of the fence. The positive aspect of an Aspen horse is the fearlessness he can come to exhibit when he truly trusts his rider or handler. For example, take a jumper who overcomes his natural fear of a jump with open spaces in it or surrounded by "frightening" objects because he has complete confidence and trust in his rider.

KEY CHARACTERISTICS

Fear of the unknown, anxiety, apprehension.

WHEN TO USE ASPEN:

- A horse is excessively spooky around objects, or fearful when asked to do something new.
- To help a horse restore lost confidence due to incorrect training or an accident.
- A horse is frightened of small, confining spaces, such as a horse trailer. (Be sure to give Aspen several times before the horse is asked to go into a small space).
- A horse is recovering from being sedated, or being tranquilized, and begins to show signs of anxiety.

Centaury (Centaurium erythraea or C. umbellatum)

PERSONALITY TYPE

The Centaury horse is quiet, willing, and usually calm. He is dominated by all other horses and does not defend himself very well. When ridden in a group situation he becomes tired more quickly than the other horses. As a foal, this type of horse is slow to wean and does not want to leave his mother even when the mare tries to push him away. He may protest the weaning process for a long time and, even when he accepts it, he will stay close to his mother if allowed to rejoin her. Because he is content to follow other horses this type of horse makes a great school horse.

KEY CHARACTERISTICS

Dominated by other horses, he works best with a group.

WHEN TO USE CENTURY

- During a foal's weaning process.
- Separating a horse from one group of horses and introducing him to a new group.
- A horse is very ill, or severely injured, and has lost the will to live.

Cherry Plum (Prunus cerasifera)

PERSONALITY TYPE

This horse endures mental and physical hardship calmly, stoically enduring great discomfort. But when no longer faced with the unpleasant or difficult situation, the Cherry Plum horse may become nervous and difficult to handle. This behavior is based on a horse's fear of the unknown. In the difficult situation, the horse knew what to expect; in the pleasant situation, he constantly expects the worst. For example, it can be seen in a show horse that is retired and turned out to pasture. He is uncomfortable venturing out into the field and stays close to the stable area, or gate, often needing a companion, or smaller enclosure, just to relax.

KEY CHARACTERISTICS

Fear of the unknown, difficulty adjusting to major changes in life.

WHEN TO USE CHERRY PLUM

- Use when making a major change in a horse's life such as retiring a show horse to pasture, or taking an ex-racehorse to use as a pleasure horse.
- Before subjecting a nervous horse to potential stress—going in the trailer, or introducing unfamiliar objects in a jumping session.
- During the first-saddling process.

Chestnut Bud (Aesculus hippocastanum)

PERSONALITY TYPE

This horse does not remember his training despite repeated attempts. He tries to avoid training by running away, or simply will not pay attention.

KEY CHARACTERISTICS

Does not learn well by experience.

WHEN TO USE CHESTNUT BUD:

- A horse does not remember his training.
- To increase a horse's attention and improve concentration.

Chicory (Cichorium intybus)

PERSONALITY TYPE

A Chicory horse is demanding. Also possessive about his handlers; he does not tolerate the person working with him giving attention to any other horse. A Chicory horse is most often a mare.

KEY CHARACTERISTICS

Possessive of attention.

WHEN TO USE CHICORY:

- A horse demonstrates jealousy of other horses.

Clematis (Clematis vitalba)

PERSONALITY TYPE

A Clematis horse lacks confidence and, because of this, is sometimes thought of as lazy. This type of horse appears to fall asleep at any given opportunity and generally responds poorly to training.

KEY CHARACTERISTICS

Inattentive.

WHEN TO USE CLEMATIS:

- To increase confidence during training.
- To improve a horse's attention and ability to concentrate on what he is being asked to do.
- Following sedation to help a horse wake up more quickly.
- To help bring a horse out of a coma, or any loss of consciousness.

Crab Apple (Malus pumila or sylvestris).

PERSONALITY TYPE

This remedy is often referred to as the "cleansing" remedy because its main action is to clear the mind of negative thoughts. An example of this is the horse who focuses his attention on the activity around him rather than keep it on what he is being asked to do.

KEY CHARACTERISTICS

An inability to stay focused. Despite many positive experiences he will continually remember one negative experience.

WHEN TO USE CRAB APPLE:

- During, or following, illness to help the body with its mind-cleansing process.
- Rehabilitating, or treating, an abused horse, to help clear out bad memories.
- A horse is distracted by outside activities and doesn't stay focused on schooling.

Elm (Ulmus procera)

PERSONALITY TYPE

An Elm horse is strong and reliable. He usually shows off his best characteristics, presenting a positive picture. An Elm horse can become exhausted or overwhelmed when severely stressed, however, this state usually lasts a short period of time. He is concerned for his rider's safety and will take excellent care of those who are lucky enough to ride him

KEY CHARACTERISTICS

Exhaustion seen in a normally energetic horse. May seem overwhelmed by training or work.

WHEN TO USE ELM:

- Give to a horse whose progress suddenly falters after he has been training normally.
- A horse becomes exhausted due to physical overwork or illness, and does not recover with appropriate rest.

Gorse (Ulex europaeus)

PERSONALITY TYPE

Gorse is associated with hope. It is used for treating a chronic illness or condition that has caused the horse to become seriously depressed.

KEY CHARACTERISTICS

Depression.

WHEN TO USE GORSE:

- Treating a horse with a debilitating, or chronic, illness to help relieve his depression.
- There are signs the horse has given up—refusing to eat, for example.

Holly (Ilex aquifolium)

PERSONALITY TYPE

A Holly horse may show signs of bad temper. He is resistant when being trained and may be aggressive toward humans. He is also distrustful of other horses.

KEY CHARACTERISTICS

Suspicion and distrust.

WHEN TO USE HOLLY:

- A horse is first entering a new relationship to establish a positive partnership with his new owner.
- A horse is suspicious about being handled despite a good education and upbringing.

Honeysuckle (Lonicera caprifolium)

PERSONALITY TYPE

This horse has difficulty adjusting to changes. These changes may include a new owner, different stable or pasture, or a new groom. This can result in training setbacks, poor behavior, or general depression.

KEY CHARACTERISTICS

Difficulty adjusting to change.

WHEN TO USE HONEYSUCKLE:

- A horse is not adjusting well to change in his life.

Hornbeam (Carpinus betulus)

PERSONALITY TYPE

The Hornbeam horse seems lethargic and mentally fatigued during training, but is full of energy at other times.

KEY CHARACTERISTICS

Unfocused on work.

WHEN TO USE HORNBEAM:

- A horse is not concentrating on training.
- Before starting a horse back into exercise following a long illness or injury.
- After a long trailer, or plane, trip to ensure a fresh mental outlook.
- A horse lacks energy and enthusiasm for train-

ing despite being fed an adequate diet and after all possible physical causes for the problem have been eliminated.

- During a horse show or competition to prevent mental fatigue and keep a horse's outlook fresh.

Impatiens (Impatiens glandulifera or I. roylei)

PERSONALITY TYPE

This horse is active, but nervous. He is usually gentle and kind and very intelligent. He is often impatient and difficult to train because he does not like repetitive movements—preferring variety and constant change. He is frequently tense and doesn't relax easily no matter how tired he is. The Impatiens horse works best alone—and does not get along well with other horses in team-driving or trail-riding situations. Sometimes this temperament results in the horse injuring himself as he proceeds on a course of action quickly without considering the possibility of injury. His nervous reaction to stress can also result in hives. Breeds often associated with Impatiens are Arabians, Saddlebreds, and Thoroughbreds.

KEY CHARACTERISTICS

Impatient, nervous, and tense.

WHEN TO USE IMPATIENS:

- The horse's temperament causes chronic digestive disorders such as mild colic, or gastric ulcers.
- The Impatiens horse constantly "stall walks," particularly when eating.
- This type of horse experiences mild tying-up or muscle cramping during exercise.
- A nervous horse overreacts to a situation causing hives.

Larch (Larix decidua)

PERSONALITY TYPE

The Larch horse is often talented but lacks confidence. His attitude may be the result of negative past experience, or just be his character.

KEY CHARACTERISTICS

Lacks confidence.

WHEN TO USE LARCH

- To help develop a confident attitude to enable a horse to perform the work asked of him.

Mimulus (Mimulus guttatus)

PERSONALITY TYPE

This horse is fearful or anxious about a given situation. This could be a training session, a horse show, or dealing with his everyday environment. He may outwardly be quiet and internalize his worry, so his concerns are often not noticed until an illness, such as stomach ulcers, results. When ill or injured the Mimulus horse is not an easy patient to manage, as he does not bear pain well, and can be difficult to rehabilitate. Physically, a Mimulus horse is often delicate in build. He also tends to sweat even when slightly anxious. He can be very sensitive to his environment doing best when kept on a strict schedule. A Mimulus horse frequently eats only small amounts of food. Fortunately, a Mimulus treatment is often successful.

KEY CHARACTERISTICS

Fear of a known situation.

WHEN TO USE MIMULUS:

- A horse cannot overcome a specific fear no matter how many times or ways retraining has been attempted.
- The "internal" worrier whose gastric ulcers continue to return despite treatment.
- On the nervous, sensitive horse, who is a poor eater.

Mustard *(Sinapis arvensis)*

PERSONALITY TYPE

With a person, Mustard is used to treat a sudden attack of deep depression that has come on with no obvious cause. The same sort of depression in a horse can be difficult to recognize because we are not with our horses twenty-four hours a day so do not know if there is any specific reason for the condition. If a horse is unresponsive to other attempts to treat depression, try Mustard. It can be combined with other Bach Flowers to achieve the best result possible.

KEY CHARACTERISTICS

Sudden depression for no obvious reason.

WHEN TO USE MUSTARD

- A horse is affected with depression for no known reason.
- A horse seems depressed perhaps because he is having difficulty progressing with training.
- In combination with other Bach Flowers to treat depression. Mustard combines well with Gorse if the depression started as the result of an illness.
- Use for severe depression combined with Sweet Chestnut. NOTE: Give this combination remedy for depression where the cause is known.

Oak *(Quercus robur)*

PERSONALITY TYPE

The Oak horse is strong and reliable, continuing his work despite being tired, injured, or ill, often until he completely breaks down. He is sometimes difficult to identify because due to his strength, he doesn't show his suffering. He is a brave horse who will show great courage and carry on under the most adverse of conditions.

KEY CHARACTERISTICS

Strong and reliable. Doesn't show he is suffering—mentally or physically.

WHEN TO USE OAK:

- A horse fits the personality type of Oak and has become chronically tired despite adequate rest.
- A horse is recovering from an illness or injury that has required extensive treatment, for example, physical therapy, and no longer tolerates the treatment.

Olive *(Olea europoea)*

PERSONALITY TYPE

This horse is exhausted both mentally and physically, perhaps from the stress of an ordeal. Even after he has been allowed to recover and rested, he tires easily when returned to work, and his appetite remains decreased no matter how tempting the food.

KEY CHARACTERISTICS

Complete mental and physical exhaustion.

WHEN TO USE OLIVE:

- A horse is exhausted all the time.
- A horse has had a long serious illness. Olive helps to restore vitality, strength, and the will to live.
- Following travel by trailer or plane if a horse has difficulty relaxing when the trip is over.
- During recovery, when a horse has suffered severe abuse, particularly starvation.

Pine *(Pinus sylvestris)*

PERSONALITY TYPE

The Pine horse tries extremely hard to do whatever is asked of him and becomes distressed or depressed when unable to do so. This personality type is very similar to Larch and Rock Water so these remedies may be considered if Pine is not helpful.

KEY CHARACTERISTICS

Tries to please; suffers when he fails.

WHEN TO USE PINE:

- A horse in training becomes upset being unable to perform as asked.
- A horse develops a bad attitude towards training.

Red Chestnut (Aesculus carnea)

PERSONALITY TYPE

This horse will remain calm and unaffected by surroundings in all situations except when separated from his companions. He becomes very agitated and suffers from severe separation anxiety.

KEY CHARACTERISTICS

Signs of anxiety when separated from other horses. Otherwise calm.

WHEN TO USE RED CHESTNUT:

- Weaning, having to separate a foal from its mother. It decreases the anxiety in both foal and dam.
- A horse that has difficulty being separated from the horse, or horses, he is attached to.

Rock Rose (Helianthemum nummularium)

PERSONALITY TYPE

This horse will overreact when faced with any difficult situation. He cannot mentally cope, so panics. Consequently, he is not responsive, or aware of anything else except getting out of that place. This type of horse frequently injures people with this overreaction. Often, the reason is because he has had some sort of terrifying experience, thus losing confidence in himself as well as trust in others.

KEY CHARACTERISTICS

Reacts to difficult or challenging situations with extreme fear and panic.

WHEN TO USE ROCK ROSE:

- A horse overreacts when frightened and stops listening to his handler. NOTE: In this case, Rock Rose works best when not combined with other Bach Flower remedies.
- A horse has had a bad experience and no longer trusts people.
- After any extremely frightening episode occurs.

Rock Water

(NOTE: This is not a plant—it is water from a natural spring.)

PERSONALITY TYPE

The Rock Water horse is strong and often dominant. Once trained, he does not forget what he has learned and reacts best to a strict schedule and consistent training regimen.

KEY CHARACTERISTICS

Inflexible to change.

WHEN TO USE ROCK WATER:

- A horse of this type must change his schedule, whether training, feeding time, or turn out. Rock Water helps to ease the transition.

Scleranthus (Scleranthus annuus)

PERSONALITY TYPE

This type of horse demonstrates inconsistent behavior—one day very co-operative and the next day refusing to do the first thing asked.

KEY CHARACTERISTICS

Erratic behavior.

WHEN TO USE SCLERANTHUS:

- A horse demonstrates irregular behavior whether in training or everyday handling.
- A horse is finicky about food—enjoying a particular type for a few days, then not eating it.

Star of Bethlehem (Ornithogalum umbellatum)

PERSONALITY TYPE

This horse has suffered some type of shock that he has been unable to fully deal with. Consequently, he is less responsive to what is going on around him. When being ridden he is not very sensitive to aids, and seems slow to learn.

KEY CHARACTERISTICS

Responds slowly to the environment around him.

WHEN TO USE STAR OF BETHLEHEM:

- Following a shock, whether mental or physical. Major shocks that can occur in the past include a difficult birth, being broken to ride, a severe injury, and surgery.

- A horse is slow to learn and not sensitive to training aids.

Sweet Chestnut (Castanea sativa)

PERSONALITY TYPE

The Sweet Chestnut horse is in mental anguish and despair. He stands with his head down and has no appetite, refusing any attempts to make him feel better. These emotions are difficult to interpret in a horse so before using this remedy, it may be necessary to muscle test to see if it is the correct one. (See *Applied Kinesiology Muscle Testing* on p. 148).

KEY CHARACTERISTICS

Extreme mental anguish and despair.

WHEN TO USE SWEET CHESTNUT:

- A horse appears to be completely dejected, holding his head down, refusing to eat, and not wanting any contact with other horses or people.
- A horse becomes depressed after the death of a longtime companion.

Vervain (Verbena officinalis)

PERSONALITY TYPE

The horse that responds to Vervain is one who is high-strung with a nervous temperament, always trying to rush through his work to get where he is going. Once this horse has finished exercise, he is frequently exhausted. Although an enthusiastic performer, the Vervain horse is not always successful because his focus is often too far ahead of where his body is. This horse tends to have a great deal of muscle tension that can also interfere with his performance.

KEY CHARACTERISTICS

High-strung, nervous, and tense.

WHEN TO USE VERVAIN:

- A horse is too nervous to ride, train, or show effectively.
- A horse is too focused on what will happen next and forgets about what is going on right now. For example: the jumper who forgets to keep his feet up in the air high enough to clear the fence he's in the process of jumping because his focus is already on the next fence.
- A horse tries to rush or hurry everywhere he is ridden.

Vine (Vitis vinifera)

PERSONALITY TYPE

The horse needing Vine is one who is thoroughly dominant. He exhibits poor manners when handled, and does not care about any disciplinary consequences. He is often a stallion—an example is the horse that was used for pasture breeding and accustomed to being the undisputed leader of a herd. When this stallion is removed from his herd and used as a show horse, his temperament stays the same and he continues his dominant behavior, biting and kicking at every opportunity. After a few weeks of treatment with Vine this aggressive behavior should decrease and make him easier to handle.

KEY CHARACTERISTICS

Dominant, not caring about the consequences of his behavior.

WHEN TO USE VINE:

- With a horse that demonstrates dominating, or bad, behavior even though he knows that he will be disciplined for it.
- Handling an over-aggressive stallion. However, it will take a few weeks before the behavior will improve.

Walnut (Juglans regia)

PERSONALITY TYPE

The Walnut horse does not adapt quickly to new circumstances or changes in his environment—a new owner, or travel, for example. Using Walnut will help break attachment to old habits so the horse can experience a smooth transition when a change must be made.

KEY CHARACTERISTICS

Does not easily adapt to change.

WHEN TO USE WALNUT:

- A horse goes to a new home or owner.
- You are changing the primary use of the horse. For example, schooling an ex-racehorse to become a riding horse.
- A young horse is having difficulty shedding the caps on his molar and pre-molar teeth. NOTE: This remedy is recommended to help ease teeth problems in general.

Water Violet (Hottonia palustris)

PERSONALITY TYPE

The Water Violet type is associated with a quiet, gentle horse who possesses great tolerance. This is the forgiving, calm horse who safely carries children or inexperienced riders around.

KEY CHARACTERISTICS

Quiet, gentle, and reliable.

WHEN TO USE WATER VIOLET:

- The kind, gentle, tolerant disposition in a horse changes. This can happen, for example, because of illness.

Wild Oat (Bromus ramosus)

PERSONALITY TYPE

The Wild Oat remedy is useful for the horse that shows great promise in his training, but never achieves the high level of performance of which he is capable. Even when changed to a different, usually easier, focus in his training regimen, he still doesn't fulfill his potential. It can be used as a 'cleansing' remedy after using a Bach Flower (or several) and before trying another one.

KEY CHARACTERISTICS

- Unable to perform up to his capabilities.

WHEN TO USE WILD OAT:

- A horse is not training or performing as well as he could.

IV Herbs

In Chapter Three I discussed the use of herbs as an alternative treatment, so please review that information (p. 39), as well as the instructions below, before giving herbs to your horse.

Herbs may be given to horses in their fresh state—just picked—or in dried form. The amount given of each herb varies. I have outlined my recommendations under the individual herb listings below. You add the herb to the horse's feed. (It is useful to have a small scale—similar to a postal scale—for measuring small amounts of herbs.)

You can also give herbs in a liquid form made as a tea from fresh and dried herbs. Herbal teas are often referred to as an infusion, lotion, or brew. The tea is made by putting 2 ounces (about 50 grams) of *fresh* herbs into a saucepan and adding 2 pints (1 liter) of boiling water. If you use *dried* herbs, use only 1 ounce (about 25 grams) to the same amount of boiling water. Cover, and let the tea steep for 20 to 30 minutes. Cool the tea and add it to the horse's feed, or administer by syringe. A standard dose of herbal tea is 1/2 pint (1/4 liter) twice a day.

(See the Poultice Section on p. 157 for use of herbal teas as a compress.)

Some herbs have an unpleasant, bitter taste that horses do not like—even when mixed with food. Mix the herbs well into the grain and, if the horse refuses to eat it, add honey, apple sauce, or extra virgin olive oil. Start with small amounts when adding herbs to a horse's diet to allow his digestive system to adjust gradually. If a side effect such as poor appetite, change in coat color or quality, diarrhea, constipation, or a decrease in water consumption occurs, it is best to stop using the herb until it can be determined if the reaction is caused by the herb or some other problem.

Medicinal herbs should not be used on an ongoing basis because, over time, the body stops responding and the herb becomes less effective. The reasons for the loss of efficacy of a herb that has been used successfully to treat a health problem is not fully understood, but some factors include the type of herb, and the body system it is affecting. Many herbs ultimately create changes at the cellular level; thus the system being stimulated becomes exhausted, and the herb's effectiveness is lost. When the herb is discontinued for a while, the affected cells are able to rest. The herb can then be resumed and is usually effective once again.

For this reason, I suggest discontinuing any medicinal herb after three months. If further treatment is still required, a different herb should be prescribed. Then, if necessary, the first herb can be given again after a two-to-three week break. If only one herb helps your horse with a certain condition, use it for three months then wait at least a one week before starting it again for another three months if necessary.

It is safe to use a mixture of herbs to treat different symptoms of a disease. Some mixtures are commercially available in a premixed blend designed for a specific problem. Mixtures of herbs may also be prescribed for specific problems.

List of Herbs

Aloe Vera

The juice of this plant is used directly on wounds to promote healing; it is also an ingredient in many wound creams. Apply the juice on wounds once a day. Many years ago, aloe was also used to treat horses as a purgative for the digestive tract, particularly in the treatment of parasites. However, the purgative action of this herb is very strong, and it can cause severe muscle spasms even when small amounts are used, so it is rarely used for this purpose today.

Arnica (Arnica montana)

Arnica can be used internally or externally. It is used internally in a homeopathic form, which is discussed in the sections on homeopathy (Chapter Three and Homeopathy Appendix V). As an herb, it is used mainly as an anti-inflammatory lotion (tincture) for bruising or inflamed areas. It is also available in cream, ointment, and balm form. Arnica lotion is used directly on the skin surface over the affected area. Do not use it on irritated skin areas or in open wounds. Arnica lotion can be diluted with water, witch hazel, or alcohol for use as a general rubdown or during a massage. Diluted arnica lotion can also be used as a final rinse to assist in the cooling-down process. For this purpose, add about 2 teaspoons (10ml) of arnica lotion to 1 gallon (4 liters) of water.

Boneset (Eupatorium perfoliatum)

Boneset was used extensively by the North American Indians, and is still included in some modern medications. It can be used as a mild immune system stimulant, a laxative, and a diaphoretic (to increase sweating). Boneset's most popular use is in the treatment of fever—especially a fever associated with some types of influenza. Give 1/4 cup (60ml) of the herb each day. Or, for a fever, make a tea from this daily dose and administer 1/4 cup (60ml) every 30 minutes for 4 doses.

Calendula (Calendula officinalis)

Calendula is used externally as an ointment or cream on injured areas or cuts. A lotion can also be made from the flowers and used to soak sore hooves, bathe swollen areas, or as a compress. To make a calendula lotion, combine about 1/2 cup (125ml) of calendula flowers with 1 pint (1/2 liter) of boiling water and strain it after it has cooled. For internal use, the loose herb is often fed to horses for digestive disorders, lymphatic problems, stress, and urinary infections. It is available in commercial herbal mixes for this purpose.

Cat's Claw (Uncaria tomentosa)

This herb from the Peruvian rainforest is taken orally. It has been widely studied and found to be effective in treating cancer by neutralizing free radicals, stimulating the immune system, as well as inhibiting the growth of some leukemia cells. To date, there are no research studies on the effects of cat's claw in treating horses with cancer. However, I am aware of many cases in which all hope had been lost and cat's claw was used as a last resort with good results. Cat's claw also impedes formation of blood clots and has anti-inflammatory properties. The dosage most often used is about 1/4 ounce (5 to 10 grams) twice a day, added to feed or fed alone if the horse likes it that way. Although cat's claw is considered non-toxic, it has been known to cause diarrhea if the dose is too high. The absorption effect is better on an empty stomach. **Caution:** *Do not give to nursing mares.*

Chamomile, German (Matricaria recutita)

Chamomile is used fresh, as a lotion or tea (you can make your own from the flowers), or dried. The lotion, or tea, can be applied to affected areas—as an anti-inflammatory and pain reducer—or added, as you would a handful of the dried flowers, to the horse's feed daily. In the case of skin allergies, chamomile lotion or tea can be applied as a rinse after a medicated bath, or by itself to help decrease itching and irritation. To make a tea using loose chamomile, add a big handful of chamomile flowers to 2 quarts (2 liters) boiling water. Allow the tea to cool and then strain it through cheesecloth. If using chamomile tea bags, use 4 bags to 2 pints (1 liter) of boiling water. To treat swollen, inflamed eyes, soak a chamomile tea bag in boiling water for 3 minutes, cool until mildly warm, and then apply the tea bag directly on the swollen area over the eye.

Clivers (Cleavers) (Galium aparine)

This herb is most helpful for supporting the lymphatic system and treating skin conditions. It acts as a diuretic and has been used to assist in treating many conditions where swelling is involved such as swollen or stocked-up legs. Clivers is often recommended to help treat bladder infections and bladder stones. It can be given orally in a dosage of 1/2 to 3/4 ounce (15 to 20 grams) twice a day. An infusion or lotion can be used to bathe skin lesions by adding 1 ounce (30 grams) of flowers to 1 pint (1/2 liter) of boiling water and allowing it to cool. Clivers can also be used in a compress.

Comfrey (Symphytum officinale)

Comfrey is most commonly used to treat bruising and connective tissue inflammation and to assist bone healing. The entire plant may be used or just the leaves. The herb is bruised, dipped in boiling water, put in cheesecloth, cooled slightly, and used as a poultice over the affected area. It is also used as a mild expectorant to treat respiratory conditions and is soothing to the digestive tract. When feeding the herb internally, you can give 4 or 5 fresh leaves, 1 ounce (30 grams) of the dried herb twice a day. Or, make a tea to be applied externally (made of 1 ounce of the herb mixed with 2 1/2 cups (1 pint) of boiling water which is steeped until it is cool) twice daily.

Dandelion (Taraxacum officinale)

This herb is useful when treating kidney, liver, and digestive disorders. It acts as a general stimulant, having a mild laxative effect and promoting liver function. Dandelion also serves as a diuretic. Horses have been known to seek out dandelions, particularly the roots which contain the highest amount of active taraxacin, the most effective ingredient in dandelion. The herb contains many vitamins and minerals, with high concentrations of vitamin A and potassium. In her book, *A Modern Horse Herbal*, Hilary Page Self suggests using dandelion as a natural electrolyte since it also contains magnesium and calcium. Feed several handfuls of fresh dandelion leaves or 5 roots a day. If using the dried leaves, feed about 1 ounce (30 grams) a day.

Devil's Claw (Harpogophytum procumbens)

This herb has become increasingly popular as an anti-inflammatory and analgesic. It is most effective when dealing with inflammation associated with bone diseases such as arthritis. (Be warned that this herb may produce a diuretic effect in some cases.) Use 1/2 ounce (15 to 20 grams) of the dried root, once a day. Caution: Do not give to pregnant mares; if the lining of the stomach is irritated or gastric ulcers are present.

Echinacea (Echinacea angustifolia; Echinacea purpurea)

This can be used internally to stimulate the immune system or externally to treat skin conditions topically. Echinacea increases white blood cell production and is very helpful when treating bacterial and viral infections. It can also be used as a stimulant to help protect a horse when there is an outbreak of disease in the area. Dosage is 1/2 to 1 ounce (15 to 30 grams) a day.

Eyebright (Euphrasia officinalis)

Eyebright is a very effective herb used to treat eye conditions such as inflammation and conjunctivitis (an infection in the eye). It also works well for injuries to the eye either as an eyewash or as a compress. To make an eye wash or compress, use 1 ounce (30 grams) of the herb added to 2 1/2 cups (500 ml) of boiling water. Allow the herb to steep for about 15 minutes, then strain out the herb and keep the liquid to use for treatments. The herb can also be given internally by adding 1 ounce (30 grams) a day to the feed. Eyebright is also available in a homeopathic form.

Fenugreek (Trigonella foenum-graecum)

This herb is often used as an appetite stimulant; but it also helps to improve a horse's general condition. It is sometimes added to disguise the taste of feed. Fenugreek is high in nutrients, particularly iron in a form that is easily absorbed by the digestive tract. The steroidal saponins it contains work well in animals to treat diabetic conditions and lower cholesterol levels. Since these saponins are similar to hormones, it is not advisable to feed them to horses suspected of having hormonal imbalances. Dosage is 1 ounce (30 grams) once a day. Fenugreek complements garlic and works well when fed along with it.

Garlic (Allium sativum)

This well-known herb can be used as an expectorant or a diuretic, or to promote sweating. It also has some antibiotic-like properties. Garlic is also fed to assist in treatment of respiratory infections, especially when mucus is present. The oil of garlic contains a form of sulfur that is excreted through the skin after garlic is eaten; the sulfur is responsible for the odor associated with those who eat it regularly. Sulfur is probably the ingredient responsible for deterring insects as well as the antiseptic or antibiotic-like properties attributed to garlic. Feed 5 to 10 freshly crushed cloves daily, or give 1/2 to 1 ounce (15 to 30 grams) of pure garlic powder daily. Another form of garlic is a concentrated aged garlic extract such as Kyolic. Some research indicates that aged garlic is superior for several reasons. Raw garlic contains a harsh, irritating compound called allicin, which can lead to gastrointestinal disorders, damage of the stomach lining, diarrhea, and anemia. The aging process eliminates these irritating effects and potential toxic properties. Another advantage of using a product like this is the uniformity of its biological value versus that of raw garlic that varies from crop to crop. Of course, when using the aged garlic you will lose out on the insect-deterring effects of raw garlic that were mentioned above. Use 1/4 ounce (5 to 10 grams) a day when feeding an aged garlic product.

Goldenseal (Hydrastis canadensis)

Goldenseal is used mainly to treat digestive disorders. The alkaloids it contains act as a laxative and are very soothing on mucus membranes. It is frequently included in herbal tonic mixtures for older horses because it stimulates the digestive system and soothes the stomach. Goldenseal can also be combined with water and used to wash ulcerated areas in the mouth. ***Caution:*** *Do not use this herb in horses without the guidance of a vet. It is poisonous if fed in too high a dosage.*

Kelp (Fucus vesiculosus)

Also known as bladderwrack, kelpware, or seawrack, this plant of the sea is used to help strengthen the body. Kelp contains iodine, sodium, and potassium as well as other elements and is helpful to support the thyroid and treat some arthritic conditions. It is usually given internally, but it can also be used as a compress to help reduce inflammation of soft tissue or bone. Feed 1/2 to 1 ounce (15 to 30 grams) in the feed daily. If your horse is being treated with pharmaceutical drugs for a thyroid condition, consult your vet before feeding kelp since the dosage of his thyroid medication may need to be monitored and perhaps altered.

Lavender (Lavendula angustifolia)

The oil of this fragrant herb has anti-microbial properties and is used in two ways. A few drops can be added to water and used as a wash to clean out wounds. In France, it is also used in this way to treat parasites on animals. As an aromatherapy, lavender is used to treat fatigue and depression, as well as to promote relaxation. (For instructions on how to use aromatherapy, see Appendix II.) In the past, lavender was given internally to horses to decrease gas and muscle spasms from colic, but many horses do not react well to lavender, and the dosage is unreliable so it is no longer used internally. Caution: If using lavender oil as aromatherapy during a competition, do not use it directly on the horse or allow the horse to ingest or lick the oil. It may cause an interaction and test false positive in a drug test.

Licorice (Glycyrrhiza glabra)

The dried root of this herb found in Europe and Asia has been used for thousands of years as an expectorant to treat coughs, and a demulcent to reduce gastric acid secretions. Another type of licorice, known as wild licorice, or American sarsaparilla, is found in the US. The root is used to treat respiratory diseases, and the leaves are used for skin lesions. (***Caution:*** *Do not give to pregnant mares as it may affect hormone levels. Do not give to horses with heart, lymph, or circulatory problems as it may affect potassium levels.*) Give 1/4 to 1/2 ounce (7 to 15 grams) daily.

Marshmallow (Althea officinalis)

This herb is effective in treating digestive and urinary disorders that involve inflammation or irritation. It contains mucilage that is very soothing, particularly to gastric ulcers, inflammation, and cystitis. Marshmallow can be fed on a regular basis to horses prone to frequent colic episodes and to horses with cystitis. It is also used as an external poultice for bruises, sprains, and skin inflammations. Powdered marshmallow is the easiest form to use for making a poultice, or when adding to the feed. Feed 1/2 ounce (15 grams) of the powdered herb a day. If you are using the dried root, best results can be obtained by boiling 4 ounces (110 grams) in 5 pints (2 1/2 liters) of water until it is reduced to 3 pints (1 1/2 liters) of water. Cool and strain the liquid. Use it as a poultice, or feed 1/2 to 1 ounce (15 to 30 grams) a day.

Meadowsweet (Filipendula ulmaria)

Meadowsweet is used to treat inflammation, reduce fevers, as an antiseptic, and a diuretic. It is also particularly helpful for treating diarrhea, since it coats the digestive tract and has astringent properties. For the best results, the entire plant should be used, not just certain parts. This herb contains salicylic acid, tannins, and mucilage. It can be used in treating conditions for which aspirin might be prescribed without the gastric irritation that can result from aspirin. Meadowsweet can be fed in the fresh form, cut up, dried, or made into a liquid. The dosage for the fresh herb is 1/4 to 1/2 cup of chopped herb a day. If giving the dried herb, feed 1/2 to 1 ounce (15 to 30 grams) a day. It can be made into a liquid by boiling 1 ounce (30 grams) of the dried herb in 2 pints (1 liter) of water for 5 minutes. Then allow it to cool, strain, and give 1/2 to 1 pint (1/4 to 1/2 liter) a day).

Nettle (Urtica dioica)

In the past, nettle was sometimes used as a component of the daily horse feed, and it is still fed in the spring to stimulate and cleanse the horse's body in many areas of the world. Its primary use today, however, is as a medicinal herb to treat bronchial and asthmatic problems. Because it stimulates circulation, it is used to treat navicular disease and laminitis too. Nettle is also popular as a tonic to treat anemia because it contains vitamin C, phosphates, and sodium. In addition, nettle is used as a conditioner because it produces a shiny dappled coat when fed regularly. Nettle stings when touched, so take care if you pick it fresh to feed to your horse. Set the fresh nettle in the sun for an hour or so and the stinging property will go away. Fresh nettle can be fed separately in small amounts, or added to the feed—give several handfuls a day. If fresh nettle is unavailable, dried nettle can be used. Give 1/2 to 1 ounce (15 to 30 grams) of the dried herb daily. (**Caution:** *Some horses have a hive-like reaction of small raised areas on the skin when fed nettle. This problem usually goes away in a day. If a horse has this reaction to nettle, discontinue feeding it.*)

Pau d'Arco (Tabecuia impetiginosa)

This herb stimulates new cell growth and can be used to treat many problems such as wounds, fungal infections, bacterial infections, anemia, and cancer. Other effects of this herb are appetite stimulation and relief from pain. Pau d'Arco is often included in herbal tonics for horses because it promotes red blood cell production and generally makes horses feel better. Best results for disease treatment are seen following 10 to 15 days of treatment. A holistic vet should be consulted to determine the proper dosage and length of treatment since both vary depending on the problem being treated.

Raspberry (Rubus idaeus)

The leaves of the raspberry bush are usually used for treating mares during and after pregnancy to tone the uterine muscles and reduce the chance of hemorrhage occurring. The fruit, when made into syrup, can be used to help reduce fever, treat a sore throat, and dissolve tarter from teeth. And cold raspberry tea is an effective treatment for diarrhea, mild stomach spasms, and mouth ulceration. Add 1 ounce (30 grams) of leaves to the feed daily. Make raspberry syrup by mixing 2 lbs (900 grams) of berries, with 2 1/2 cups (500 ml) of white wine vinegar, then sealing the mix in an airtight container for 5 days. Mix 1 ounce (30 grams) of this with 1 1/4 cups (300ml) of water and give orally twice a day, or to get rid of tarter, apply the mixture on a toothbrush and brush daily. Raspberry tea is made by steeping 1 ounce (30 grams) of leaves in 2 1/2 cups (600ml) water and adding to horse's feed once a day.

St. John's Wort (Hypericum perforatum)

For horses, this herb is only used externally. The flowers are used to make an oil for treating inflamed areas on the skin. Always dilute the oil or tincture, using only a few drops to a bowl of water to wash a wound. St. John's Wort should not be given internally because it causes photosensitivity in horses. Horses that consume St. John's Wort often break out on their white-colored hair areas with wounds that look like sunburn.

Slippery Elm (Ulmus rubra; Ulmus fulva)

This herb is used internally to treat gastric inflammation, colic, and diarrhea. Its high mucilage content helps to coat and soothe the digestive tract. Slippery elm is frequently mixed with yogurt and given to foals suffering from diarrhea. Dosage of the powdered herb is 2 to 4 tablespoons a day. Use the lower dosage for foals. Externally, slippery elm is useful to treat wounds and inflamed or infected areas in a poultice form. To make a poultice, mix the herb with boiling water until a paste is formed, allow it to cool slightly, then apply directly on the affected area, and cover with a bandage. For the best result, change the poultice every 2 hours.

Tea Tree Oil (Melaleuca alternifolia)

This oil has become a common ingredient in many horse products. It can be helpful when treating bacterial and fungal skin infections, and it also repels insects. Tea tree oil has also been used as an essential oil (see Aromatherapy Appendix II) and as a component of massage oil for strained muscles. **Caution:** *Never use pure tea tree oil on a horse. I recommend using great care when using products containing tea tree oil since many horses react to it by blistering on the skin where it is applied. This frequently occurs even when tea tree oil is applied in a very dilute form. Always try any product containing tea tree oil on a small area first and wait about 30 minutes to see if the horse has a reaction to it before continuing to apply the product.*

Valerian (Valerian officinalis)

The cut or powdered root of this herb is used for medicinal purposes with horses, mainly to calm the nervous system, thus acting as a sedative. It is particularly useful as a sedative because when correctly dosed it does not affect a horse's ability to think and perform. It is also an effective antispasmodic and laxative, and can help to relieve stomach spasms, flatulence, constipa-tion, as well as bronchial conditions. Give 1/2 ounce (15 grams) daily.

Witch Hazel (Hamamelis virginiana)

This well-known herb is used to control hemor-rhage, both internal and external; to treat gastric upsets, insect bites, and burns; and as a com-press for eye inflammation. It is a handy reme-dy to keep on hand to control bleeding of minor injuries and to provide relief for injured, swollen eyes. When witch hazel is properly prepared, it contains tannins, which seem to act on the veins to reduce bleeding. However, preparation of true witch hazel distillate, extract, or oint-ment, is time consuming. As a result, most com-mercially available witch hazel is prepared using a process that removes the tannins. If possible, get witch hazel from a herbalist who prepares it in the proper manner.

Yucca (Yucca filamentosa)

Yucca contains saponin and is used as a stimu-lant as well as a treatment for arthritic condi-tions. It is readily available as a commercially prepared product or can be bought from herbal suppliers. I recommend using the yucca powder or liquid form (dose according to label direc-tions) over the pelleted variety. The powder (2 teaspoons daily) is more pure than the pellets and has a higher amount of saponin in it. The liquid contains a consistently high quantity of saponin and is easy for the horse to digest and assimilate. If you cannot find pure yucca, buy powder that is not "clumping" and is labeled as at least 75 percent pure and give according to label directions. NOTE: Yucca may test "false-positive" in a drug test.

Yunnan Paiyao

This Chinese patent herb is very effective in controlling hemorrhage, even in cases of severe injury. For short-term use it is safe. However, do not use this herb for more than two weeks since it can cause permanent kidney damage. It is available as liquid or capsules. In most cases 1 ounce (30 grams) should be given orally once a day, but in cases of severe hemorrhage, the dose can be repeated in 4 hours for a total of 2 doses in one day. The liquid dose is 1 fluid ounce (28ml) orally; capsule dose is 4 capsules.

V Homeopathics

I discussed homeopathy at some length in Chapter Three (p. 40) so please review that section before using any of the remedies I list below.

Homeopathic remedies come in pills or liquid form, with pills being the most common. Since homeopathic pills are usually made with a sugar base, most horses eat them readily. Alternatively, pills can be dissolved in 1 tablespoon (15ml) of water and then given the same way as a liquid homeopathic.

Liquid homeopathics can be given using a syringe in the mouth. Always administer a homeopathic remedy with a clean syringe and use that syringe for administering that specific homeopathic medicine. Clean after each use. Replace it with a new sterile one for each different remedy you administer.

I find a syringe easier, but many horses are difficult to medicate this way. If your horse objects, put the remedy in the grain. Although some veterinary homeopaths feel that homeopathics should not be given at the same time as food, many horses will not take them any other way. Personally, I have found similar efficacy whether homeopathics are given separately, or with food. On the other hand, I have noticed poor efficacy with homeopathics when they are given to horses that struggle a lot when medicated. I have not seen any studies on this issue but I theorize that the decreased efficacy could result from a physiological change caused by the release of epinephrine (adrenaline) during the struggle.

Liquid homeopathics may also be dropped on to a sugar cube (or cubes) and administered easily this way.

In between uses of homeopathics, store them carefully. Homeopathic remedies are sensitive to light, heat, and microwaves. Keep them in a cool dry place, out of direct sunlight. Do not leave them in your car, briefcase, or bag, where temperatures may rise. Keep lids on tightly so they will not absorb moisture, which could change the potency or strength of the medication. Before using a homeopathic liquid, check the bottle to make sure no contamination has occurred. Hold the bottle up to the light and look for floating flakes or debris that indicate that the bottle is no longer usable.

Unlike other medications, there are two factors to consider when using homeopathics—potency and dosage. As I discussed in Chapter Three, potency refers to the level of dilution of the remedy. Dosage refers to the amount of the remedy and the frequency in which it is given. There are many different brands of homeopathics so I recommend following the dosage suggested on the label. If you are using homeopathics packaged for humans, find the recommended dosage for an adult human on the label and multiply it by 10 for a 1,000-pound (approx. 450 kgs) horse.

Specific homeopathic recommendations are listed in Part Three, the *Horse Ailments* section of this book. While I suggest potencies, remember that these are just guidelines. If you are unable to obtain the suggested potency, it is more important that the horse receive the homeopathic medication than it is to give exactly the same potency I recommend. However, when prescribing homeopathics yourself, you should remember to give only the lower potencies (no higher than 30c). When using the lower potencies, there is a good safety margin so that you can't hurt your horse if you select the incorrect homeopathic. With the higher potencies, such as 200c or 1M, the incorrect remedy could cause harm. A higher potency should be prescribed by a homeopathic vet.

(NOTE: I have suggested remedies with higher potencies in a couple of cases in Part Three. These cases are exceptions to the rule. And, for a few other health problems, I have recommended a higher potency but ask that you check with a homeopathic vet before giving the remedy.)

Homeopathics have a wide range of application. The homeopathics listed are not limited to the uses mentioned here.

Caution: *Homeopathic remedies should only be given one at a time unless otherwise indicated.*

List of Homeopathics

Aconitum Napellus

Often used in horses to treat influenza and respiratory problems. Also used to treat hoof problems, particularly laminitis and inflammation of the coffin joint. Use three times a day, though if necessary in acute cases, you can start by repeating the dosage every 30 minutes for up to 6 doses in acute cases. Low potencies of 3c or 6c work well in most cases. In severe cases, 30c can be used. It is sometimes effective with mild gas colic, but check with a homeopathic vet before treating.

Antimonium Crudum

Used in horses to treat hives. Works best when symptoms include itching, irritability, and restlessness, and when bathing with hot or cold water aggravates hives. Use 6c potency three to four times a day.

Apis Mellifica

Works well on cases involving swelling or edema. Very effective in reactions to insect bites or hives that involve itching. Also helps treat joint and tendon problems with swelling and sensitivity. Use 3c or 6c potencies. For insect reactions and hives, dose four times a day. For other situations dose three times daily. Urination may increase because apis acts as a mild diuretic.

Arnica Montana

Used in cases of injury where inflammation and bruising are present. This excellent anti-inflammatory can be used in low potencies of 12X or 30X, or 6c to 30c, for minor injuries two to three times a day. For more severe cases, high potencies of 1M to 50M may be prescribed by your homeopathic vet.

Arsenicum Album

Used to treat injuries involving the lower limbs when swelling and muscle spasms are involved.

Allergies that cause coughing and itching, and burning skin with rough, scaly patches also often respond well to this remedy. Use 30C potency twice a day.

Belladonna

Most commonly used in horses to treat very painful colic involving muscle spasms and gas. Also used to treat laminitis when the pulse in the leg is greatly elevated. Use 30C potency every 30 minutes for 3 dosages, then follow up three times a day. Check with your homeopathic vet before using for colic.

Bryonia

This remedy is particularly effective when treating respiratory conditions involving coughing such as Chronic Obstructive Pulmonary Disease (COPD). Bryonia is also used to treat liver conditions, especially those in which the liver is enlarged and pain is present. It is used in cases where arthritis is affecting the legs from the knees to the hooves, and heat and/or swelling is present. Mares suffering from ovulation pain often respond well to Bryonia as well as mares that are irritable during estrus. Can be used to ease discomfort in mares with distended painful mammary glands. Use potencies of 3C, 6C or 12C two to three times a day.

Calcarea Carbonica

This is a very useful remedy for horses, especially when treating digestive disorders. Use it when a horse has a history of mild digestive upsets that occasionally progress into a minor colic. Horses that respond best to Calcarea carbonica often eat dirt, manure, or sand; consume a lot of salt; and will sometimes lose their appetites when stressed or over-exercised. These horses will often refuse warm mashes (such as bran mash), eating them only when the mash has cooled. Calcarea Carbonica can also help horses that rub their tails. Use it as a remedy when you cannot pinpoint any other cause for this. The usual potency is 6C or 12C twice a day. This remedy can also be used to help calm a horse, but should not be given on a constant basis for that purpose. Use for calming 3 days at a time, three to four times a day in the 30C potency.

Calcarea Fluorica

Made from fluoride of lime, this remedy is most often used with horses for problems associated with the feet. Use it to treat navicular disease and pedal osteitis (inflammation of the coffin bone). Also used to treat cases of thrombus. Do not use Calcarea Fluorica excessively; a potency of 3C given once a week for 4 to 6 weeks is sufficient.

Carbo Vegetabilis

Made from vegetable charcoal, this remedy is used most commonly for digestive problems in horses. It works well when colic occurs after exercise or is caused by excessive gas. It is useful when the horse's manure is odd smelling, or has an unpleasant odor. It is also helpful for treating frequent nosebleeds that originate from the nose or sinus region. Chronic gum infections also respond well to Carbo Vegetabilis. Use a potency of 3C to 12C for acute conditions and 30C for chronic conditions, twice a day.

Eyebright (Euphrasia)

Used to treat inflammation of the eye. This homeopathic form of the herb eyebright works well in treating chronic conjunctivitis, and is available in a commercial form that is put directly onto the eyes. Use the oral form in a potency of 3C to 12C twice a day. Use the commercial form for direct eye application according to directions.

Hekla Lava

This is an excellent remedy for horses with hoof problems associated with bone abnormalities such as arthritis and navicular disease. Also used to treat ringbone. Hekla Lava is particularly effective when treating problems affecting the jaw and sinus areas, such as pain caused from an infected molar. Use a potency of 3C or 6C three times a day.

Hepar Sulphuris Calcareum

Used to treat problems associated with the hoof, mainly navicular disease, pedal osteitis, and joint inflammation in the fetlock, pastern, or hoof. This remedy is also useful in the treatment of chronic ulcers on the cornea of the eye. Low potencies of 6C or 12C are most often used in horses twice a day.

Hypericum

Made from the herb St. John's Wort. This remedy works well when treating injuries to nerves. It reduces pain and promotes healing and is frequently used following surgery or to relieve spasms following an injury. Puncture wounds and bite wounds respond well to treatment with Hypericum. Use a potency of 3C or 6C three times a day.

Ipecacuanha

Used for digestive upsets, particularly colic and diarrhea. Cases in which it is most effective are those that involve spasmodic colic. Often in these cases the abdominal pain will cause the horse to stretch his hind legs out behind him. Diarrhea symptoms that are helped with Ipecacuanha are extreme straining with pain, accompanied by no appetite or thirst. This remedy works well alone for digestive upsets or when combined with Calcarea Carbonica or Carbo Vegetabilis. Use a potency of 30C. A higher potency may be prescribed by a homeopathic vet.

Kali Bichromicum

Use to relieve discomfort from gastric ulcers. An overly nervous or stressed horse with a chronic case of gastric ulcers may respond well to this remedy. Kali Bichromicum is also help to treat a stiff horse whose joints are audible when he moves. Use 3C, 6C, 12C, or 30C two or three times a day. This homeopathic does not store well, so keep out of extreme heat and cold. If you purchase it in liquid form be sure that the liquid is clear before you administer it.

Lachesis

Used in horses for injuries, particularly those involving excessive hemorrhaging or bite wounds. Occasionally this remedy helps foals with a tendency toward contracted tendons. For emergencies, use 6C or 12C in one single dose. For severe hemorrhaging, up to 200C can be used in a single dose. For foals with contracted tendons, use one dose of 3C once a week for three weeks.

Ledum

Very effective for treating puncture wounds and spider bites. Use 6C, 12C or 30C three to four times daily.

Lycopodium

Frequently used in horses to treat respiratory infections, especially those with a cough or involving pneumonia. Works particularly well in cases that are worse from 4 pm to 8 pm. Use a potency of 6C or 12C once a day.

Magnesia Phosphorica (Tissue Salt No. 8)

Used mainly to treat muscle spasms. Muscle spasms associated with nerve inflammation such as sciatica, respond particularly well. It can be combined with other remedies, such as Arnica, to treat injuries or with some of the colic remedies such as Carbo Vegetabilis to help spasmodic colics. Use a potency of 6C or 12C up to three times a day.

Nux Vomica

This remedy is useful for horses who are very sensitive to change, such as a horse who becomes nervous when moved to new surroundings or when going to a show. It is also helpful for horses that don't eat well when nervous. Nux Vomica helps treat the liver and is indicated as the first remedy to use when liver enzymes are elevated. It can be helpful in supporting liver functions when a horse has a chronic illness, such as cancer. Nux Vomica is also helpful following severe stress. Useful for mild colic but check with your homeopathic vet first. Use a potency of 6C, 12C, or 30C two times a day.

Phosphorus

Horses are very responsive to this remedy for a variety of problems. It is used to slow hemorrhaging and is effective for this purpose when injuries occur or if surgery must be performed. Phosphorus supports the liver and is one of the most effective remedies to treat respiratory viruses in horses. Even chronic respiratory cases often respond well to Phosphorus. This remedy is also useful to treat pulmonary hemorrhage. Use a potency of 6C, 12C or 30C twice a day, except in the case of hemorrhage when phosphorus should be given every 15 minutes up to a total of 6 doses.

Podophyllum

Works well in horses with diarrhea that contains mucus but is not associated with pain. Some horses with intermittent diarrhea respond well to this remedy. Use a potency of 6C twice a day. If treating a foal, use 30C twice a day.

Psorium

Used in horses to treat irritated gums or around sore teeth. Psorium is occasionally effective with horses that have a dry cough that recurs seasonally. It can be used in tincture form to rub sparingly on the affected gum area. When treating a cough, your homeopathic vet may suggest a high potency such as 200C or higher, given once every 2 weeks.

Rhus Toxicodendron

Some cases of arthritis respond very well to this remedy, especially when there is swelling and heat associated. This remedy can be used to treat scar tissue so it is often a good preventive treatment following injuries or surgery. Rhus Toxicodendron can improve some neurological conditions and sometimes help symptoms associated with Equine Protozoal Myeloencephalitis (EPM). Use a potency of 3C twice a day for arthritic symptoms. Use 3C, 6C, or 12C twice a day for scar tissue. A potency of 30C given two to three times a day works best for neurological conditions.

Ruta Graveolens

Used to treat conditions involving joint inflammation, sprains, or bone bruises. It is very effective as a follow-up treatment to Arnica for treating sprains or bruises. Injuries involving the flexor tendons respond especially well to this remedy. Use a potency of 3C or 6C twice a day.

Silicea

This remedy can be used to treat a variety of problems in horses. It is frequently used when pain is associated with the knees. Other conditions that respond well are fistulous withers and chronic abscesses. Horses with a tissue reaction or damage from a vaccination may be helped by this remedy. Use a potency of 6C, 12C, or 30C twice a day.

Sulfur

This remedy can be very effective for respiratory and liver problems. Respiratory conditions that respond best to sulfur are those involving a productive cough with a purulent discharge from the nose. A fever may be present and breathing may be difficult when lying down. Use this remedy with caution—it is best by a homeopathic vet. If that is not possible, use a low potency such as 6C, once a day.

Thuja Occidentalis

This remedy works well when treating warts and some tumors. Consult a homeopathic vet about using Thuja to treat a tumor. Some tumors that respond well to this remedy are those on pedicles or stalks and those that are soft and spongy. Significant improvement of symptoms can occur when Thuja is added to the treatment for Lyme Disease and periodic ophthalmia. Treatment for warts can include both the tincture form on the warts and the homeopathic form orally. Potencies to use are 3C, 6C, 12C, or 30C two or three times a day.

Urtica Urens

This remedy works well for problems originating in the spleen, particularly immune-system reactions. It is also used to treat hives, especially cases that return at the same time every year. Urtica is helpful in reducing the flow of milk after weaning in mares that are not drying up quickly. This remedy is effective when treating a herpes virus that has been suppressed and is causing muscle soreness. Use a potency of 3C or 6C once or twice a day.

Other Homeopathic Products

BHI, a company based in Germany, markets homeopathic products throughout Europe and the United States. They publish their own guide *Materia Medica* for the use and applications of their products. Products that are particularly effective for horses are BHI Arthritis and BHI Zeel, both of which treat bone problems by relieving symptoms and encouraging healing. These products are a mix of homeopathic remedies that are effective for this purpose. Another product, BHI Traumeel, is a cream that works well as an anti-inflammatory. Although very effective, it can be messy to use over large areas.

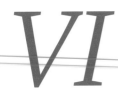

VI Product Suppliers

Please note: At the time of this writing, the companies listed below supply one or more products that are acceptable within the guidelines of this book. This does not necessarily mean that the authors recommend all products made by, or sold by, these companies.

Product quality can change from year to year; companies can change management or policies or standards. We urge you to keep this in mind, to be continually alert, and to read labels and product brochures carefully, even for products you have been using for a long time.

There may be other fine suppliers or new companies not listed here. Our not listing certain suppliers does not necessarily mean that we wouldn't recommend them if we knew about them.

USA

Advanced Biological Concepts
301 Main Street, PO Box 27
Osco, IL 61274
Tel: 800-373-5971, Fax: 309-522-5570
Web: www.a-b-c-plus.com
E-mail: helfter@netexpress.com
Excellent source for electrolytes; free-choice trace minerals; clay-based poultices with herbs; vitamins (including Ester C); herbal mixes; salts; yucca; MSM; antioxidants (including coenzyme Q10); biotin and methionine; and colloidal silver.

Arbico Environmentals
18701 North Lago Del Oro Parkway
Tucson, AZ 85739
Tel: 520-825-9785, Fax: 520-825-2038.
Web: www.arbico.com
E-mail: info@arbico.com
Specialize in environmentally sound pest control using beneficial insects.

Avena Botanicals
219 Mill Street
Rockport, ME 04865
Tel: 207-594-0694
Web: www.avenaherbs.com
E-mail: avena@avenaherbs.com
Herbs offered in various preparations, including Heal-All Salve; some homeopathic remedies

Bio-Magnetic Resources

539 Accord Station
Accord, MA 02018-0539
Tel: 800-890-3618
Web: www.biomagnetic.com
E-mail: customerservice@biomagnetic.com
Manufacture alternative health care and oriental medicine supplies.

BioScan

6 Walden Road
Carrales, NM 87048
Tel: 800-388-2712, Fax: 505-867-6102
Web: www.bioscanlight.com
E-mail: info@bioscanlight.com
Carry a line of products that combine light therapy with magnetic pulsation to detect and treat a variety of health problems.

Bio-Vet Inc.

PO Box 155
Baraboo, WI 53913
Tel: 800-246-8381, Fax: 608-356-7882
Web: www.bio-vet.com
E-mail: Bio-Vet@sauk.com
Makers of microbial supplements.

Chamisa Ridge, Inc.

PO Box 23294
Santa Fe, NM 87502
Tel: 800-743-3188
Web: www.chamisaridge.com
E-mail: info@chamisaridge.com
Carry a line of natural horse care products; Hilton Herbs; Bach Flower Essences—including Rescue Remedy; colloidal silver; probiotics; essential oils for aromatherapy; and homeopathics.

DAC

Direct Action Company
PO Box 2205
Dover, OH 44622
Tel: 800-921-9121
Web: web.tusco.net/dac
E-mail: dac@tusco.net
Manufacturers of vitamins, minerals, oils, yucca, digestive aids, electrolyte mixes, biotin, glucosamine, chondroitin, and other custom horse supplements.

Dr. Brennan's Equine Emergency Homeopathic Kit

965 Bobcat Court
Marietta, GA 30067
Tel: 770-612-0318
A selection of homeopathic remedies for emergency care of horses.

A Drop in the Bucket

586 Round Hill Rd.
Greenwich, CT 06831
Tel: 888-783-0313, Fax: 203-625-8345
Web: www.bucket.simplenet.com
E-mail: bucket586@aol.com
Carry herbs, herbal mixtures, homeopathics, flower essences, lasers, natural insect repellents, probiotics, and preparations containing glucosamine, chondroitin, MSM, yucca, coenzyme Q10, and shark cartilage.

Ellon Botanicals, Inc.

401 Kings Highway
Winona Lake, IN 46590
Tel: 800-4-BE-CALM
Web: www.ellonbotanicals.com
Manufacturers and distributors of the Bach Flower remedies, including Rescue Remedy (Calming Essence).

Equilite

20 Prospect Avenue
Ardsley, NY 10502
Tel: 914-693-2553, Fax: 914-693-4956
Web: www.equilite.com
E-mail: info@equilite.com
Source of probiotics; supplements containing chondroitin, glucosamine, shark cartilage, and garlic; herbal poultices, flower essences; and homeopathics.

Health Freedom Resources

1533 Long Street
Clearwater, FL 33755
Tel: 727-443-7711, Fax: 727-442-4139
Web: www.healthfree.com
E-mail: healthfree@healthfree.com
Source of Flora Source (an acidophilus supplement), herbal first aid salves, and herbal poultices.

Heel Inc.

11600 Cochiti, SE
Albuquerque, NM 87123
Tel: 800-621-7644
Fax: 505-275-0578
Web: www.heelbhi.com
Manufacturer of the BHI (Biological Homeopathic Industries) product line that includes BHI Traumeel, BHI Arthritis, and BHI Zeel.

Hilton Herbs (see UK list and Chamisa Ridge entry above)

Jerry Teplitz Enterprises, Inc.

228 North Donnawood Drive, Ste. 204
Virginia Beach, VA 23452
Tel: 800-77-RELAX , Fax: 757-431-1503
Web: www.teplitz.com
E-mail: teplitz@compuserve.com
Carry books, tapes, and other products on stress reduction.

Kyolic Garlic

Wakunaga of America Co., Ltd.
23501 Madero
Mission Viejo, CA 92691
Tel: 800-421-2998, Fax: 949-458-2764
Web: www.kyolic.com
Manufacturer high-potency garlic in capsule, tablet, and liquid forms.

Morinda Inc.

Tel: 800-445-8596
Web: www.tahitian-juice.com
Source of Tahitian Noni.

Morrills' New Directions

21 Market Square
Houlton, ME 04730
Tel: 800-368-5057; in Maine, call 800-649-0744
Web: www.morrills.com
E-mail: morrills@ainop.com
Carry MSM, coenzyme Q-10, acidophilus, Ester C, glucosamine, chondroitin, shark cartilage, colloidal minerals, homeopathics, Bach Flower Remedies, herbal preparations, natural pest controls, and other natural care and grooming products.

NaturVet

Garmon Corporation
27461-B Diaz Road
Temecula, CA 92590
Tel: 888-628-8783, Fax: 909-695-2978
Web: www.naturvet.com
E-mail: naturvet@naturvet.com
Manufacture a variety of supplements including glucosamine, chondroitin, MSM, and yucca.

Nelson Bach USA, Ltd.
Wilmington Technology Park
100 Research Drive
Wilmington, MA 01887-4406
Tel: 800-319-9151, Fax: 978-988-0233
Web: www.nelsonbach.com
E-mail: info@nelsonbach.com
Manufacture and distribute Bach Flower Remedies, including Rescue Remedy, homeopathics, and aromatherapy products.

Norfields
632 3/4 N. Doheny Drive
Los Angeles, CA 90069
Tel: 800-344-8400, Fax: 310-278-4170
Web: www.norfields.com
E-mail: info@norfields.com
Manufacture magnetic health care products.

Nutramax Laboratories
2208 Lakeside Blvd.
Edgewood, MD 21040
Tel: 800-925-5187
Web: www.nutramaxlabs.com
Makers of Cosequin® (contains glucosamine and chondroitin) and Comal®Q10 (coenzyme Q10).

Nutribiotic, Inc.
133 Copeland St.
Suite C
Petaluma, CA 94952
Tel: 707-263-0411
Web: www.nutribiotic.com
E-mail: info@nutribiotic.com
Makers of Citricidal (an extract of the pulp, seed, and inner rind of grapefruit) products for disinfection and control of intestinal parasites.

Respond Systems
20 Baldwin Drive
Branford, CT 06405
Tel: 800-722-1228, Fax: 203-481-2456
Web: www.respondsystems.com
E-mail: doreen@respondsystems.com
Manufactures pulse magnetic field therapy units and laser therapy equipment.

The Vitamin Shoppe
4700 Westside Avenue
North Bergen, NJ 07047
Tel: 888-880-3055, Fax: 800-852-7153
Web: www.vitaminshoppe.com
E-mail: clarify@vitaminshoppe.com.
Carry vitamins, herbs, homeopathics, and Bach Flower remedies at discounted prices.

Vitamins.com
2924 Telestar Court
Falls Church, VA 22042
Tel: 800-741-8273
Web: www.vitamins.com
E-mail: feedback@vitamins.com
Carry natural supplements, herbs, homeopathics, and Bach Flower remedies.

Zand Herbal Formulas
1722 14th St., Ste. 230
Boulder, CO 80302
Tel: 800-371-8420
Web: www.zand.com
E-mail: info@zandboulder.com
Manufactures herbal formulas for animals and people.

UK

Aero Marketing
3 Squires Close
Somersham
Cambs PE28 3HT
Tel: 01487 841055
Aerobic oxygen supplies.

Ainsworths Homeopathic Pharmacy
36 New Cavendish Street
London W1M 7LH
Tel: 0207 935 5330
Fax: 0207 486 4313
Web: www.ainsworths.com
Homeopathic remedies.

Animal Alternatives
PO Box 289
Richmond
Surrey TW10 7XH
Tel: 0208 940 3725
Fax: 0208 332 2054
E-mail: info@animal-alternatives.co.uk
Web: www.animal-alternatives.co.uk
Nutraceuticals and probiotics.

Bayhouse Aromatics
St George's Road
Brighton
West Sussex
BN2 1EE
Tel: 01273 601109
Fax: 01273 601174
Aromatherapy supplies.

Bee Health Ltd
Sneatondale Honey Farm
Race Course Road
East Ayton
Scarborough YO13 9HT
Tel: 01723 864001
Fax: 01723 862455
Bee health products based on propolis.

Bio Pathica
PO Box 217
Ashford
Kent TN23 6ZU
Tel: 01233 636678
Fax: 01233 638380
Heel and BHI homeopathic products.

The Dr Edward Bach Centre
Mount Vernon
Sotwell
Wallingford
Oxon
OX10 0PZ
Tel: 01491 834678
Bach flower remedies; information and education.

Cloudcraft Books
16 Wheelers Walk
Pagan Hill
Stroud
Glos GL5 4BW
Tel/Fax: 01453 753403
Book supplier specialising in holistic horse care and training.

East West Herbs Ltd
Langston Priory Mews
Kingham
Oxon OX7 6UP
Tel: 01608 658862
Fax: 01608 658816
E-mail: office@eastwestherbs.co.uk
Web: www.eastwestherbs.com
Dried herbs, herbal tinctures, Chinese herbs.

The Fragrant Earth Company Ltd
Orchard Court
Magdalene Street
Glastonbury
Somerset BA6 9EW
Tel: 01458 831216
Fax: 01458 831361
E-mail: all-enquiries@fragrant-earth.com
Web: www.fragrant-earth.com
Aromatherapy supplies.

Galen Homeopathics

Lewell Mill
West Stafford
Dorchester
Dorset DT2 8AN
Tel: 01305 263996
Fax: 01305 250792
Homeopathic remedies.

Helios Homeopathic Pharmacy and Manufacturers

89-97 Camden Road
Tunbridge Wells
Kent TN1 2QR
Tel: 01892 537254/536393 (24 hours)
Fax: 01892 546850
E-mail: pharmacy@helios.co.uk
Web: www.helios.co.uk
Homeopathic remedies.

Herbal Apothecary

103 High Street
Syston
Leicester LE7 1GQ
Tel: 0116 260 2690
Fax: 0116 260 2757
E-mail: herbaluk@aol.com
Web: www.herbalapothecary.net
Dried herbs, tinctures, and creams.

Hilton Herbs Ltd

Downclose Farm
North Perrot
Crewkerne
Somerset TA18 7SH
Tel: 01460 78300
Fax: 01460 78302
E-mail: helpline@hiltonherbs.com
Web: www.hiltonherbs.com
Mail order medicinal herbs and a wide range of natural healthcare products and remedies for horses, dogs and other animals, including some for humans; offers a valuable helpline service.

Natural Animal Feeds Ltd

Penrhos
Raglan
Monmouthshire NP15 2DJ
Tel: 01600 780 256
Fax: 01600 780 536
Herbal and nutraceutical products.

Neal's Yard Remedies

29 John Dalton Street
Manchester M2 6DS
Tel: 0161 831 7875
Fax: 0161 835 93322
E-mail: mail@nealsyardremedies.com
Web: www.nealsyardremedies.com
Aromatherapy oils, natural medicines, herbs, flower and homeopathic remedies.

Nelson Veterinary & Equine Ltd

3 The Elliott Centre
Elliott Road
Cirencester
Glos GL7 1YS
Tel: 01285 655122
Fax: 01285 655133
E-mail: nve@nve.co.uk
Web: www.nve.co.uk
Probiotics.

A Nelson & Co. Ltd

Broadheath House
83 Parkside
London
SW19 5LP
Tel: 0208 780 4200
Fax: 0208 780 5893
Web: www.anelson.co.uk
Homeopathic pharmacy/mail order.

Nutri Centre
7 Park Crescent
London W1N 3HE
Tel: 0207 4365 122
Flower remedies.

Ozvet
Cactus World Ltd
Church Farm
Fulmer
Bucks SL3 6HD
Tel: 01753 660809
External treatments based on tea tree oil from Australia.

Phyto Products Ltd
Park Works
Park Road
Mansfield Woodhouse
Notts NG19 8EF
Tel: 01623 644334
Fax: 01623 657232
E-mail: info@phyto.co.uk
Dried herbs.

Savant Distributions Ltd
15 Iveson Approach
Leeds LS16 6LJ
Tel: 0113 230 1993
Fax: 0113 230 1915
E-mail: savant@mail.com
Web: www.savant-health.com
Equine nutritional supplements.

Tisserand Aromatherapy Products Ltd
Newton Road
Hove
East Sussex BN3 7BA
Tel: 01273 325666
Fax: 01273 208444
E-mail: info@tisserand.com
Web: www.tisserand.com
Aromatherapy oils.

Weleda UK Ltd
Heanor Road
Ilkeston
Derbyshire DE7 8DR
Tel: 0115 9448200.
Freefax: 0800 132069
Web: www.weleda.co.uk
Anthroposophic and homeopathic remedies.

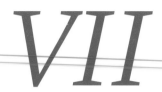

Books and Videos

These books and videos specifically address the topics raised in this book. With a few exceptions, books on breeds and training are not listed, since this book is focused on natural care rather than those topics.

HORSE CARE BOOKS

Aromatherapy for Horses (Threshold Picture Guide No. 40) by Caroline Ingraham, Kenilworth Press (UK), Half Halt Press (US), 1997.

The Aromatherapy Kit: Essential Oils and How to Use Them by Charla Devereux, Charles E. Tuttle Co., Inc., 1993.

Bach Flower Remedies by Edward Bach, M.D., and F.J. Wheeler, M.D., Keats Publishing, 1952, 1979.

Bach Flower Remedies for Horses and Riders by Martin J. Scott with Gael Mariani, Kenilworth Press (UK), Half Halt Press (US), 1999.

Bach Flower Therapy: Theory and Practice by Mechthild Scheffer, Thorsons Publishers, 1981, 1984.

Beating Muscle Injuries by Jack Meagher, Lynnewood Publishing Associates, PO Box 8296, Lynn, MA 01904, Tel: 781-596-1238, 1985, and Cloudcraft Books Ltd (UK), 1998.

Conditioning Sport Horses by Hilary M. Clayton, B.V.M.S., Ph.D., M.R.C.V.S., Sports Horse Publications, 1991.

Discovering Homeopathy: Medicine for the 21st Century by Dana Ullman, M.P.H., North Atlantic Books, 1991.

Equine Acupressure by Nancy Zidonis and Amy Snow, Tall Grass, third edition 1999.

Equine Atlas of Acupuncture Loci by Peggy Fleming, D.V.M., 21412 Field of Dreams Lane, Dade City, FL 33525, Tel: 352-583-2400, Fax 352-583-4007.

Equine Massage by Jean Pierre Hourdebaight, Howell Book House, 1997.

Everybody's Guide to Homeopathic Medicines by Stephen Cummings, M.D., and Dana Ullman, M.P.H., Jeremy P. Tarcher, 1991.

Feeding and Nutrition: The Making of a Champion by John Kohnke, B.V.Sc., R.D.A., Birubi Pacific, 1992.

For the Good of the Horse by Mary Wanless, Trafalgar Square Publishing (US), Kenilworth Press (UK), 1997.

For the Good of the Rider by Mary Wanless, , Trafalgar Square Publishing (US), Kenilworth Press (UK), 1998.

Getting in TTouch: Understand and Influence Your Horse's Personality (published in the UK *as Getting in Touch with Horses*) by Linda Tellington-Jones, Trafalgar Square Publishing (US) and Kenilworth Press (UK), 1995.

Grooming to Win by Susan Harris, IDG Books Worldwide, 1991.

A Guide to Equine Nutrition by Keith Allison, J.A. Allen & Co. Ltd, 1995.

Hands-On Energy Therapy for Horses and Riders by Clare Wilde, Kenilworth Press (UK), Trafalgar Square Publishing (US), 1999.

The Herb Book by John Lust, Bantam Books, 1974.

Herbal Handbook for Farm and Stable by Juliette de Bairacli-Levy, Rodale Press, 1976.

Herbs for Horses (Threshold Picture Guide No.27) by Jenny Morgan, Kenilworth Press (UK), Half Halt Press (US), 1993.

Homeopathy (Threshold Picture Guide No.44) by Christopher Day, Kenilworth Press (UK), Half Halt Press (US), 2000.

Improve Your Horse's Well-Being: A Step-by-Step Guide to TTouch and TTEAM Training by Linda Tellington-Jones, 1999, Trafalgar Square Publishing (US) and Kenilworth Press (UK), 1999.

An Introduction to the Tellington-Jones Equine Awareness Method by Linda Tellington-Jones and Ursula Bruns, Breakthrough Publications, Inc., 1988.

Massage for Horses (Threshold Picture Guide No.38) by Mary Bromiley, Kenilworth Press (UK), Half Halt Press (US), 1996.

The Magical Staff by Matthew Wood, North Atlantic Books, 1992.

A Modern Horse Herbal by Hilary Page Self, Kenilworth Press (UK), Half Halt Press (US), 1996.

Natural Remedies (Threshold Picture Guide No.35) by Christopher Day, Kenilworth Press (UK), Half Halt Press (US), 1996.

Original Book of Horse Treats: Recipes You Can Make at Home for Your Horse by June V. Evers, Horse Hollow Press, 1994.

Pocket Manual of Homoeopathic Materia Medica with Repertory by William Boericke, M.D., B. Jain Publishers, New Delhi, India, 1992.

Rodale's Illustrated Encyclopedia of Herbs by Claire Kowalchik and William H. Hylton, Editors, Rodale Press, 1987.

Seven Herbs: Plants as Teachers by Matthew Wood, North Atlantic Press, 1986.

Straight Forward Riding by Lesley Ann Taylor and Carol Brett, Balance, 1998

The Tellington TTouch: A Breakthrough Technique to Train and Care for Your Favorite Animal by Linda Tellington-Jones with Sybil Taylor, Viking Penguin, 1992.

The Treatment of Horses by Homeopathy by G. Macleod, C.W. Daniel 1977 (revised 1993).

Tyler's Herbs of Choice: The Therapeutic Use of Phytomedicinals by James E. Robbers, Ph.D. and Varra E. Tyler, Ph.D., Sc.D., 2nd Edition, Haworth Press, 1999.

Veterinary Acupuncture: Ancient Art to Modern Medicine, edited by Allen M. Schoen, D.V.M., American Veterinary Publications, Inc., 1994.

HOLISTIC HEALTH AND NATURAL LIVING

Alternatives in Healing by Simon Mills, M.S., and Steven J. Finando, Ph.D., Plume/NAL, 1988.

Alternatives for the Health Conscious Individual (newsletter), Mountain Home Publishing, P.O. Box 829, Ingram, TX 78025; phone 512-367-4492.

A Cancer Battle Plan by Anne E. Frähm with David J. Frähm, Pinion Press, 1992.

Common-Sense Pest Control: Least Toxic Solutions for Your Home, Garden, Pets, and Community by William Olkowski, Ph.D., Sheila Daar and Helga Olkowski, Taunton Press, 1991.

Echo, Inc. (Educational Concern for Hydrogen Peroxide) [newsletter], P.O. Box 126, Delano, MN 55328.

The Fall of Freddie the Leaf by Leo Buscaglia, Holt, Rinehart & Winston, 1983.

The Family News (quarterly newsletter on oxygen therapies), 9845 N.E. Second Avenue, Miami Shores, FL 33138; phone 800-284-6263.

Free Radicals, Stress and Antioxidant Enzymes —A Guide to Cellular Health (booklet) by Peter R. Rothschild, M.D., Ph.D., and William J. Fahey, University Labs Press, 1991.

Health and Healing by Andrew Weil, M.D., Houghton Mifflin 1983, 1998.

How to Heal the Earth in Your Spare Time by Andy Lopez, published by The Invisible Gardener, 29169 Heathercliff Road, Suite 216-408, Malibu, CA 90265; phone 302-457-6658.

Kindred Spirits: How the Remarkable Bond Between Humans and Animals Can Change the Way We Live by Allen M. Schoen, DVM, Broadway Books, 2001.

Love, Miracles, and Animal Healing: A Veterinarian's Journey from Physical Medicine to Spiritual Understanding by Allen M. Schoen, DVM, and Pam Proctor, Simon & Schuster, 1995.

The Natural Dog by Mary L. Brennan, D.V.M. with Norma Eckroate, Plume Books, 1994.

Natural Health, Natural Medicine by Andrew Weil, M.D., Houghton Mifflin, 1990.

The New Natural Cat by Anitra Frazier with Norma Eckroate, Plume Books, 1990.

Nontoxic, Natural and Earthwise by Debra Lynn Dadd, Jeremy P. Tarcher, 1990.

Perfect Health: The Complete Mind/Body Guide by Deepak Chopra, M.D., Harmony Books, 1991.

Prescription for Nutritional Healing by James F. Balch, M.D., and Phyllis A. Balch, C.N.C., Avery Publishing Group, 1990.

A Quick Guide to Food Additives by Robert Goodman, Silvercat Publications, 1981, 1990.

Spontaneous Healing by Andrew Weil, M.D., Alfred A. Knopf, Inc., 1995.

Switched-On Living: Easy Ways to Use the Mind/Body Connection to Energize Your Life by Jerry V. Teplitz, J.D., Ph.D., with Norma Eckroate, Hampton Roads Publishing, 1994.

Vibrational Healing by Richard Gerber, M.D., Bear & Co., 1988.

Your Body Doesn't Lie by John Diamond, M.D., Warner Books, 1980, (also published under the title *Behavioral Kinesiology*, Harper & Row, 1979).

VIII Associations and Organizations

HOLISTIC VETERINARY

Academy of Veterinary Homeopathy

751 Northeast 168th Street
North Miami Beach, FL 33162-2427
Tel: 305-652-1590, Fax: 305-653-7244
Web: www.acadvethom.org
E-mail: avh@naturalholistic.com

Trains and certifies veterinary homeopaths. Send a self-addressed, stamped envelope for a list of qualified veterinary homeopaths in your area or fax-on-demand at 305-653-3337.

American Holistic Veterinary Medical Association

2218 Old Emmorton Road
Bel Air, MD 21015
Tel: 410-569-0795, Fax: 410-559-7774
Web: www.altvetmed.com
E-mail: AHVMA@compuserve.com

Professional organization that serves as a forum to explore alternative veterinary health care. Publishes a quarterly journal for members. Send self-addressed stamped envelope for list of holistic veterinarians in your area.

American Veterinary Chiropractic Association

623 Main St.
Hillsdale, IL 61257
Tel: 309-658-2920, Fax: 309-658-2622
Web: www.animalchiro.com
E-mail: AmVetChiro@aol.com

Professional organization that promotes veterinary chiropractic through courses and certification. Send a self-addressed, stamped envelope for a list of certified practitioners.

APACHE (Association for the Promotion of Animal Complementary Health Education)

Archers Wood Farm
Coppington Road
Sawtry
Huntingdon
Cambridgeshire
England PE17 5XT
Tel: 07050 244196
E-mail: apache@avnet.co.uk
Web: www.avnet.co.uk

British Association for Homeopathic Veterinary Surgeons
Chinham House
Stanford-in-the-Vale
NR Faringdon, Oxon
England SN7 8NQ
Tel: 01367-710324
Web: www.bahvs.com

British Institute of Homeopathy
Cygnet House
Market Square
Staines
Middlesex
England
TW18 4RH
Tel: 01784 440467
Web: www.britinsthom.com
E-mail: britinsthom@compuserve.com
Homeopathy/Bach courses and training.

*British Institute of Homeopathy
In the USA:*
520 Washington Blvd.
Suite 423
Marina Del Rey, CA 90292
Tel: 310-577-2235
E-mail: bihus@thegrid.net

*British Institute of Homeopathy
In the Germany:*
Spannskamp 28
22527 Hamburg
Germany
Tel: 49 40 54767248

International Association of Veterinary Homeopathy
Sonnhaldenstr. 24
CH-8370
Switzerland

International Veterinary Acupuncture Society
PO Box 271395
Fort Collins, CO 80527-1395
Tel: 970-266-0666, Fax: 970-266-0777
Web: www.ivas.org
E-mail: ivaoffice@aol.com
Professional organization fosters research on acupuncture in veterinary medicine. Call or write for information and lists of veterinary acupuncturists in the United States and other countries.

National Center for Homeopathy
801 N. Fairfax, #306
Alexandria, VA 22314
Tel: 877-624-0613, Fax: 703-548-7792
Web: www.homeopathic.org
E-mail: info@homeopathic.org
Directory of homeopaths, including veterinarians. Offers a catalog of books and annual courses.

Society for Animal Flower Essence Research (SAFER)
Pengraig Fach
Nr Blaenycoed
Carmarthen
Dyfed SA33 6EU
England
Tel: 01296 281761
E-mail: bachexpress@hotmail.com
Promotes the understanding and use of flower essences for animal treatment.

Tellington TTouch Equine Awareness Method (TTEAM) and *Tellington TTouch*
P.O. Box 3793
Santa Fe, NM 87501-0793
Tel: 800-854-TEAM, Fax: 405-455-7233
Web: www.lindatellingtonjones.com

In the UK:
TTEAM Secretary U.K.
Sunnyside House
Stratton Audley Road
Fringford, Bicester
Oxon, England OX6 9ED
Tel: 01869-277730

In Germany:
TTEAM Gilde
Bibi Degn
Hassel 4
57589 Pracht
Germany
Tel: 02682-8886

TREATMENT OPTIONS

Immune Augumentative Therapy for Cancer
c/o Martin Goldstein, DVM
RR 4, Box 262-B
Rte. 123
South Salem, NY 10590
Tel: 914-533-6066

ENVIRONMENTAL AND HOLISTIC HEALTH ORGANIZATIONS

Bio-Integral Resource Center
P.O. Box 7414
Berkeley, CA 94707
Tel: 510-524-2567, Fax: 510-524-1758
Web: www.birc.org
E-mail: birc@igc.org
A non-profit organization that researches and promotes information on the least toxic methods of pest management.

International Bio-Oxidative Medicine Foundation
P.O. Box 891954
Oklahoma City, OK 73189
Tel: 405-478-4226
Promotes the use of hydrogen peroxide therapy and gives referrals to practitioners who use it.

Price-Pottenger Nutrition Foundation
P.O. Box 2614
La Mesa, CA 91943-2614
Tel: 800-366-3748, Fax: 619-574-1314
Web: www.price-pottenger.org
E-mail: info@price-pottenger.org
Educational organization dedicated to providing scientific information on nutrition and health. Call or write for a catalog of books, pamphlets, and tapes.

Illustration Credits

Index